M000250159

Latina/o American Health and Mental Health

Recent Titles in Race, Ethnicity, Culture, and Health Series

Mexican American Psychology: Social, Cultural, and Clinical Perspectives
Mario A. Tovar

Better Health through Spiritual Practices: A Guide to Religious Behaviors
and Perspectives That Benefit Mind and Body
Dean D. VonDras, PhD, Editor

Latina/o American Health and Mental Health

Practices and Challenges

Leticia Arellano-Morales and Erica T. Sosa

Race, Ethnicity, Culture, and Health
Regan A. R. Gurung, Series Editor

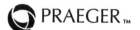 PRAEGER ™

An Imprint of ABC-CLIO, LLC
Santa Barbara, California • Denver, Colorado

Copyright © 2018 by Leticia Arellano-Morales and Erica T. Sosa

All rights reserved. No part of this publication may be reproduced, stored in a retrieval system, or transmitted, in any form or by any means, electronic, mechanical, photocopying, recording, or otherwise, except for the inclusion of brief quotations in a review, without prior permission in writing from the publisher.

Library of Congress Cataloging-in-Publication Data

Names: Arellano, Leticia M., author. | Sosa, Erica T., author.
Title: Latina/o American health and mental health : practices and challenges / Leticia Arellano-Morales and Erica T. Sosa.
Description: Santa Barbara, California : Praeger, [2018] | Series: Race, ethnicity, culture, and health | Includes bibliographical references and index.
Identifiers: LCCN 2017031181 (print) | LCCN 2017033824 (ebook) | ISBN 9781440854903 (ebook) | ISBN 9781440854897 (hard copy : alk. paper)
Subjects: | MESH: Mental Disorders—ethnology | Community Mental Health Services | Hispanic Americans | Attitude to Health—ethnology | Cultural Characteristics | Culturally Competent Care—methods | United States—epidemiology | Latin America—ethnology
Classification: LCC RC451.5.H57 (ebook) | LCC RC451.5.H57 (print) | NLM WA 305 AA1 | DDC 616.89008968/073—dc23
LC record available at https://lccn.loc.gov/2017031181

ISBN: 978-1-4408-5489-7 (print)
       978-1-4408-5490-3 (ebook)

22 21 20 19 18   1 2 3 4 5

This book is also available as an eBook.

Praeger
An Imprint of ABC-CLIO, LLC

ABC-CLIO, LLC
130 Cremona Drive, P.O. Box 1911
Santa Barbara, California 93116-1911
www.abc-clio.com

This book is printed on acid-free paper ∞

Manufactured in the United States of America

To our beloved Latina/o community, may our book help create positive changes and empowerment.

We thank our editor, Dr. Regan A. R. Gurung, for his patience and support. We also thank Debbie Stone for her assistance with our book and her eye for detail.

To my family, Jose and Janina, I love you to the moon and beyond. Thank you for enhancing my life and always inspiring me. To my parents, Frank and Stella, I love you. Thank you for always supporting me and for teaching me about *amor* and *caridad*.

—Leticia Arellano-Morales

To my mother, Maria; my sisters, Andrea, Veronica, and Stephanie; and my brothers-in-law, Jonas and Seth. Thank you for constantly inspiring and supporting me in all I do. To my niece, Brielle, and nephew, Micah. May the changes we make today create a better world and brighter future for you and for all children.

—Erica Sosa

Contents

Series Foreword

There are clearly many different cultural approaches to health, and it is of great importance for health care workers and the administrations that support them to be culturally aware. Knowing about the different approaches to health can also help the lay consumer be better apprised of cultural differences that in turn can lead to a reduction in stereotyping or prejudicial attitudes toward behaviors that may be seen as different from the norm. This book represents the second in a series of titles each designed to focus on a subgroup representing the diversity of America.

Each book is designed to provide a comprehensive introduction to a particular group of people. What is the history of that group in America? What is the diversity within the group? What are the unique mental, physical, or socioeconomic issues associated with the group. It is important to acknowledge that many cultural variations exist within ethnic communities. Knowing how different cultural groups approach health and having a better understanding of how factors such as acculturation are important can help clinicians, health care workers, and others with an interest in how lifestyle decisions are made be more culturally competent. The efforts to increase cultural competency in the treatment of mental and physical health are promising but the wider health care arena and the general public need to pay attention to the causes of health disparities and the role played by multicultural approaches to health. We need a better connection between health care and the community so that individuals can seek out treatments that best fit their cultural needs and the manifold health disparities can be reduced.

Regan A. R. Gurung
Ben J. and Joyce Rosenberg Professor of Human
Development and Psychology
University of Wisconsin, Green Bay

Preface

In the United States, there are 56.6 million Latina/os, and they currently comprise 17.6% of the total U.S. population (U.S. Census Bureau, 2015). As the largest ethnic minority group, Latina/os are expected to increase to 119 million and represent 28.6% of the total U.S. population by 2060. Regarded as the "browning of America" the continued growth and diversity of Latina/os (Casas, Alamilla, Cabrera, & Ortega, 2015) is compounded by their social and economic inequities and requires continued attention to their health and mental health needs and treatment outcomes. Indeed, their exponential growth requires innovative approaches to advance work to effectively study, understand, and serve the fastest-growing U.S. ethnic minority group (Adames & Chavez-Dueñas, 2017).

Despite health initiatives to eliminate health disparities and improve the nation's health, there is ample research indicating that Latina/os continue to experience health and mental health disparities. Thus, health and mental health providers, policymakers, researchers, and scholars face the daunting task of not only developing ample facilities, resources, and personnel to eliminate their health and mental health disparities, but also face the challenge of creating pathways to secure their self-empowerment and liberation (Buki & Piedra, 2011). A preliminary step in this process requires a basic recognition of the vast heterogeneity of Latina/os and the recognition that they are multiracial and multidimensional and not a monolithic group. Their significant heterogeneity contributes to differences in their levels of acculturation, socioeconomic status, regional locations, insurance, and other sociocultural factors that shape their health and mental health.

We review current works to explicitly highlight significant and complex within-group differences among Latina/os. We also review data from the Pew Research Center and various epidemiological studies regarding Latina/o adults and children to help the reader understand the impact of multiple forms of marginalization. As do other scholars, we call for the use of strength-based approaches that focus on their resilience rather than deficit-based perspectives that are often applied to Latina/os (Adames & Chavez-Dueñas, 2017; Falicov, 2014). Social justice and ecological perspectives are also warranted to eliminate the health and mental health disparities of Latina/os. Thus, an understanding of Latina/o health and mental health will require a more in-depth understanding of the factors that shape the barriers, health and mental health practices, and beliefs of diverse Latina/os to allow for culturally responsive prevention, interventions, and treatment outcomes.

Our overall goal is to help prepare a vast array of professionals to effectively serve Latina/os by understanding their complex health and mental health needs. A main tenet of our book is to highlight the diversity, perseverance, and resilience of Latina/os, rather than focusing on deficiencies and stereotypes. Unlike other works, *Latina/o American Health and Mental Health: Practices and Challenges* simultaneously addresses the health and mental health of Latina/os, as holistic views of health and illness do not differentiate between psychological and physical health. It is our perspective that addressing both areas through ecological perspectives will provide the reader with an increased understanding of the interplay between the health and mental health of Latina/os. We propose that innovative approaches with Latina/os require conceptualizations that recognize how race/ethnicity, gender, sexuality, immigration status, identity, and social class simultaneously shape the experiences of Latina/os, as well as their health and mental health.

Chapter 1 provides a demographic overview of Latina/os to enable the reader to appreciate the significant diversity of Latina/os and the factors that contribute to projections of their increased growth. We also provide data regarding the socioeconomic status of Latina/os and how various Latina/o heritage groups may fare better than others. Because Latina/o heritage groups differ in their immigration patterns and sociopolitical histories, we review the diverse immigration histories of diverse Latina/o heritage groups. We also address other factors related to immigration, including the geographic concentrations of diverse Latina/o heritage groups and issues relative to immigrant adults and children. Lastly, we review salient cultural values of Latina/os and issues relative to gender socialization and sexual identity.

Chapter 2, "Patterns of Chronic Disease," discusses various health issues that impact different segments of the Latina/o population. The heterogeneous nature of Latina/os is demonstrated within the varying health behaviors and health issues of each Latina/o heritage group. For example, we discuss the issue of the Latina/o Paradox and how despite their relatively lower incomes and education levels and decreased access to resources, foreign-born Latina/os exhibit better health outcomes than their U.S.-born counterparts. This chapter also explores health issues among Latina/o adults and children and highlights critical issues that warrant increased attention. Throughout this chapter, we present various models that explain disease and apply these models to Latina/os. We also review existing epidemiological studies and highlight the need for more epidemiological research that specifically focuses on Latina/os.

Chapter 3, "Health Care Access and Delivery among Latina/o Populations," explores access to health care among Latina/os. For example, we discuss how Latina/os are less likely to have a usual provider and are less likely to access health care services than their White/European American counterparts. Unfortunately, these differences are further impacted among Latina/os by their country of origin and immigration status. Thus, we highlight the importance of understanding these trends and explore health care access among Latina/o heritage groups. We also examine barriers to accessing health care, including differences in access by nativity status and language barriers. Additionally, this chapter includes a brief discussion of how health care is accessed and utilized among higher-risk individuals, such as Latina/os with one or more chronic diseases. Also, because diabetes and HIV are two chronic diseases that impact Latina/os, we address how Latina/os must navigate the health care system and their unique barriers. Lastly, we provide recommendations for addressing the barriers to care and improving access to health care among Latina/os.

Chapter 4, "Community Efforts for Health Promotion in Latina/o Communities," examines community-based initiatives for health promotion in Latina/o communities. Given the number of Latina/os who experience difficulties accessing the health care system, finding alternative routes for delivering health promotion and disease prevention services is critical. Within Latina/o communities, language, family, and religion are often paramount. Accordingly, these elements are potential points of entry and support for health promotion delivery in the Latina/o community. Thus, we discuss a variety of approaches including promotora-based models, faith-based initiatives and family-based approaches to health. Additionally, we examine various approaches that are utilized for some of the most prevalent health issues that currently impact Latina/os, such as diabetes, obesity, and cancers.

Chapter 5, "Nontraditional Health Practices," includes a discussion of nontraditional approaches for health used by Latina/os. The use of complementary and alternative medicine is relatively common among

Latina/os. This chapter explores various nontraditional approaches to health such as *curanderos* and alternative medicine. Implications of these practices and the lack of communication about these practices with health care providers are also addressed. For example, greater knowledge of *curanderismo* and other nontraditional health care practices can enable practitioners to become better informed and enable them to easily discuss these practices with their Latina/o patients and increase patient trust and comfort disclosing such information.

Chapter 6, "Prevalence of Mental Health Disorders," presents a brief overview of the protective and risk factors that impact the mental health of Latina/os. We also review epidemiological studies to identify the prevalence of mental health disorders among Latina/o children and adolescents and how demographic and sociocultural factors are associated with these mental health disorders. We also review smaller studies to address important cultural and psychosocial variables that impact Latina/os' mental health, particularly depression, suicide, and substance use among adolescents. Lastly, because it is equally important to understand prominent idioms of distress among Latina/os, we review empirical studies that focus upon *susto* (fright), *nervios* (nerves), and *ataque de nervios* (attack of nerves).

Chapter 7, "Mental Health Barriers among Latina/os," explores access to mental health care among Latina/os. We discuss how Latina/os may rely on primary care settings to meet their mental health needs and avoid the stigma of mental illness. We particularly highlight how Latina/o heritage groups differ in their access and utilization of mental health care services by country of origin, nativity, and language. We also explore the various individual, cultural, organizational, and societal factors that contribute to these mental health barriers and provide recommendations to address them. For example, we address how cultural value orientations are often prominent among Latina/o interpersonal relationships and influence the clinical encounter. In addition, we highlight how mental health interventions with Latina/os must reflect cultural sensitivity through clinical approaches and program activities that build on the cultural strengths of Latina/os.

Chapter 8, "Culture-Specific Interventions and Community Efforts," provides a general overview of the psychological strengths of Latina/os and intervention frameworks/guidelines for clinical work with Latina/os. For example, we review several guidelines and models that are multidimensional, systemic, and holistic, rather than simply recommending techniques for the generic Latina/o client. We review the debate regarding evidence-based programs and treatments and cultural adaptations for Latina/os, such as cognitive behavioral therapy. We also address culture-specific treatments and community mental health efforts with Latina/os, such as the use of *promotoras*, gender-specific groups, and interventions with Latina/o youth to highlight how these approaches address the mental health needs of diverse Latina/os.

Chapter 9, "Nontraditional Mental Health Practices," includes a general discussion of the role of indigenous healers and spiritual and indigenous practices of Latina/os. We highlight how worldviews among Latina/os often reflect that the body, mind, and spirit are interconnected and that illness is derived from disequilibrium from various sources, including natural, social, spiritual, or psychological disturbances (Avila & Parker, 1999). We provide a general overview of *Curanderismo*, *Santería*, and *Espiritismo* and their application to Latina/o mental health. In addition, we review issues of spirituality and social justice, such as *mujerista* psychology and address treatment implications and recommendations for integrating indigenous forms of healing within the therapeutic process.

Lastly, Chapter 10, "Future Considerations," provides recommendations based on the data presented throughout the book. We explore opportunities for increasing cultural competency in health care and mental health care and explore ways to promote health using culturally tailored approaches for Latina/o heritage groups. We also discuss opportunities for advancing practice, research, and policy to support Latina/o health. For example, we explore how the current political landscape influences opportunities to conduct research for underserved and vulnerable groups such as Latina/os, but more importantly, why conducting this research is more important than ever before.

REFERENCES

Adames, H. Y., & Chavez-Dueñas, N. Y. (2016). *Cultural foundations and interventions in Latino/a mental health: History, theory and within group differences.* New York: Routledge.

Avila, E., & Parker, J. (1999). *Woman who glows in the dark: A curandera reveals traditional Aztec secrets of physical and spiritual health.* New York: Tarcher/Putnam.

Buki, L. P., & Piedra, L. M. (Eds.). (2011). *Creating infrastructures for Latino mental health.* New York: Springer.

Casas, J. M., Alamilla, S. G., Cabrera, A. P., & Ortega, S. (2015). The browning of the United States from generalizations to specifics: A mental health perspective. In H. Grey & B. N. Hall-Clark (Eds.), *Cultural considerations in Latino American mental health* (pp. 1–30). New York: Oxford University Press.

Falicov, C. J. (2014). *Latino families in therapy: A guide to multicultural practices* (2nd ed.). New York: The Guilford Press.

U.S. Census Bureau. (2015). Projections of the size and composition of the U.S. population: 2014 to 2060. Retrieved from https://www.census.gov/content/dam/Census/library/publications/2015/demo/p25-1143.pdf

Chapter 1

Introduction

We are at the crossroads in Latino mental health. The future well-being of our nation rests in our ability to promote the mental and physical health in this population. In many ways, the task before us is daunting, yet history reminds us of the endless possibility of human ingenuity to use the tools at hand and realize the most seemingly impossible goals.

—Buki and Piedra, 2011, p. ix

There are currently 56.6 million Latina/os within the United States, and they comprise 17.6% of the total population (U.S. Census Bureau, 2016). As the largest ethnic minority group, Latina/os are expected to increase to 119 million and represent 28.6% of the total U.S. population by 2060 (Colby & Ortman, 2014). As the fastest-growing ethnic minority group, they face formidable social and economic barriers. Unfortunately, despite their representation within the U.S. population, Latina/os are often neglected, misunderstood, and inappropriately served within health and mental health settings (Buki & Piedra, 2011; Casas, Alamilla, Cabrera, & Ortega, 2015). Moreover, their increased growth is occurring during heightened social tensions, political rhetoric, intense anti-immigrant sentiments and policies, as well as human rights violations. We concur with Buki and Piedra's (2011) assessment that the United States is at a crossroads, and health and mental health providers, policymakers, and scholars face the daunting task of not only developing ample facilities, resources, and personnel to eliminate their health and mental health disparities, but also face the challenge of creating pathways to secure their self-empowerment and liberation.

A main tenet of our book is to highlight the diversity, perseverance, and resilience of Latina/os, rather than to focus on deficiencies and stereotypes. In doing so, the current chapter provides a demographic overview of Latina/os to enable the reader to appreciate the diversity of Latina/os and the factors that contribute to their increased growth projections, such as their nativity, age, and marital status, among others. Much of these data are derived from current reports from the Pew Research Center regarding Latina/os. In addition, data regarding the socioeconomic status (SES) of Latina/os is provided. We also address factors related to immigration, including their geographic concentration and issues relative to immigrant adults and children. The last section addresses salient cultural values of Latina/os and issues relative to gender socialization and gender identity.

Because of historical racial mixing, Latina/os are indeed a heterogeneous group and are regarded as multiracial or *mestizos* (Ramirez, 1998). Their diversity is evidenced within their ethnicity, physical appearance, traditions, cultural practices, and Spanish language dialects (Gallardo, 2012; Santiago-Rivera, Arredondo, & Gallardo-Cooper, 2002). Identity among Latina/os is multidimensional and multifaceted. Thus, it is prudent for health and mental health providers to recognize the multidimensional nature of their identity that is influenced by various factors, such as their gender, physiology or racial identity (Adames & Chavez-Dueñas, 2017). Pan-ethnic terms such as *Hispanic* or *Latino* are often used, but they obscure the diversity among Latina/os and are not racial categories because of the multiple ethnic and racial heritages of Latina/os (Arredondo et al., 2014), nor do they consider place of birth or generation status (Casas et al., 2015).

The term *Hispanic* is an umbrella term created by the federal Office of Management and Budget to categorize all persons of Spanish origin, regardless of race (Alcoff, 2005). However, this term is often rejected by Latina/os because of the genocide perpetrated by the Spaniards. Because it emphasizes a White European colonial heritage, *Hispanic* also excludes other important heritages of Latina/os, such as their indigenous, mestizo, slave, non-European, and non-Spanish-speaking heritages (Delgado-Romero, Galvan Hunter, & Torres, 2008). Furthermore, the term does not allow for gender identity (Casas et al., 2015). Conversely, the term *Latino* is also an umbrella term to emphasize roots in Latin American countries and the use of the Spanish language, but debate and controversy also exists regarding this term. Critics argue that *Latino* also obscures the diverse histories and sociopolitical realities of U.S. Latina/os (Gloria & Segura, 2004), while others indicate that it is culturally inclusive (Gallardo, 2012) and can garner solidarity (Oboler, 2005). While we recognize the limitations of the term *Latina/o*, we use this term to recognize the breadth and depth of the Latina/o population in the United States (Gallardo, 2012) but reference specific Latina/o heritage groups whenever possible to allow for a greater understanding of these diverse heritage groups.

Indeed, the use of self-identifying terms varies by generational status, nationality, SES, gender, and personal preference (Casas et al., 2015; Gloria & Segura, 2004). For instance, preferences for terminology among Latina/os are often associated with national forms of self-identification, such as *Dominicano, Cuban*, or *Peruvian*; sociopolitical views, such as *Xicana* or *Boricua* (Delgado-Romero et al., 2008; Gallardo, 2012); as well as other inclusive terms such as *Latin@* or *Latinx* (Adames & Chavez-Dueñas, 2017; Reichard, 2015) as gender-neutral terms. In addition, Latinos may self-identify as *American* to emphasize that they are simply Americans or *Spanish* to acknowledge their Spanish ancestry.

Indeed, it is important for health and mental health providers to recognize that extensive diversity exists among Latina/os because of their national origin, geographic region, education, income, acculturation, physiology, and other salient factors (Betancourt & Flynn, 2009). Further, their diversity is amplified by genetic, cultural, political, and religious/spiritual influences (Gans et al., 2002). Latina/os include Mexican Americans, Puerto Ricans, Cubans, Central Americans, South Americans, Dominicans, or other Latina/o ethnic groups, regardless of race. They represent individuals of Native American, African, Asian, and European ancestry and originate from more than 25 countries in the Northern and Southern hemispheres, Central America, as well as the Caribbean (Arredondo et al., 2014; Borrell & Crawford, 2009).

The diversity of Latina/os stems from centuries of European conquest, genocide, and oppression among indigenous peoples, including the Taínos and Caribs in the Caribbean and the Aztecs, Mayas, and Incas in Latin America (see Adames & Chavez-Dueñas, 2017), and ties with other indigenous groups in the Northern and Southern hemispheres. In addition, the diversity of Latina/os is also attributed to the African diaspora in the Americas, as the Spanish imported more than 10 million African slaves to Latin America. Other slaves, such as Asians, were brought to South America (Arredondo et al., 2014). Nonetheless, despite their history of oppression and conquest, Latina/os are descendants of strong and advanced civilizations and remain resilient (Adames & Chavez-Dueñas, 2017).

DEMOGRAPHIC OVERVIEW OF LATINOS

As previously indicated, there are currently 56.6 million Latina/os in the United States, comprising 17.6% of the total population (U.S. Census Bureau, 2016). Between 1970 and 2000, the Latina/o population increased by 368%, as compared with an increase of 138% among the general U.S. population (U.S. Census Bureau, 2008). Within the past decade, Latina/os also accounted for more than half of the growth within the U.S. population. Although their previous growth was due to their immigration rates, the projected growth of Latina/os is based upon their fertility rates and younger age. Statistical profiles of Latina/os (Stepler & Brown, 2016) indicate that Mexicans are the largest heritage group (64%), followed by Puerto Ricans (9.6%), Salvadorans (9.6%), Cubans (3.7%), Dominicans (3.2%), and all other Latina/os (see Table 1.1). Combined, Mexicans and Puerto Ricans comprised 74% (40,691,275) of the U.S. Latina/o population in 2014.

Nativity and Citizenship

The population growth of Latina/os significantly increased, by 70.6%, between 1980 and 2014. In terms of nativity, 65% of Latina/os are U.S.-born, and 35% are foreign-born (see Table 1.2). However, demographic trends indicate that immigration from Latin America declined since 2010, as the percentage of foreign-born Latina/os declined from 40% in 2000 to 35% in 2013 (Stepler & Brown, 2016), including foreign-born Latina/os from Ecuador, Mexico, and Nicaragua. As indicated in Table 1.1, among Latina/o heritage groups, Venezuelans (69%), Peruvians (65%), Guatemalans (63.5%), and Colombians (63.5%) have the highest foreign-born rates, while Mexicans (33%) have the lowest foreign-born rates (López & Patten, 2015). Contrary to stereotypes of Latina/os, 76% of Latina/os are U.S. citizens, of which 11.7% are naturalized U.S. citizens. Among Latina/o heritage groups, Puerto Ricans (99%), Cubans (76%), and Mexicans (75%) have higher citizenship rates. Conversely, Hondurans and Guatemalans have lower citizenship rates (50%) (López & Patten, 2015).

Marital Status

There is significant diversity in the marital status of Latina/os in terms of nativity and heritage group. For example, 46.1% of Latina/os are married, 37.8% are never married, 9.0% are divorced, 3.6% are widowed, and 3.5% are separated (Stepler & Brown, 2016). There are also nativity differences among Latina/os, as 56.2% of foreign-born Latina/os are married, versus 36.5% of U.S.-born Latinos. Similarly, 27.3% of foreign-born Latina/os are never married, versus 47.7% of U.S.-born Latina/os. Among Latina/o heritage groups, Argentineans (58%) and Venezuelans (54%) are more likely to be married, while Hondurans (39%) and Puerto Ricans (36%) are less likely to be married (López & Patten, 2015).

Table 1.1 Nativity by Latina/o Heritage Group, 2014

	Total	Percent	U.S.-Born	Foreign-Born	% Foreign-Born
Mexican	35,371,314	64.0	23,741,580	11,629,734	32.9
Puerto Rican	5,319,916	9.6	5,236,903	83,058	1.6
Salvadoran	2,100,433	3.8	860,454	1,239,979	59.0
Cuban	2,045,970	3.7	878,694	1,167,276	57.1
Dominican	1,763,651	3.2	804,618	959,033	54.4
All Other Spanish/ Hispanic/ Latino	1,683,332	3.0	1,412,145	271,187	16.1
Guatemalan	1,324,694	2.4	490,464	834,230	63.0
Colombian	1,046,332	1.9	382,153	664,179	63.5
Honduran	812,731	1.5	296,951	515,780	63.5
Spaniard	753,538	1.4	643,473	110,065	14.6
Ecuadorian	659,166	1.2	258,695	400,471	60.8
Peruvian	614,151	1.1	215,130	399,021	65.0
Nicaraguan	414,136	0.7	175,838	238,298	57.5
Venezuelan	302,778	0.5	94,362	208,416	68.8
Argentinean	268,099	0.5	105,238	162,861	60.7
Panamanian	189,748	0.3	106,008	83,740	44.1
Chilean	149,113	0.3	64,636	84,477	56.7
Costa Rican	140,581	0.3	66,928	73,653	52.4
Bolivian	110,101	0.2	41,752	68,349	62.1
Uruguayan	67,226	0.1	22,021	45,205	67.2
Other Central American	47,233	0.1	24,519	22,714	48.1
Other South American	38,639	0.1	20,235	18,404	47.6
Paraguayan	27,590	<0.05	6,773	20,817	75.5
Total	55,250,517	100	35,949,570	19,300,947	34.9

Note: Hispanic origin is based on self-described ancestry, lineage, heritage, nationality group or country of birth.

Source: Stepler, R., & Brown, A. (2016). *Statistical portrait of Hispanics in the United States, 2014*. Washington, DC: Pew Research Center.

Table 1.2 Latina/o Population by Nativity: 1980–2014

	1980	1990	2000	2010	2014	Percent change 2000–2014
U.S.-born	10,600,760	14,046,463	21,072,230	31,912,465	35,949,570	70.6
Foreign-born	4,174,320	7,790,388	14,132,250	18,817,105	19,300,947	36.6
Citizen	1,258,080	2,042,452	3,917,885	5,544,860	6,477,524	—
Noncitizen	2,916,240	5,747,936	10,214,365	13,272,245	12,823,423	—
Total	**14,775,08**	**21,836,85**	**35,204,48**	**50,729,57**	**55,250,51**	**8.9**

Percent Distribution

	1980	1990	2000	2010	2014	Share of total change 2000–2014
U.S.-born	71.7	64.3	59.9	62.9	65.1	74.2
Foreign-born	28.3	35.7	40.1	37.1	34.9	25.8
Citizen	8.5	9.4	11.1	10.9	11.7	—
Noncitizen	19.7	26.3	29.0	26.2	23.2	—
Total	**100.0**	**100.0**	**100.0**	**100.0**	**100.0**	**100.0**

Source: Stepler, R., & Brown, A. (2016). *Statistical portrait of Hispanics in the United States, 2014.* Washington, DC: Pew Research Center.

Fertility

Among all racial and ethnic groups, Latinas demonstrate the highest birth rates, 80 births per 1,000 women of childbearing age (15–44), followed by African American (64%), White/European American (59%), and Asian American (56%) women. High birth rates among Latinas are partly explained by the high share of foreign-born Latinas (Livingston & Cohn, 2012). Among women of reproductive age who gave birth in 2014, 7% of Latinas gave birth, compared to African American (6.2%), Asian American (6.1%), White/European American (5.8%), and Other (5.8%) women. Foreign-born Latinas have higher birth rates as compared with U.S.-born Latinas (7.9% and 6.4%, respectively) (Stepler & Brown, 2016). There are also differences in fertility rates among Latina/o heritage groups. Among Latinas ages 15 to 44, Guatemalan (9%) and Salvadoran (8%) women demonstrate higher birth rates, while Venezuelan (5%) and Colombian (5%) demonstrate lower birth rates (López & Patten, 2015).

However, while Latinas demonstrate the highest birth rates among all racial and ethnic groups, a report from the Pew Research Center indicates interesting trends in birth rates among Latinas (Livingston & Cohn, 2012), indicating sharp decreases in birth rates among both U.S.-born and foreign-born Latinas between 1990 and 2010. For example, among U.S.-born Latinas of childbearing age, the birthrate decreased from 82.4 in 1990 to 65.4 in 2010, resulting in a 21% decrease. Greater changes are also observed among foreign-born Latinas, as their birth rates declined from 136.9 in 1990 to 96.3 in 2010, resulting in a 30% decline (see Table 1.3). These trends also indicate that among all foreign-born women, Latinas demonstrate the most dramatically decreased birth rates. Livingston and Cohn (2012) suggest that the decreased birth rates of foreign-born Latinas are largely due to their economic distress, as their poverty and unemployment significantly increased after the start of the Great Recession.

Age

Census data indicate that Latina/os are the youngest ethnic minority group, with a median age of 28 years, as compared with a mean age of 37 among the general population (Stepler & Brown, 2016). There are nativity differences among Latina/os, as the mean age of U.S.-born Latina/os is 19, as compared to 41 among immigrant Latina/os (Patten, 2016). Patten suggests that the Latina/o population is defined by its youth, as 32% (17.9 million) are younger than 18 years of age, 26% are Millennial adults (18–33), 22% are Generation X (34–49), 22% are Boomers (50–68), and 19% are 69 years of age and older. In addition, 47% of U.S.-born Latina/os

Table 1.3 Birth Rates by Race/Ethnicity and Nativity of Mother, 1990 and 2010

Births per 1000 Women, Ages 15–44

	2010	1990	% Change 1990–2010
All women	64.0	71.2	−10%
U.S.-born	58.9	66.5	−11%
Foreign-born	87.8	112.8	−22%
U.S.-born women			
White/European American	57.3	60.1	−5%
Black/African American	61.3	86.2	−29%
Latina/Hispanic	65.4	82.4	−21%
Asian American	32.0	42.7	−25%
Foreign-born women			
White/European American	87.2	95.1	−8%
Black/African American	89.9	112.1	−20%
Latina/Hispanic	96.3	136.9	−30%
Asian American	68.3	78.5	−13%

Note: Percent change calculated before rounding. Whites/European Americans, Blacks/ African Americans, and Asians include only non-Latina/os. Asian Americans include Pacific Islanders. Latinas are of any race.
Source: Livingston, G., & Cohn, D. (2012). *U.S. birth rate falls to a record low: Decline is greatest among immigrants*. Washington, DC: Pew Research Center.

are Millennials or younger. Among Latina/o heritage groups, Cubans are oldest, with a median age of 40, followed by Argentineans (37), and Peruvians (36), while Mexicans are youngest, with a median age of 26, followed by Hondurans, Guatemalans, and Dominicans with a median age of 28 (López & Patten, 2015) (see Figure 1.1).

English and Spanish Proficiency

Despite stereotypes that Latina/os solely speak Spanish, Latina/os demonstrate English proficiency, as 68% of Latina/os, ages five and older, speak only English in their homes or "speak English very well." Among Latina/o adults, 25% are English-dominant, 38% are Spanish-dominant, and 36% are bilingual. There are also differences in English proficiency among Latina/o heritage groups, as 83% of Puerto Ricans, 75% of Argentineans, and 70% of

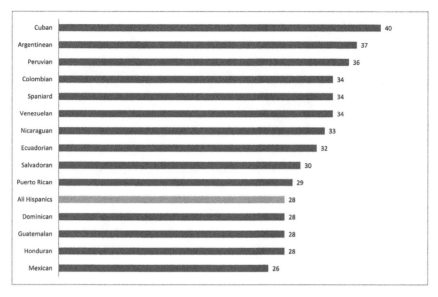

Figure 1.1 Median Age of Latina/o Heritage Groups, 2013.

Note: Median age for the general U.S. population is 37.
Source: López, G., & Patten, E. (2015). *The impact of slowing immigration: Foreign-born share falls among 14 largest U.S. Hispanic origin groups.* Washington, DC: Pew Research Center.

Venezuelans are proficient in English (see Figure 1.2). However, only 48% of Hondurans and 45% of Guatemalans are proficient in English (López & Patten, 2015). Similarly, 73% of Latina/os ages five and older speak Spanish at home, and Salvadorans (89%) report the highest share, followed by Dominicans, Hondurans, and Guatemalans (88%) (López & Patten, 2015). However, it is important to note that Latina/os throughout Latin America speak languages and dialects other than Spanish. For example, according to the Archive of Indigenous Languages of Latin America (n.d.), between 550 and 700 indigenous languages are spoken in Latin America. In particular, there are approximately 8.5 million Quechua speakers in Peru, Brazil, Bolivia, Argentina, Ecuador, and Colombia and three million Guarani speakers in Paraguay. Similarly, there are approximately 1.3 million speakers of Kekchi in Guatemala and 1.3 million Nahua speakers in Mexico.

Religious Affiliation

There are also notable differences in religious affiliation among Latina/os, as the number of Catholics has continually decreased within past decades

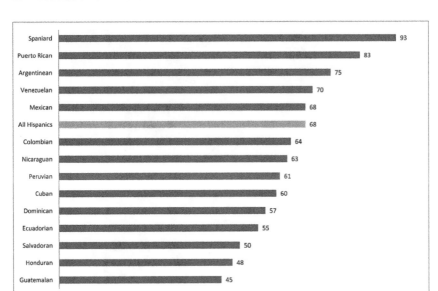

Figure 1.2 Percent of Latina/os Ages Five and Older with English Proficiency, by Latina/o Heritage Group, 2013.

Note: Total U.S. share is 92%. Latinos who speak English proficiently are those who speak only English at home or, if they speak a non-English language at home, indicate that they can speak English "very well."
Source: López, G., & Patten, E. (2015). *The impact of slowing immigration: Foreign-born share falls among 14 largest U.S. Hispanic origin groups.* Washington, DC: Pew Research Center.

(see Figure 1.3). For example, the 2013 National Survey of Latinos and Religion (Pew Research Center, 2014) indicates that almost half (55%) of Latina/o adults identify as Catholic, a 12% decline from 2010. Approximately 22% identify as Protestant, and 18% do not identify a religious affiliation. Among Latina/o heritage groups, Mexicans (61%) and Dominicans (59%) are likely to identify as Catholic. Conversely, Salvadorans are more likely to identify as evangelical Protestants than Mexicans, Cubans, and Dominicans. Similarly, 60% of foreign-born Latina/os identify as Catholic, versus 48% of U.S.-born Latina/os. The decline of Catholic affiliation is also more pronounced among younger Latina/os, as 45% of Latina/os under the age of 30 identify as Catholic (45%), as compared with 64% of Latina/os ages 50 and older (64%). Interestingly, younger men with higher levels of educational attainment identify as religiously unaffiliated (Pew Research Center, 2014). The 2013 National Survey of Latinos and Religion also indicates that among Latina/os who changed their religious affiliations, 55% gradually "drifted away" from their childhood religion and 52% no longer

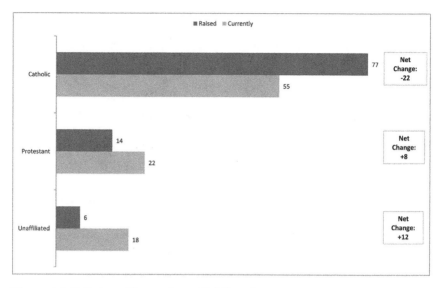

Figure 1.3 Religious Change from Childhood to Present Day among Latina/os, by Percentages.

Source: Pew Research Center. (2014). The shifting religious identity of Latinos in the United States: Nearly one-in-four Latinos are former Catholics. Washington, DC: Pew Research Center.

believe in the teachings of their childhood religion. Among former Catholics who are currently Protestants, 49% report that it is important for them to locate a church that "reaches out and helps its members more" (Pew Research Center, 2014).

SOCIOECONOMIC STATUS OF LATINA/OS

Socioeconomic factors also influence the social, physical, and psychological well-being of Latina/os. These factors merit consideration to understand the epidemiological and psychological issues of Latina/os (Casas et al., 2015), particularly as the economic and social disparities of Latina/os are reflected in their limited access to adequate medical and psychological care. Likewise, the socioeconomic disadvantages of Latina/os, particularly immigrants, also contribute to their increased exposure to occupational and environmental hazards, long work hours, lack of employer benefits, and limited occupational mobility throughout their lifetime (Andrade & Viruell-Fuentes, 2011). Similarly, residence in poor and unsafe neighborhoods and food insecurity also create chronic stressors that compromise the health and mental health of Latina/os (Vega, Rodriguez, & Gruskin, 2009).

Education

Latina/os demonstrate the highest dropout rate among all major racial and ethnic groups and reached 1.5 million in 2001 (Fry, 2014). In 2014, Latina/os demonstrated the highest dropout rate (6.0%), followed by African Americans (4.6%), White/European Americans (3.3%), and Asian Americans (1.5%). There are also nativity differences among Latina/os, as foreign-born Latina/os demonstrate higher high school dropout rates (11.2%) than U.S.-born Latina/os (4.9%) (Stepler & Brown, 2016). Furthermore, 35% of Latina/os aged 25 and older have less than a high school education, as compared with 7.9% of White/European Americans and 15.5% of African Americans. There are greater educational disparities among foreign-born Latina/os, as 47.8% have less than a high school education, as compared with U.S.-born Latina/os (18.9%). However, despite increased trends indicating decreased dropout rates, educational disparities among Latina/os remain, as they are less likely to enroll in a four-year college, attend academically selective colleges, and attend full time (Krogstad, 2016). They also demonstrate greater enrollment within community colleges or public two-year schools, and their enrollment is higher than any racial/ethnic group (48%). However, only 30% of Whites/European Americans, 32% of Asian Americans, and 36% of African Americans attend public two-year colleges (Krogstad, 2016).

Latina/os also lag behind other racial/ethnic groups in their college completion. The Pew Research Center (Krogstad, 2016) indicates that although college enrollment significantly increased, from 22% in 1993 to 35% in 2014, among Latina/os between the ages of 18 to 24, their overall college completion rates are alarming. For instance, 63% of Asian Americans within this age group completed their college degree, followed by 41% of White/European Americans, and 22% of African Americans, but only 15% of Latina/os between the ages of 18 and 24 completed their college degree in 2014 (Krogstad, 2016). Among adults who earned a Bachelor's degree or higher, there are similar trends, Asian Americans have the highest rates (51.7%), followed by White/European Americans (33.6%), and African Americans (19.8%). Regrettably, Latina/os have the lowest percentage of adults who earned a Bachelor's degree or higher (14.4%) (Stepler & Brown, 2016). There are also nativity differences in college completion rates, as U.S.-born Latina/os report higher college completion rates (18.8%) than foreign-born Latina/os (10.8%) (see Table 1.4). Among Latina/o heritage groups, Venezuelans report the highest percentage of educational attainment, as 50% earned a Bachelor's degree or higher. Conversely, Salvadorans attained the lowest percentage of educational attainment, as only 8% earned a Bachelor's degree or higher, followed by Hondurans and Guatemalans (9% each) (López & Patten, 2015).

Table 1.4 Median Household Income, Percent of Poverty, and Share without Health Insurance among Latina/o Heritage Groups, 2013

	Bachelor's Degree or More	Education Some College	H.S. Diploma or Less	Median Household Income	% of Poverty Line	Share Without Health Insurance
Argentinean	41%	26%	33%	$63,000	11%	21%
Colombian	33%	30%	38%	$50,900	16%	25%
Cuban	25%	24%	51%	$40,500	20%	25%
Dominican	17%	26%	58%	$33,900	28%	21%
Ecuadorian	19%	25%	56%	$48,000	19%	31%
Guatemalan	9%	15%	75%	$38,200	28%	45%
Honduran	9%	18%	74%	$36,080	28%	46%
Mexican	10%	22%	68%	$40,000	26%	31%
Nicaraguan	19%	29%	52%	$50,000	17%	31%
Peruvian	31%	31%	38%	$53,000	13%	26%
Puerto Rican	18%	30%	53%	$38,900	27%	14%
Salvadoran	8%	18%	74%	$44,060	20%	37%
Venezuelan	50%	28%	22%	$56,270	18%	26%

Source: López, G., & Patten, E. (2015). *The impact of slowing immigration: Foreign-born share falls among 14 largest U.S. Hispanic origin groups.* Washington, DC: Pew Research Center.

Employment

Among persons 16 years of age and older who were not in the labor force in 2014, Latina/os reported the lowest rates of unemployment, at 33% (foreign-born Latina/os, 30.8%; U.S.-born Latina/os, 34.9%), as compared with African Americans (38.1%), White/European Americans (37.7%), Other (37.5%), and Asian Americans (35.4%). However, their high rates of employment do not immediately translate into greater economic benefits such as employer-supplied benefits, upward mobility, and decreased economic exploitation. For example, it is speculated that while 66% of Latina/os were employed, they lacked health insurance because of their employment in occupations that do not offer affordable health care. For example, only 2.2% of Latina/os were employed in science and engineering occupations in 2014 (Stepler & Brown, 2016). Census data indicate that the five main occupations among Latina/os include office and administrative support (11.9%), installation, repair, and production (11.1%), sales (10.1%), construction and extraction (9.1%), and building and grounds cleaning and maintenance (8.9%). There are nativity differences among Latina/os, as the five main occupations of foreign-born Latina/os include building and grounds cleaning and maintenance (13.7%), installation, repair, and production (13.6%), construction and extraction (13.3%), food preparation and serving (10.1%), and transportation and material moving (9.2%). However, among U.S.-born Latina/os, their five main occupations include office and administrative support (15.8%), sales (12.8%), management and business (9.6%), installation, repair, and production (8.7%), and food preparation and serving (7.7%) (Stepler & Brown, 2016).

Poverty

Unfortunately, Latina/os live in poverty and experience economic disparities. For instance, in 2010 the Pew Hispanic Center (Lopez & Velasco, 2011) reported that the highest number of children who lived in poverty were Latina/os (6.1 million [37.3%]), as compared with White/European American (30.5%), and African American children (26.6%). Among these Latina/o children, 4.1 million were children of immigrant parents, while 2.0 million had U.S.-born parents. More recent data indicate that 14.9% of the U.S. population lives below the poverty line (Stepler & Brown, 2016). Among racial/ethnic groups, African Americans have the largest percentage of individuals living below the poverty line (26.3%), followed by Latina/os (23.5%), Asian Americans (11.8%), and White/European Americans (10.3%) (Stepler & Brown, 2016). Among Latina/o heritage groups, Guatemalans, Hondurans, and Dominicans demonstrate the highest proportion of persons living below the poverty line (28% each), while Argentineans have the lowest proportion (11%) (see Table 1.4). The 2014 median household income for Latina/os was $42,200, but the median household income for the U.S. population was significantly higher, at $53,200 (López & Patten, 2015).

There are nativity differences among Latina/os; U.S.-born Latina/os earned $47,400, as compared with $39,000 among foreign-born Latina/os (Stepler & Brown, 2016). Interestingly, Argentineans demonstrate the highest median household income, at $63,000, while Dominicans and Hondurans demonstrate lower median household incomes ($33,900 and $36,080, respectively) (López & Patten, 2015). Other indicators of poverty also include welfare income and food stamps. For example, in 2014, 3.9% of Latina/os received welfare income, as compared with 2.7% of the U.S. population, and 22.4% of Latina/os received food stamps, as compared with 13.2% of the U.S. population (Stepler & Brown, 2016).

Insurance Coverage

Census data also indicate that Latinos are uninsured. Latina/os comprise the highest percentage of uninsured persons within the United States (23.7%) and surpass the percentage of the total uninsured population (12.0%) and all ethnic/racial groups, including African Americans (14.6%), Asian Americans (10.4%), and White/European Americans (8.2%) (Stepler & Brown, 2016). There are also similar nativity trends, a higher percentage of foreign-born Latina/os are uninsured (41.7%) compared to U.S. born Latina/os (14.0%) (Stepler & Brown, 2016). Prior to the implementation of the Affordable Care Act in 2013, Hondurans and Guatemalans had the largest percentage of uninsured persons (46% and 45%, respectively) while Puerto Ricans had the smallest percentage of uninsured persons (14%) (López & Patten, 2015).

Geographical Locations of Latina/os

Most Latina/os (76%) reside within nine states, including Arizona, California, Texas, Colorado, Florida, Illinois, New Mexico, New Jersey, and New York (Ennis, Rios-Vargas, & Albert, 2011). In addition, 50% of Latina/os reside in just three states—California, Texas, and Florida. However, Latina/o heritage groups tend to concentrate in specific geographical regions of the United States for various reasons, including geography, history, socioeconomic, and political factors (Casas et al., 2015). Census data (Ennis et al., 2011) indicate that California, Texas, Arizona, Illinois, and Colorado are five states with large Mexican populations (one million or more), while Puerto Ricans are concentrated in New York, Florida, New Jersey, Pennsylvania, and Massachusetts (see Figure 1.4). Cubans are concentrated in Florida,

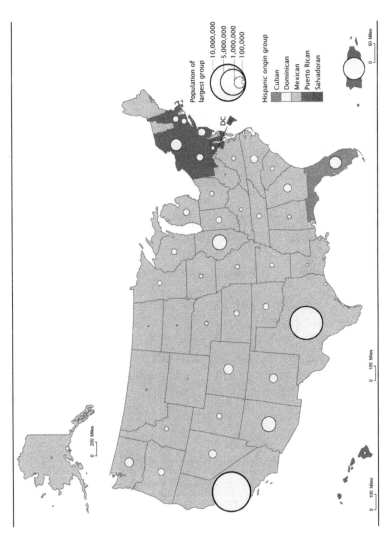

Figure 1.4 Distribution of Latina/o Heritage Groups by State, 2010.

The area of each circle is proportional to the population of the largest Hispanic origin group in a state. The legend presents example symbol sizes from the many symbols shown on the map.

Source: Ennis, S. R., Rios-Vargas, M., & Albert, N. G. (2011). The Hispanic population: 2010. https://www.census.gov/prod/cen2010/briefs/c2010br-04.pdf

California, New Jersey, New York, and Texas. Dominicans are concentrated in New York, New Jersey, Florida, Massachusetts, and Pennsylvania, while Guatemalans are concentrated within California, Florida, New York, Texas, and New Jersey. Lastly, Salvadorans are concentrated in California, Texas, New York, Virginia, and Maryland, and other Latina/os with less than one million persons are concentrated in California, Florida, Texas, New York, and New Jersey (Ennis et al., 2011).

Demographic changes are also evident within other states (see Figure 1.5), as the Latina/o population increased significantly in the South and Midwest, and the population in these areas more than doubled between 2000 and 2010 (Ennis et al., 2011). These new relocation patterns among Latina/os in new destinations are attributed to a hostile political climate in the Southwest and increased employment opportunities and increased job security within meat and poultry processing and nondurable manufacturing plants in rural areas (Crowley & Lichter, 2009). Sáenz and Morales (2015) identified 20 new Latina/o destination states (i.e., states in which Latina/o populations drastically increased between 1980 and 2010, with an unprecedented growth of 245%). These states within the Midwest, South, and Northeast include the following: Alabama, Arkansas, Delaware, Georgia, Iowa, Kansas, Kentucky, Maryland, Minnesota, Missouri, Nebraska, New Hampshire, North Carolina, North Dakota, Oklahoma, Rhode Island, South Carolina, South Dakota, Tennessee, and Wisconsin (see Table 1.5). In one decade alone, between 2000 and 2010, the population of Latina/os

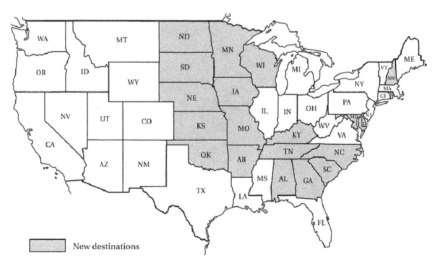

Figure 1.5 Population Growth between 2007 and 2014.

Source: Sáenz, R., & Morales, M. C. (2015). *Latinos in the United States: Diversity and change.* Malden, MA: Polity Press.

Table 1.5 Latina/o Population Changes in Latina/o New Destination States and Other States, 2000–2010

Latino Population			Latino % Change	% of 2000–2010 State Growth Due to Latinos	% of State Population Latino	
States	**2000**	**2010**	**2000– 2010**		**2000**	**2010**
Alabama	75,830	185,602	114.8	33.0	1.7	3.9
Arkansas	86,866	186,050	114.2	40.9	3.2	6.4
Delaware	37,277	73,221	96.4	31.4	4.8	8.2
Georgia	435,227	853,689	96.1	27.9	5.3	8.8
Iowa	82,473	151,544	83.7	57.5	2.8	5.0
Kansas	188,252	300,042	59.4	67.9	7.0	10.5
Kentucky	59,939	132,836	121.6	24.5	1.5	3.1
Maryland	227,916	470,632	106.5	50.9	4.3	8.2
Minnesota	143,382	250,258	74.5	27.8	2.9	4.7
Missouri	118,592	212,470	79.2	23.8	2.1	3.5
Nebraska	94,425	167,405	77.3	63.4	5.5	9.2
New Hampshire	20,489	36,704	79.1	20.1	1.7	2.8
North Carolina	378,963	800,120	111.1	28.3	4.7	8.4
North Dakota	7,786	13,467	73.0	18.7	1.2	2.0
Oklahoma	179,304	332,007	85.2	50.8	5.2	8.9
Rhode Island	90,820	130,655	43.9	937.7[a]	8.7	12.4
South Carolina	95,076	235,682	147.9	22.9	2.4	5.1
South Dakota	10,903	22,119	102.9	18.9	1.4	2.7
Tennessee	123,838	290,059	134.2	25.3	2.2	4.6
Wisconsin	192,921	336,056	74.2	44.3	3.6	5.9
New destination states	2,650,279	5,180,618	95.5	32.9	3.6	6.4
All other states	32,655,539	45,296,976	38.7	64.4	15.7	19.9
Total	35,305,818	50,477,594	43.0	55.5	12.5	16.3

[a] Because of population loss of non-Latinos, the total population of Rhode Island increased by only 4,248 between 2000 and 2010, while the Latino population grew by 38,835 during this period.

Source: Sáenz, R., & Morales, M. C. (2015). *Latinos in the United States: Diversity and change.* Malden, MA: Polity Press.

doubled from 2.7 million in 2000 to 5.2 million in 2010. For instance, between 2000 and 2010 the population of Latina/os in South Carolina increased by 147.9% (See Table 1.5). Unfortunately, many of these new destination areas lack the necessary infrastructure to meet the needs of immigrant Latina/os and the unprecedented growth in their population.

IMMIGRATION EXPERIENCES OF LATINA/O HERITAGE GROUPS

Latina/o heritage groups differ in their immigration patterns and sociopolitical histories, including exposure to social, material, and political inequality (Guarnaccia et al., 2005a). However, Latin America and the Spanish Caribbean share similar histories of colonization imperialism and a contentious relationship with the United States. Grey and Hall-Clark (2015) note that the influence of the U.S. military, and political, and economic interests shaped the lives of Latina/os and contributed to their loss of land, economic exploitation, conflict, and distrust of the U.S. government. In particular, their second-class citizenship and history of colonization is evident, particularly as U.S. political doctrines and military interventions regarding land, politics, and trade resulted in economic and political dominance in Latin America and adversely impacted the physical and psychological well-being of Latina/os (Organista, 2007). Consequently, many Latina/os fled their native countries in search of economic prosperity and safety for their families (p. xix). In addition, the drug trade, guerilla warfare, violence, and civil wars in Latin America also impacted its citizens, as well as individuals within the United States. Thus, poverty, violence, and instability prompted numerous Latina/os to leave their countries of origin (Grey & Hall-Clark, 2015). The immigration history of each specific Latina/o heritage group has implications for its reception and subsequent economic or social integration, as well as their lack of integration into the United States. These histories reflect their current social and economic position as well as their access to resources (Andrade & Viruell-Fuentes, 2011; Arellano-Morales et al., 2015).

Geographical distinctions among Latina/o heritage groups are often due to their distinct immigration experiences, and current economic factors influence the regions in which different Latina/o heritage groups reside. Competition for resources, anti-Latina/o sentiments, and political rhetoric also shape the experiences of Latina/os and shape their physical and mental health. Thus, we discuss the immigration experiences of diverse Latina/o heritage groups to provide a context of their sociopolitical histories. For instance, while a significant number of Latina/os immigrated within the past few decades, we remind the reader that they are not a newly arrived group in the United States, as their presence within the Americas predates the arrival of the Spaniards and other Europeans (Andrade & Viruell-Fuentes, 2011).

Mexican Americans

Mexicans are the largest Latino heritage group (64%), and there are currently 35,371,314 Latina/os of Mexican heritage in the United States (Stepler & Brown, 2016). They have unique patterns of immigration because similar to Native Americans, Mexicans were native to what is currently regarded as the Southwest United States. The indigenous history of Mexico (i.e., Aztecs, Toltecs, Mayans, Zapotecs, Tarascans, Purepechas, and many others) predates the arrival of Spanish conquistadores during the 15th century that resulted in forced colonization and genocide. Consequently, the mixture of Europeans and indigenous persons resulted in *mestizos*. In terms of Mexico's history with the United States, it is marked by conflict that includes war, substantial loss of land, and continuous exploitation of labor (Organista, 2007).

Because of the Mexican War and 1848 Treaty of Guadalupe Hidalgo, approximately half of Mexico was ceded to the United States. Despite receiving dual citizenship under this treaty, most Mexicans lost their substantial land holdings because of heavy taxation and seizure, the encroachment of American settlers, and other dishonest activities (Organista, 2007). Unfortunately, many elite and peasant Mexicans found themselves poor, disenfranchised, and exploited. Events such as the Mexican revolution, economic decline, and political turmoil contributed to large waves of immigration into the United States. For instance, approximately 750,000 Mexicans immigrated between 1900 and 1930. In addition, the need for cheap labor and decreased immigration restrictions contributed to increased immigration among Mexicans during the past century (Galarraga, 2007).

According to Organista (2007), the history of Mexican labor is one that is marked by cyclical patterns that reveal exploitation during labor shortages and the abuse of their civil rights during periods of economic recession (p. 17). For instance, the loss of basic human rights was demonstrated within the repatriation of approximately one million Mexican Americans during the Depression in the early 1930s (Balderrama & Rodríguez, 1995). Because of the assumption that Mexicans were a tax burden and also seized jobs from Americans, they were indiscriminately repatriated, as were their U.S.-born children. The shortage of labor due to WWII resulted in the importation of Mexicans for agricultural labor through the *Bracero Program*. Between 1942 and 1964, approximately five million braceros entered the United States from Mexico as laborers (Organista, 2007). However, because of the large number of immigrants entering the United States, anti-Mexican hysteria also resurfaced and under the directives of the U.S. Immigration Service, *Operation Wetback* was developed. Approximately 3.8 individuals of Mexican descent, including the U.S.-born children were deported. Decades later, the passage of Arizona Senate Bill 1070, received considerable attention and generated considerable controversy, as one of the strictest anti–illegal immigration laws within the United States, and allows for the racial profiling of Latinos and the deportation of unauthorized immigrants. In addition, the first 100 days of Trump's presidency hallmarks significant criminalization of Latina/o immigrants, increased raids, and deportations.

Puerto Ricans

The history of Puerto Rico is also manifested by a legacy of conquest. Spanish conquistadors landed on the island of Puerto Rico (originally known as Boriquen), in 1493 and subsequently conquered the indigenous Taínos. Regrettably, the Taínos were soon annihilated as a result of forced labor, disease, and violence. African slaves were imported because of the decreased number of Taínos, and marriages between African slaves, Spaniards, and Taínos created the rich composition of Puerto Ricans (Organista, 2007). Four centuries later, Puerto Rico became a U.S. territory in 1898 as a result of the brief Spanish–American War and the Foraker Act of 1900. As a commonwealth, Puerto Rico has a history of conflict and subordination with the United States. Heavy taxation, credit restrictions, and economic exploitation resulted in political turmoil and violence during the subsequent decades. As a commonwealth, the island of Puerto Rico has its own constitution and elected governor. However, while the Jones Act of 1917 granted Puerto Ricans U.S. citizenship, they remain politically and economically disenfranchised, since they are unable to vote in national elections and lack representation within the U.S. House and Senate (Organista, 2007).

Because Puerto Ricans are U.S. citizens, they are able to freely travel between the island and mainland without restrictions. As such, they are regarded as a *commuter nation* (Adames & Chavez-Dueñas, 2017). According to Canino and Stolberg (2001), there were various factors that contributed to their immigration to the mainland, including encouragement from the island government, island overpopulation, and low airfares to the United States. The immigration patterns of Puerto Ricans to the U.S. mainland are classified into three distinct periods. During the first period (1900–1945), most Puerto Ricans arrived in New York City. However, smaller groups also settled in Hawaii, California, Arizona, and Ohio. During the second period (1946–1964), also known as the *Great Migration*, the largest numbers of Puerto Ricans (approximately 887,000), settled in New York, New Jersey, Connecticut, Chicago, Pennsylvania, and other areas (Canino & Stolberg, 2001; Organista, 2007). The last period, regarded as the *revolving-door migration*, began in 1965. This period was characterized by fluctuating immigration patterns and greater dispersal into other areas of the United States. However, according to the Pew Research Center (Cohn, Patten, & Lopez, 2014), a large wave of immigration has occurred since 2010, as 144,000 Puerto Ricans left the island between 2010 and 2013 in search of economic opportunities on the mainland. These recent immigrants differ from earlier immigrants in that they are more likely to live in the South, especially in Florida, and to have lower household incomes and a greater likelihood of living in poverty. Puerto Ricans are the second largest Latino heritage group and represent 9.6% of Latinos, with 5,319,961 Puerto Ricans residing in the U.S. mainland (Stepler & Brown, 2016).

Cubans

Unlike the immigration histories of Mexican Americans and Puerto Ricans, the immigration experiences of Cubans are quite diverse and include four distinct waves of immigration. After the Spanish–American War, Cuba became an independent island in 1898. However, the United States held substantial economic interests in Cuba prior to Castro's regime. Economic exploitation resulted in an anti-American sentiment among its populace, and eventually led to the Cuban Revolution. While Fidel Castro's regime was initially regarded with optimism because of changes in health care and education, he became a dictator and persecuted his opponents (Organista, 2007). The hostility between Castro and the United States resulted in the first wave of 200,000 affluent and well-educated White Cuban immigrants who settled in south Florida between 1959 and 1962. These exiles were regarded as *Golden Exiles* because the majority were White Cuban professionals, entrepreneurs, and landowners. Because they fled communism, they encountered a positive reception, which was not granted to any other Latina/o heritage group throughout U.S. history, and this support helped facilitate their economic prosperity (Adames & Chavez-Dueñas, 2017). For example, they received unprecedented support through the 1966 Cuban Adjustment Act, that provided both direct and indirect assistance to facilitate their labor market integration, including certification of professional credentials, a college loan program, and bilingual education (Tienda & Sánchez, 2013), as well as an accelerated citizenship process. In addition, the Cuban Refugee Program provided approximately one billion dollars between 1965 and 1976 to help facilitate their economic and political prosperity (Adames & Chavez-Dueñas, 2017).

The second wave of Cuban immigration, between 1960 and 1970, was the largest, as it included 260,600 Cubans who were relatives of prior exiles. Because of the coordinated airlifts between the U.S. and Cuban government, these exiles also received refugee status. Because these exiles were brought to the United States from Cuba by airplane, this wave of immigration was regarded as the *Freedom Flights* (Adames & Chavez-Dueñas, 2017). The third wave of immigrants in 1980 differed significantly from the prior waves of immigrants. Regarded as *Marielitos*, because they sailed from the Port of Mariel, these Cuban exiles were not well received. Unfortunately, they arrived during an economic recession and comprised blue-collar workers (75%) and dark-skinned Black Cubans (Organista, 2007). Unlike their counterparts, they were housed in temporary detention camps and flown to military detention centers. They were also screened for "dangerousness" because of apprehension that they were criminals or mentally ill. The fourth wave of immigration began in 1994 with the rafter crisis and the numerous Cuban *balseros* (rafters) who attempted to enter the United States. This event initiated a rapid change in U.S. policy under President Clinton. The new policy required the U.S. Coast Guard to intercept *balseros* and redirect them to Guantánamo Bay according to the provisions of the Wet Foot/Dry Foot agreement. If they are caught at sea (wet foot) they are returned to Cuba but once they touch land (dry foot), they are granted permanent residency (Guzmán & Carrasco, 2011).

Cuban immigration to the United States increased dramatically with President Obama's renewed relations with Cuba in 2014. According to the Pew Research Center (Krogstad, 2017a), 24,278 Cubans entered the United States in fiscal year 2014, and the number of Cubans who entered the United States in fiscal year 2015 increased significantly, by 78% ($N=43,159$). In addition, 56,406 Cubans entered the United States in fiscal year 2016 (Krogstad, 2017a). Current data suggest that 2,045,970 Cubans reside in the United States, and represent 3.7% of Latinos, making them the fourth-largest Latino heritage group (Stepler & Brown, 2016).

Dominicans

As with Puerto Rico, the Dominican Republic was under Spanish rule and also experienced a contentious relationship with the United States. For example, Christopher Columbus first colonized the Dominican Republic in 1492. Because of the demise of the indigenous Caribitaino and Arawak, the Spanish imported African slaves to the Caribbean (Adames & Chavez-Dueñas, 2017). The United States also occupied the Dominican Republic between 1916 and 1924 during World War I. Despite sporadic migrations among middle-class Dominicans in the 1950s during President Rafael

Trujillo's dictatorship, large waves of immigration began after the civil war and subsequent U.S. intervention (Guzmán & Carrasco, 2011). The first wave of immigration began in the 1960s, as 10,000 Dominicans feared for their safety following President Trujillo's assassination and the election of Juan Bosch. Fears of communism prompted the United States to reoccupy the Dominican Republic in 1965. The continued political unrest contributed to the second large wave of immigration among largely blue-collar workers between 1968 and 1973 who settled mostly in the Northeast. The third wave of immigration took place during the 1980s and 1990s, due to the Dominican economic crisis (Adames & Chavez-Dueñas, 2017). In addition to settlements in New York and Boston, Dominicans also settled in Miami. Current estimates suggest that 1,763,651 Dominicans reside in the United States and represent 3.2% of Latinos.

Central Americans

Immigrants from Central America (i.e., Costa Rica, El Salvador, Guatemala, Honduras, Nicaragua, and Panama) who immigrated to the United States before the 1970s were largely persons from middle- or upper-class backgrounds, as well as displaced farmers and workers, due to industrialization, changes in agriculture, political unrest, and increased foreign interventions (Andrade & Viruell-Fuentes, 2011). After the 1970s, political turmoil and violence, poverty, economic threats, oppression, and egregious human rights abuses created the first large waves of immigrants from Central America, beginning with Salvadorans, followed by Guatemalans in the early 1980s, as well as Nicaraguans and Hondurans in the mid-1980s (Engstrom & Piedra, 2005; Organista, 2007). Many immigrants included individuals from rural areas with lower levels of education (Andrade & Viruell-Fuentes, 2011). Organista (2007) suggests that because their lives were interrupted by intense civil wars, they are considered "cross-fire refugees" (p. 33). Accordingly, more than a million Central Americans fled to the United States to escape guerilla warfare, violence, and other traumatic activities. For example, Engstrom and Piedra (2005) indicate that "the terms *massacre*, *death squads*, *torture*, and *disappearance* are commonly associated with political violence in Central America" (p. 175), as an estimated 300,000 Central Americans were killed and numerous others experienced injury and trauma.

In addition, these Central American countries were characterized by extreme poverty, high mortality rates, and vast disparities among the poor and wealthy. Despite the political turmoil and violence within many of these countries, the U.S. federal government failed to acknowledge the political persecution of refugees from El Salvador, Honduras, and Guatemala and failed to provide political asylum and government assistance as political refugees. However, the U.S. provided Nicaraguan refugees with increased support because it recognized their persecution from communist Sandinistas (Engstrom & Piedra, 2005; Guzmán & Carrasco, 2011). However, for political reasons, the United States failed to initially grant them political asylum and government assistance as political refugees.

Unfortunately, their lack of federal assistance and classification as political refugees did not facilitate their reception and incorporation into the United States. However, the efforts of immigrant-rights groups and class-action lawsuits resulted in the provision of *Temporary Protected Status* by the Justice Department to Salvadorans who arrived prior to September 1990. Their temporary protected status is time-limited and does not offer a pathway to permanent resident status but requires acts of Congress to gain extensions (Tienda & Sánchez, 2013). Congress also passed the Nicaraguan Adjustment and Central America Relief Act of 1997 to confer legal permanent resident status to registered asylees (and their dependents) from Nicaragua, Cuba, El Salvador, and Guatemala who resided in the United States for at least five consecutive years before December 1, 1995. In addition, because of natural disasters, such as Hurricane Mitch and Salvadoran earthquakes, Central American refugees also received temporary protected status until 2013 (Tienda & Sánchez, 2013).

South Americans

Immigration from South American predates the late 18th century, before Latin American wars for independence, but the first major wave included almost half a million immigrants from South America after WWII, between 1951 and 1977 (Andrade & Viruell-Fuentes, 2011; Oboler, 2005). As with other Latin American countries, immigration from South American countries (Argentina, Bolivia, Chile, Colombia, Ecuador, Paraguay, Peru, Uruguay, and Venezuela) was also shaped by U.S. foreign and economic policies. For example, the Cold War and fear of communism contributed to economic and political instability, as the United States supported corrupt regimes and dictators to support its economic and strategic interests in South America (Guzmán & Carrasco, 2011). This also resulted in the international migration of South American professionals between the 1960s and mid-1970s (Andrade & Viruell-Fuentes, 2011). The exodus of these middle- and upper-class professionals was regarded as "the brain drain" due to the need for doctors, nurses, physicians, scientists, and engineers in the United States (Oboler, 2005). In addition, the modernization in agriculture resulted in the loss and displacement of thousands of peasants and small farmers.

The second large wave of immigration is attributed to the forced migration and political exile of South Americans who fled their homelands in Chile, Argentina, Uruguay, and Paraguay from the mid-1970s through the 1980s because of the terror created by dictators (Oboler, 2005). While these dictatorships eventually ended at the conclusion of the 20th century, South Americans continue to immigrate to the United States because of widespread poverty (Andrade & Viruell-Fuentes, 2011), economic instability, and drug violence in Colombia, Peru, and Ecuador. For instance, hyperinflation and massive underemployment accelerated Peruvian immigration during the 1990s, and prolonged political instability, armed conflict, and drug violence triggered Colombian emigration over the latter half of the 20th century. Although the early waves of Colombian immigrants largely included upper-class professionals, members of the working class also immigrated to the United States (Tienda & Sánchez, 2011).

SUMMARY

Latina/os are not a monolithic group and demonstrate diverse immigration patterns and sociopolitical histories. Their countries of origin also demonstrate divergent relationships with the United States, although most Latin American countries have experienced a history of conflict with the United States. Thus, health and mental health providers must be well informed of their clients' sociopolitical histories, particularly their Latina/o clients, as they shape their well-being. Further, such awareness of these variables should contribute to humane and respectful attitudes toward Latinos in clinical work with Latina/os.

LATINA/O IMMIGRANTS WITHIN THE UNITED STATES

Latina/os have a long-standing history of immigration to the United States but their immigration patterns have changed in the past decade. For instance, in 2000, Mexico alone accounted for a third (34%) of recent immigrants, an 11% increase from 1970. Combined with other immigrants from Central and South America (13%), Latina/os comprised 48% of all recent arrivals in 2000 (Pew Research Center, 2015a). However, the share of recent arrivals from Mexico decreased significantly, to only 15% in 2013, but the share of recent arrivals from Central and South America remained constant (13%), indicating that Latina/os solely comprised 28% of all recent arrivals. Demographic trends indicate that immigration from Latin America has declined since 2010, and the percentage of foreign-born Latina/os declined from 40% in 2000 to 35% in 2013 (López & Patten, 2015), including Ecuadorian, Mexican, and Nicaraguan immigrants.

Unauthorized Latina/o Immigrants

Several labels, that are often derogatory, are ascribed to unauthorized Latina/os, such as *illegal alien* or *illegal*. Instead, Latina/os scholars call for the use of humane terms. While the term *undocumented immigrant* is often used, the use of the term *unauthorized immigrant* is preferred (Arredondo et al., 2014). An unauthorized immigrant is a person who entered the United States without authorization or arrived with a visa and remained after it expired (Pew Research Center, 2015b). According to the Pew Research Center, there are an estimated 11.3 million unauthorized U.S. immigrants (Krogstad, Passel, & Cohn, 2017), and Mexico also is the largest (49%) source of U.S. unauthorized immigrants (Passel & Cohn, 2014). However, the number of unauthorized Mexican immigrants declined from 6.4 million in 2009 to 5.6 million in 2014, largely because of family reunification. Economic and political factors contribute to decreased immigration rates among Latina/os, such as the U.S. economic recession and deterioration of the U.S. job market, as well as stricter enforcement of immigration laws and deportations (Pew Research Center, 2015b). However, among other Latina/o heritage groups, El Salvador (675,000) has the second highest percentage of unauthorized immigrants, followed by Guatemala (525,000), Honduras (350,000), the Dominican Republic (170,000), and Colombia (150,000) (Passel & Cohn, 2014). In addition to experiencing political turmoil and violence, poverty, economic threats, oppression, and egregious human rights abuses within their countries of origin (Engstrom & Piedra, 2005), unauthorized Latina/o immigrants also face significant risk during their perilous journey to the United States, such as extortion, sexual assault, kidnapping, human trafficking, and forced disappearance (Stinchcomb & Hershberg, 2014). Unfortunately, these tumultuous experience contribute to their increased rates of post-traumatic stress disorder (PTSD) and other related disorders.

As with adults, unaccompanied Latina/o children also make treacherous journeys to the United States in search of a better life, safety, and family reunification (Adames & Chavez-Dueñas, 2017; Stinchcomb & Hershberg, 2014). The number of unaccompanied Latina/o minors has drastically increased. For example, of the 68,541 unaccompanied minors in 2014, a total of 51,705 (75%) were from the "Northern Triangle" countries of Central America, including El Salvador, Guatemala, and Honduras. The number of unaccompanied minors from these Northern Triangle countries also drastically increased between 2011 and 2014, as the U.S. Customs and

Border Protection apprehended 15,949 unaccompanied minors in 2011 and 68,541 unaccompanied minors in 2014, a striking 429% increase (Stinchcomb & Hershberg, 2014).

Tragically, unaccompanied minors who are detained by government officials may also experience degrading and frightening conditions during their detainment. For example, in 2014 government officials were ill prepared to deal with the arrival of large numbers of unaccompanied minors, and many children experienced human rights violations, such as being housed in warehouses without access to food, water, or showers (Adames & Chavez-Dueñas, 2017). Unfortunately, not all unaccompanied minors receive political asylum and are forced to return to their home countries. For example, among unaccompanied minors from the Northern Triangle, only 14% received asylum in 2013 (Stinchcomb & Hershberg, 2014).

The process of immigration is often stressful for Latina/o immigrants (Arbona et al., 2010; Cavazos-Rehg, Zayas, & Spitznagel, 2007; Goodkind, Gonzales, Malcoe, & Espinosa, 2008; Sullivan & Rehm, 2005), and the physical journey to the United States is often dangerous or fatal for unauthorized Latina/o immigrants. Unauthorized Latina/os experience language limitations, limited access to resources, trauma, social isolation, and vulnerability including fear of deportation, and human rights violations (Cavazos-Rehg et al., 2007; Díaz-Lázaro, Verdinelli, & Cohen, 2012; Sullivan & Rehm, 2005). Latina/o immigrants often reside in crowded or unsafe neighborhoods, experience poverty and economic exploitation, and are often employed in occupations that are unsteady, physically unsafe, and low paying (Cavazos-Rehg et al., 2007; Eggerth, DeLaney, Flynn, & Jacobson, 2012).

Latina/o immigrants are frequently regarded as second-class citizens and perceived as criminals or "social pariahs" who drain the economy (Sullivan & Rehm, 2005). Dehumanizing portrayals of Latina/o immigrants in the media and the larger political discourse may implicitly encourage violence and harassment against undocumented Latina/o immigrants (Ayón & Becerra, 2013). Regrettably, unauthorized Latina/os face increased risk of health and psychological disorders because of prolonged exposure to stress and constant fear of deportation (American Psychological Association, Presidential Task Force on Immigration, 2012; Cavazos-Rehg et al., 2007; Fussell, 2011). Because they are criminalized, unauthorized Latina/os are fearful of seeking critical services, such as police assistance or medical care (Adames & Chavez-Dueñas, 2017). Punitive and restrictive anti-immigration laws, such as Arizona's Senate Bill 1070, and other legislation in Alabama and Georgia have amplified hate crimes against Latina/os, among both unauthorized and U.S. citizens. Lamentably, President's Trump anti-immigrant rhetoric also contributes to increased hostility toward Latina/os and other immigrant groups.

As of this writing, the Deferred Action for Childhood Arrivals (DACA) remains vulnerable, as critics argue that it creates amnesty and provides social and economic benefits to more than 750,000 young unauthorized individuals (Krogstad, 2017b). While DACA allows unauthorized Latina/os under the age of 31 to apply for a driver's license, attend school, and obtain a work permit, it is not a direct pathway to citizenship. The Development, Relief, and Education for Alien Minors (DREAM) Act is bipartisan legislation that aims to create a pathway to citizenship for unauthorized children if they meet the following criteria: Arrival to the United States as a minor (younger than the age of 16), continuous residency in the United States for at least five years, good moral character, and a high school diploma or GED. Additional provisions include serving in the military or graduating from a four-year university ("The DREAM ACT", n.d.).

Mixed-Status Families

The aggressive enforcement of immigration policies impacts not only individuals but Latina/o families as well (Enriquez, 2015), as approximately five million children have at least one unauthorized parent (Adames & Chavez-Dueñas, 2017; Capps, Castañeda Chaudry, & Santos, 2007). Families that include both U.S. citizens and authorized family members are regarded as *mixed status*. Unfortunately, mixed-status families, particularly immigrant Latina mothers, are also the targets of countless hate groups and elected officials who equate them with vermin and opportunists (Romero, 2011). For example, the hate group Mothers Against Illegal Aliens (MAIA) asserts that Mexican immigrant mothers are opportunistic breeders who have numerous illegitimate children to gain access to public resources and citizenship and consequently injure "legitimate" White children in the process (Romero, 2011). What is lost in this nativist rhetoric and criminalization of mixed status Latina/o families is the reality that they must contend with the stressors of living with the fear of policing programs, raids, detention, and deportation. Unfortunately, these stressors create adverse emotional, relational, financial, and academic consequences for Latina/o immigrant parents and their children (Brabeck & Xu, 2010; Capps et al., 2007; Chaudry et al., 2010).

The constant fear of deportation and separation from their family members also negatively impacts the health and mental health of mixed-status families (Adames & Chavez-Dueñas, 2017; Brabeck & Xu, 2010; Capps et al., 2007). Furthermore, families who experience deportation experience significant hardships, including difficulty coping with economic and psychological stressors. Children experience feelings of abandonment, emotional trauma, psychological duress, and mental health problems (Baum, Jones, & Barry, 2010; Capps et al., 2007; Chaudry et al., 2010). For example, The National Council of La Raza (NCLR; Capps et al., 2007) examined three communities (New Bedford, MA, Grand Island, NE, and Greeley, CO) that experienced large-scale workplace raids and impacted 912 Mexican, Guatemalan, Honduran, and Salvadoran immigrant workers. In the immediate aftermath of the raids, their children ($N=506$), who were largely citizens (66%), were temporarily or permanently separated from their parents.

The NCLR reports that these Latina/o immigrant workers and their families experienced feelings of abandonment, trauma, fear, isolation, depression, family fragmentation, limited supervision, and economic hardships (Capps et al., 2007). In particular, the combination of fear, isolation, and economic hardship also led to depression, separation anxiety disorder, PTSD, school absences, and suicidal thoughts. Lamentably, very few individuals sought mental health care for themselves or their children (Capps et al., 2007). These findings support prior studies indicating that parental deportation causes increased emotional and behavioral distress among Latina/o children, including sleep problems, depression, anxiety, and poorer grades (Allen, Cisneros, & Tellez, 2015; Baum et al. 2010; Brabeck & Xu 2010; Chaudry et al., 2010; Dreby 2012; Zayas, Aguilar-Gaxiola, Yoon, & Rey, 2015), as well as the loss of supportive school networks, strained relationships with parents, and violence (Gulbas et al., 2016).

CULTURAL VALUES AMONG LATINA/OS

Today's Latinos/as are the descendants of remarkably advanced, fascinating, and resilient civilizations, rich in racial and cultural diversity. Their legacy is alive today in the strong traditional values that were an integral part of their cultures.

—Adames and Chavez-Dueñas, 2017, p. 28

Latina/o families are fluid and dynamic and in a state of transformation because of social, political, and economic forces. In addition, factors such as acculturation shape Latina/o families. Thus, family configurations among Latina/os are diverse, and transformations are taking place with the blending of religions, spiritual practices, social classes, generations, and ethnicities, as well as same-sex unions and marriages (Arredondo et al., 2014). Furthermore, the parenting styles of Latina/os are diverse and impacted by acculturation and enculturation. For instance, parents with lower levels of acculturation may demonstrate greater control over their children, while parents with higher levels of acculturation may demonstrate greater egalitarianism (see Falicov, 2014 for a discussion of Latina/o parenting styles).

Latina/os share strong commonalities, such as the use of Spanish, a collectivistic orientation that emphasizes the importance of the family and extended family members, and strong community ties. Comas-Díaz (2006) suggests that most Latinos embrace a relational worldview that is central to their identity, well-being and healing. This relational orientation also shapes their identity based on various collective contexts, such as their identity in relation to family, ancestors, community, ethnicity, spirituality, and environment (p. 437). For instance, a core aspect of Latina/o culture is *familismo* (familism), characterized by family loyalty, cooperation, and family interdependence that involves family obligations, emotional and financial support, and personal involvement with others (Delgado et al., 2008; Falicov, 2009b, 2014). Co-parents or *compadres* may play an important role within family life and obtain kinship through religious ceremonies, such as baptisms, communions, and weddings (Falicov, 2009b, 2014; Santiago-Rivera et al., 2002). In addition, family and personal relationships are guided by *respeto* (respect), such as appropriate deferential behavior toward others. *Respeto* involves differential behavior based upon age, gender, or SES. For example, a son who demonstrates *respeto* toward an elder demonstrates that he is *una persona bien educada,* meaning that his parents taught him the importance of respect within interpersonal relationships (Gloria & Segura-Herrera, 2004). *Personalismo* is the tendency to prefer personal contact and the avoidance of conflict or confrontation (Adames & Chavez-Dueñas, 2017; Añez et al., 2008; Santiago-Rivera et al., 2002), and a style of communication that includes personal warmth and genuineness that transpires through *platicando* (small talk) (Adames & Chavez-Dueñas, 2017; Gloria & Segura-Herrera, 2004). Similarly, *amabilidad* (amiable) refers to politeness and civility within one's demeanor and interactions with others (Adames & Chavez-Dueñas, 2017). *Dignidad* (dignity) refers to the belief that individuals are inherently worthy and deserve respect (Adames & Chavez-Dueñas, 2017; Santiago-Rivera et al., 2002). Similarly, *confianza* (trust) is the development of trust, intimacy, and familiarity that facilitate the expansion of interpersonal social networks, as trust is needed within these relationships (Adames & Chavez-Dueñas, 2017). While the endorsement of these cultural variables varies among Latina/os, as a function of their acculturation and enculturation, as well as their ethnic identity, caution is warranted regarding assumptions that they apply to all Latina/os (Gloria & Segura-Herrera, 2004).

Gender

Adherence to gender roles also varies among Latina/os, as these cultural values are fluid and shaped by various factors, such as acculturation, SES, education, and family composition (Santiago-Rivera et al., 2002). Nonetheless, Latina/o scholars indicate that great importance is given to gender roles among men and women and that these gender roles are often shaped by religious beliefs and values (Diaz, Mivelle, & Gil, 2013). The area of Latina/o gender roles, particularly *machismo*, is controversial because of the stereotypical and negative portrayals of Latino men that have dominated the literature, as well as portrayals of passive Latinas. Latino masculinity, is significantly more complex than the negative set of behaviors and traits (aggression, sexism, chauvinism, alcoholism, and hypermasculinity) that are often presented in the literature (Arciniega, Anderson, Tovar-Blank, & Tracey, 2008; Diaz et al., 2013; Torres, Solberg, & Carlstrom, 2002).

Furthermore, a wide range of masculine expressions incorporate elements of machismo (Torres et al., 2002). Thus, these narrow perspectives of Latino men fail to recognize how SES, economic independence, and acculturation significantly impact how gender roles are internalized or manifested behaviorally (Fallon & Bauza, 2015). For example, Mirandé, Pitones, and Diaz (2011) examined notions of masculinity among Latino day laborers and Chicano men. They observed that machismo and traditional masculinity were not culturally based phenomena but rather class-based, as polar views were observed between the two samples of Latinos. Day laborers were more likely to endorse traditional beliefs that reinforced the primacy of men and subordination of women, while their counterparts were more likely to endorse nontraditional gender roles. Recent conceptualizations of machismo suggest that it includes both negative and positive qualities, such as *caballerismo*. Arciniega and colleagues (2008) suggest that the concept of machismo is bidimensional and includes positive qualities, such as *caballerismo*. Originating in medieval codes of honor, *caballerismo* (horseman) includes being chivalrous, family-centered, nurturing, and emotionally connected. Research suggests that Latino men understand that their role as men includes respect for women and their autonomy, politeness, and nurturance of the family, but they also experience conflicting messages about masculinity (Arciniega et al., 2008; Diaz et al., 2013). Regrettably, discrimination and gender role conflict among Latinos often creates vulnerability to depression, anxiety, and substance use (Negi, 2013).

Marianismo is often regarded as the counterpart of machismo and has strong origins in the colonial period and Catholicism. Spaniards placed a strong emphasis on women's chastity, purity, and subservience, particularly as the Virgin Mary symbolized an important image of womanhood (Adames & Chavez-Dueñas, 2017). In addition, *marianismo* is supported by the cultural values of *simpatia*, *respeto*, and *familismo* (Castillo, Perez, Castillo, & Ghosheh, 2010; Piña-Watson et al., 2016). Recent empirical studies regarding *marianismo* indicate a multidimensional construct that includes the following dimensions: being virtuous and chaste, family and spiritual pillars, subordination to others, and self-silencing to maintain harmony (Castillo et al., 2010; Piña-Watson et al., 2016). Endorsement of *marianismo* varies among Latinas, according to their education, acculturation, economic independence, urban/rural residence, and other factors (Falicov, 2014; Faulkner, 2003).

Commitment to these elements of *marianismo* may create positive and negative consequences for women. For example, research indicates that Latinas who do not endorse these traditional views, such as chastity, may experience conflict with their mothers, community members, or partners, while Latinas who subscribe to chastity are regarded as good women (Faulkner, 2003). Recent studies indicate elements of *marianismo*, such being a family pillar, virtuous and chaste, and spiritual pillar are positively associated with positive academic attitudes and higher educational goals of Mexican American adolescents (Piña-Watson et al., 2016). However, despite the ongoing shift of gender roles, Latinas continue to experience distress due to familial, parental, acculturative, socioeconomic, employment, and racism-related stressors (Goodkind et al., 2008), as well as sexual harassment (Waugh, 2010) and intimate partner violence (Cho, Velez-Ortiz, & Parra-Cardona, 2014; Flores, 2004, Sabina, Cuevas, & Zadnik, 2015). Similarly, despite their educational advancement and professional achievements, Latina professionals also experience hostile work environments, tokenism, limited mentoring opportunities, and glass ceilings (Comas-Diaz, 1997).

Increased attention is also needed regarding lesbian, gay, bisexual, transgender, queer, questioning, intersex, asexual, and ally (LGBTQIA) Latina/os. Estimates suggest that LGBTQIA Latina/os comprise 15% of all adults and 17% of all LGBTQIA adults (Pastrana, Battle, & Harris, 2017), and approximately one million LGBTQIA Latina/o immigrants reside in the United States (Garcia, 2013). Because heterosexuality is often inherent in Latina/o culture, scholars prefer the term *Latinx* to identify the numerous persons of Latin American descent whose gender identities fluctuate among different points of the gender spectrum (Reichard, 2015), as the "x" erases gender (Pastrana et al., 2017). Adames and Chavez-Dueñas (2017) note that views of gender are grounded in a historical, cultural, and political context.

In addition, they suggest that gender norms, gender identity, and gender expression among Latina/os are shaped by their history and colonization, as observed by incidents of homophobia, heterosexism, and transphobia within the Latina/o community.

Lamentably, because heterosexuality is often inherent, homosexuality among Latina/o families is not always accepted. Thus, it is common for LGBTQIA Latina/os to hide their sexual identity from their families, colleagues, and society at large because of fears of rejection and isolation (Espín, 2012). Espín (2012) suggests that families may quietly tolerate a LGBTQIA family member but that their tolerance constitutes denial rather than acceptance of their sexuality. Flores (2013) also suggests that the coming-out process of LGBTQIA Latina/os may be experienced as "cultural suicide" because of the risk of family loss and community marginalization (p. 109). Thus, they are at risk for multiple forms of discrimination because of their gender, ethnicity, and sexuality, including physical and verbal abuse that may result in depression, isolation, and suicide (Flores, 2013; Morales, 2013), risky sexual behaviors and use of illegal drugs (Ryan, Huebner, Diaz, & Sanchez (2009), as well as suicidal ideation, anxiety, and exile from family (Díaz et al., 2001). LGBTQIA Latina/o immigrants may also leave their native countries to avoid violence and persecution (Cerezo, Morales, Quintero, & Rothman, 2014).

Recent scholarship suggests that the strength and saliency of family support impacts the coming-out process of LGBTQIA Latina/os, and being out to others is influenced by age, country of origin, connections to the LGBTQIA community, belief in the importance of sexual orientation, and family support (Pastrana, 2015). On average, LGBTQIA Latina/os come out to others at the age 15, a majority (92%) are out to their friends and family, and a majority (91%) feel supported by their families (Battle, Pastrana, & Daniels, 2013). It is also important to note that while LGBTQIA Latina/os experience significant challenges, they nonetheless demonstrate resilience and coping strategies that enable them to thrive (Gray, Mendelsohn, & Omoto, 2015), such as cultivating social networks, creating their own identities, and creating their own family structures to augment traditional family formations (Cerezo et al., 2014; Espín, 2012; Pastrana, 2015; Pastrana et al., 2017). Census data also indicate that LGBTQIA Latina/o same-sex couples fare better than their opposite-sex counterparts, as they demonstrate greater incomes and higher educational levels, and are more likely to engage egalitarian relationships (Pastrana et al., 2017). Also, approximately 29% of same-sex LGBTQIA Latina/o couples are raising children, including 22.6% of Latino same-sex couples and 41.5% of Latina same-sex couples (Pastrana et al., 2017).

CONCLUSION

The diversity of Latina/os dictates the need to for an increased understanding of their economic and sociopolitical realities. Indeed Latina/o heritage groups differ because of their migration patterns and sociopolitical histories, and their current social status, regional location, and social reception potentially affect their exposure to stressors that impact their physical and mental health. The impact of multiple forms of marginalization, both within and outside their families and communities, also shape their physical and mental health, and call for social justice within interpersonal, community, and institutional levels. Therefore, by conceptualizing that race/ethnicity, gender, sexuality, immigration status, and social class simultaneously shape the experience of Latina/os, health and mental health practitioners, researchers, and policymakers are able to develop an increased understanding of this diverse population.

Chapter 2

Patterns of Chronic Disease

For too long, Latino health research has been an afterthought, given attention only after the health of the non-Hispanic white and African American populations were studied. At one point, when Latinos were a small minority, this oversight might have been understandable.

—David E. Hayes-Bautista, 2002, p. 217

The health of Latina/os, the fastest-growing ethnic minority group, will directly impact our overall nation's health. As mentioned in Chapter 1, the presence of Latina/os is rapidly increasing, and Latina/os are projected to represent approximately 28.6% of the total U.S. population by 2060 (U.S. Census Bureau, 2015). Thus, the health of Latina/os is more important now than ever before to our nation's health. The presence of Latina/os not only necessitates the increased need for health-related research, but immediate interventions as well, to address important health issues. Given the complex and multifaceted health issues that impact Latina/os, comprehensive research is critical to inform evidence-based methods that are culturally sensitive to Latina/o communities.

The health profile of Latina/os differs from that of the general population. Leading causes of death for Latina/os in 2014 differ from those of African American and White/European American adults. For instance, cancer is the leading cause of death among Latina/os (21.5%), followed by heart disease (20.1%), and accidents/unintentional injuries (7.3%) (Centers for Disease Control and Prevention, 2015b). In addition, stroke is the 4th leading cause of death among Latina/os, followed by diabetes at 5th, and chronic liver disease and cirrhosis at 6th. By contrast, cirrhosis is not among the top 10 leading causes of death for White/European Americans or African Americans (see Table 2.1; Centers for Disease Control and Prevention, 2015b). In this chapter, we examine chronic conditions that are leading causes of death among Latina/os. Understanding the etiology of cancer, cardiovascular disease, and diabetes, specifically, as well as how these diseases vary in their prevalence among different Latina/o heritage groups, will help elucidate underlying mechanisms of these diseases. In addition to these leading causes of death, we also discuss injuries and maternal and child health, since these areas are important health concerns for Latina/os, as they pose important policy implications. Lastly, we present research regarding risk factors and how these risk profiles differ by Latina/o heritage groups, when available, in hopes of providing direction for the development of targeted programs for each Latina/o heritage group.

Throughout this chapter, we also present various models explaining disease and apply these models to Latina/os. We also include a discussion of how health research informed by models developed for White/European American populations do not appear to apply to Latina/os, leading researchers to conclude that there is a Latina/o paradox. Understanding the most burdensome diseases, especially by heritage group, can help identify priorities among these specific Latina/o heritage groups and their region of residence, to improve their health. We review existing epidemiological studies

Table 2.1 Total Deaths and Percentages for the 10 Leading Causes of Death among Latina/os

Causes of Death (based on ICD-10)	Rank	Deaths	% of Total Deaths
All causes		169,387	100.0
Malignant neoplasms	1	36,447	21.5
Diseases of heart	2	34,021	20.1
Accidents (unintentional injuries)	3	12,429	7.3
Cerebrovascular diseases	4	8,713	5.1
Diabetes mellitus	5	7,795	4.6
Chronic liver disease and cirrhosis	6	5,658	3.3
Alzheimer's disease	7	4,934	2.9
Chronic lower respiratory diseases	8	4,795	2.8
Influenza and pneumonia	9	3,875	2.3
Nephritis, nephrotic syndrome, and nephrosis	10	3,273	1.9

Note: ICD-10 = *International Classification of Diseases*, 10th ed.
Source: Centers for Disease Control and Prevention, 2015b.

and highlight the need for more epidemiological research focused on Latina/o communities. Finally, when available, we highlight research on protective factors that are associated with a decreased risk of disease development among Latina/os.

The data for this chapter are derived from several epidemiological studies that include Latina/o participants, such as the National Health Interview Survey, the National Health and Nutrition Examination Survey, and the Multi-Ethnic Study of Atherosclerosis (MESA) (Dixon, Sundquist, & Winkleby, 2000; Naimi, Nelson, & Brewer, 2010). However, most data are derived from the Hispanic Community Health Study/Study of Latinos (HCHS/ SOL) (Daviglus et al., 2012, 2016; Daviglus, Pirzada, & Talavera, 2014; LaVange et al., 2010; Penedo et al., 2016; Pinheiro et al., 2009; Schneiderman et al., 2014; Sorlie et al., 2010). The multicenter cohort study gathered valuable data on cardiovascular diseases and sampled Latina/os across heritage groups, allowing for comparisons by country of origin. These data are complemented by other population-based epidemiological studies that collectively and repeatedly examined Latina/os. These data allow us to identify patterns and trends among Latina/os, unlike other studies that simply compare Latina/os with other racial/ethnic subgroups, and thus do not explain these patterns by Latina/o heritage group.

EPIDEMIOLOGICAL STUDIES OF LATINA/O ADULTS

Many early epidemiological studies that included Latina/os either did not collect data on country of origin or primarily included Latina/os of Mexican descent, limiting the potential analysis of within-group differences by country of origin or by geographic residence. Despite these limitations, these epidemiological studies continue to provide valuable data to examine and describe the general health status of Latina/os. Health studies that comprise large Latina/o samples include the National Health Interview Survey (NHIS) and the National Health and Nutrition Examination Survey (NHANES).

The National Health Interview Survey

The NHIS is designed to investigate the health of the U.S. population; however, large Latina/o samples enable researchers to use the data to inform Latina/o health. The NHIS is one of the major data-collection programs conducted through the National Center for Health Statistics (1999); it monitors the nation's health using personal household interviews. U.S. Census Bureau employees interview all adult members of the household who are home during the time of the interview, and a reliable family member can provide information on behalf of adults who are not at home. Interviewers use laptop computers to help facilitate data collection.

The National Health Interview Survey includes the U.S. civilian noninstitutionalized population and the sampling framework is constructed around U.S. Census data. As part of this endeavor, four racial and/or ethnic groups are included in the survey. The sample of Latina/os is identified as representative of the U.S. population across geographic areas where these heritage groups reside—Southwestern states, New York City, and Florida. Additionally, the three major Latina/o heritiage groups—Mexican Americans, Puerto Ricans, and Cuban Americans—are sampled for representation through the survey.

The different editions of the NHIS included different types of questionnaires. From 1982 to 1996, the survey included two parts—the Core questionnaire and current health topics. The Core questionnaire included basic health and demographic questions. Since 1997, the NHIS has included the Core questionnaire and Supplements. The Core questionnaire gathers health and demographic information on the household (includes everyone who resides in the household), the family (additional demographic information on each family member in the household), a sample adult (randomly selected adult living in the household), and a sample child (randomly selected child). The questionnaires on the sample adult and child collect information on health status, health care services, and health behaviors. Supplements gather information on specific health issues of interest and are implemented as many times as deemed necessary based on the health topic of interest.

The National Health and Nutrition Examination Survey

NHANES is designed to assess the health and nutritional status of adults living in the United States. While its goal is not specifically to examine Latina/o health, as one of the largest and longest-running national sources of objective health and nutrition data, this survey provides valuable data that can be used by researchers to investigate Latina/o health. NHANES is conducted in cycles by the National Center for Health Statistics and collects extensive data on dietary intake and nutritional status of individuals as well as on physical examinations, clinical and laboratory tests, and personal interviews (National Center for Health Statistics, 2014).

As with the National Health Interview Survey, NHANES aims to obtain a nationally representative sample and surveys a large proportion of Latina/os. NHANES oversamples persons 60 years and older, African Americans and Latina/os (National Center for Health Statistics, 2014). More specifically, between 1999 and 2006, Mexican Americans were oversampled; between 2007 and 2010, all Latina/os were oversampled. For this reason, the data set can solely inform studies investigating Latina/o health issues between the 2007 and 2010 survey years. Years 1999–2006 can be used to analyze Mexican American health issues. Unfortunately, samples of other Latina/o heritage group samples were too small during those years to make reliable estimates.

Researchers collect data in the participant's home and mobile centers. Researchers collect health interviews in the participant's home, including demographic information, socioeconomic data, and dietary and health-related issues. Mobile centers are used to conduct medical (e.g., blood pressure), dental, and physiological measurements and laboratory tests (e.g., blood and urine testing). Research teams, including a physician, medical and health technicians, and dietary and health interviewers, collect data in English or Spanish. The data can be used to provide estimates of chronic conditions, such as cardiovascular diseases and diabetes, and risk factors associated with these conditions.

The Hispanic Health and Nutrition Examination Survey

Informed by the NHANES and to specifically identify Latina/o health status in the United States, researchers created the Hispanic Health and Nutrition Examination Survey (HHANES) and implemented the survey between 1982 and 1984 (National Center for Health Statistics, 2015b). The HHANES collected data on the three largest Latina/o heritage groups that resided within traditional geographic areas. As with the NHIS, the three Latina/o heritage groups included Mexican Americans, Puerto Ricans, and Cubans and geographic areas included southwestern states, Florida, and the New York City metropolitan area.

Data collected through the HHANES included information on specific health behaviors such as alcohol consumption, drug abuse, and dietary intake using a 24-hour dietary recall. Data were also collected on anthropometric measures, electrocardiograms, oral health screenings, blood pressure readings, radiographs, and other tests. The survey also collected demographic information and socioeconomic variables. The HHANES was the first ethnic-specific survey conducted by the National Center for Health Statistics and required researchers to translate instruments that were solely available in English and also required the recruitment of Spanish-speaking interviewers. A single Spanish-language instrument was developed despite the differing dialects of the three heritage groups included in the sample— Mexican Americans, Puerto Ricans, and Cubans.

The Multi-Ethnic Study of Atherosclerosis

The Multi-Ethnic Study of Atherosclerosis (MESA) is also an epidemiological study that specifically investigates cardiovascular diseases and characteristics of subclinical cardiovascular disease (Allison et al., 2008). MESA aims to identify cardiovascular disease risk before clinical signs and symptoms are detectable and also aims to identify associated risk factors. This national study is funded through the National, Heart, Lung, and Blood Institute at the National Institutes of Health. The longitudinal study tracks approximately 6,814 asymptomatic men and women aged 45 to 84. MESA also seeks to sample across diverse ethnic groups. Therefore, approximately 22% of the sample is Latina/o but specific Latina/o heritage groups are not identified. Other ethnic groups include African Americans and Asian Americans, primarily of Chinese descent.

Researchers collect data on each participant across five examinations. The data include blood pressure, anthropometry, electrocardiography, urine collection, blood samples, and questionnaire data on demographics, socioeconomic and psychosocial status, medical and family history, medication use, dietary intake, smoking, and physical activity. Researchers also collect additional measures at each examination related to cardiovascular disease risk (see Table 2.2).

Each of the aforementioned data sources can inform the understanding of Latina/o health. However, their limitations should be acknowledged when used to make conclusions regarding the health profile of a heterogeneous ethnic minority group such as Latina/os. Most importantly, the data sets do not contain data on specific Latina/o heritage groups other than Mexican Americans, Puerto Ricans, and Cuban Americans. Additionally, since the purpose or aim of these studies was not to analyze Latina/o health and the unique risk profiles of Latina/os, the data sets do not typically include critical variables that might better inform research in this area (i.e., acculturation, acculturative stress, cultural values, etc.).

Hispanic Community Health Study/Study of Latinos

The Hispanic Community Health Study/Study of Latinos (HCHS/SOL) is a multicenter community-based cohort study, funded by the National Heart, Lung, and Blood Institute and six other National Institutes of Health centers and offices. The HCHS/SOL examined the risk and protective factors for chronic disease among U.S. Latina/o adults. Moreover, the HCHS/SOL aimed to quantify morbidity and mortality of chronic diseases among Latina/o adults (Sorlie et al., 2010).

The sampling method for the HCHS/SOL aimed to fulfill two objectives related to Latina/o health and aimed to support prevalence estimates of

Table 2.2 Sample of Epidemiological Studies to Inform Latina/o Health

Survey or Study Title	Latina/o Subgroups Identified	Description of Data	Years of Data Collection
Hispanic Community Health Study/ Study of Latinos	Mexican Americans, Puerto Ricans, Cuban Americans, Dominicans, Central/South Americans	Data collected through interviews and extensive clinical exams	2008–present
Hispanic Health and Nutrition Examination Survey	Mexican Americans, Puerto Ricans, Cuban Americans	Data collected through examination, such as anthropometrics, oral health, health behaviors, and other lab tests	1982–1984
Multi-Ethnic Study of Atherosclerosis	Latina/os examined collectively	Data collected through physical exams and include clinical data on subclinical cardiovascular disease and risk factors	2002–2012
National Health Interview Survey	Mexican Americans, Puerto Ricans, Cuban Americans	Data collected through household interviews and include measurements on health status, health care access, national health objectives	1957–present
National Health and Nutrition Examination Survey	Mexican Americans, Puerto Ricans, Cuban Americans, Dominicans, Central/South Americans, Other	Data collected through interviews and physical examinations. Designed to assess the health and nutritional status of adults and children in the United States.	1960–present

baseline risk factors for Latina/os as well as by Latina/o heritage group. Additionally, the resulting sample needed to support evaluation of relationships between risk factors and disease outcomes during follow up (LaVange et al., 2010). The HCHS/SOL included four communities—the Bronx, Chicago, Miami, and San Diego. Researchers used a probability-based sampling

strategy to recruit participants from geographically diverse neighborhoods using face-to-face recruitment methods.

The HCHS/SOL is a prospective, population-based cohort study. Data
were collected on health status, disease burden, immigration, acculturation,
environment, health care access, and several risk factors associated with cardiovascular diseases. Additional details regarding the methods are reported
elsewhere (Sorlie et al., 2010). Researchers collected baseline data using an
examination that took seven hours to complete. They assessed dietary intake
using one 24-hour dietary recall during the baseline data collection and a
second 24-hour dietary recall six weeks after baseline data collection.
Researchers used annual follow-up phone calls to assess health status. When
a participant reported an event, the researchers obtained medical records
and compared the clinical event against predetermined criteria.

FACTORS THAT IMPACT THE HEALTH OF LATINA/OS

The social determinants of health help to identify why certain groups
are at higher risk of disease and how certain environments of vulnerable
populations, such as where they work, reside, and play impact their health
(Centers for Disease Control and Prevention, 2017). Social determinants
include aspects of living conditions that are not traditionally associated with
health, such as the aspects of social and economic opportunities that can
indirectly impact health. Social determinants of health include the neighborhood and built environment; health and health care; social and community context; education; and economic sustainability (Office of Disease
Prevention and Health Promotion, 2017). Each of these social factors is
theorized to contribute, at least in part, to differing health outcomes. Healthy
People 2020, our nation's roadmap for improving U.S. health includes social
determinants of health as a main goal—create social and physical environments that promote good health for all.

Social determinants of health are often discussed in the context of health
disparities. Health disparities research is significant because it helps identify underlying causes for differences in health outcomes between different
groups based on the group's characteristics, such as geographic location,
age, gender, and race/ethnicity. Healthy People 2020 seeks to eliminate or
reduce health disparities. Social determinants of health can theoretically
serve as a vehicle to eliminate health disparities. Because it is theorized that
health disparities are caused, in part, by unjust differences in social determinants of health, improving conditions for underserved groups and
directly addressing the social determinants of health should theoretically
lessen current gaps in health outcomes.

Chapter 1 provided Latina/o demographic profiles and when possible, presented variations by Latina/o heritage group. When applying the social determinants of health to Latina/os, we find a system of sociodemographic factors that places Latina/os at high risk for health problems (see Figure 2.1). The first determinant in social determinants of health is economic stability. Economic stability includes underlying factors such as poverty, employment, food insecurity, and housing instability. Latina/os do not fare well in any of these areas. As discussed in Chapter 1, Latina/os are more likely to live in poverty than White/European Americans, as approximately 23.5% of Latina/os live in poverty (Stepler & Brown, 2016). Chapter 1 also addressed how while Latina/os tend to have lower unemployment rates compared to White/European Americans (Stepler & Brown, 2016), they

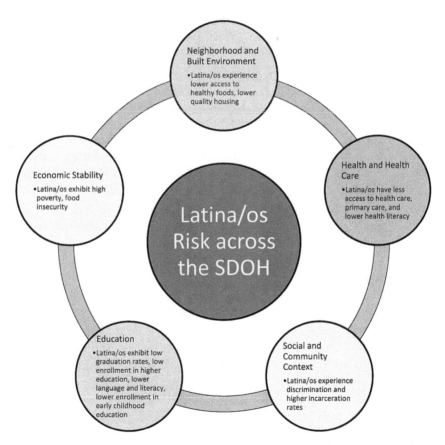

Figure 2.1 Latina/os' Risk Across the Social Determinants of Health (SDOH).
Source: Modified from the Office of Disease Prevention and Health Promotion, 2017.

are more likely than both White/European Americans and African Americans to lack health insurance.

Food insecurity is defined as limited or uncertain availability of nutritionally adequate and safe foods or limited or uncertain ability to acquire acceptable foods in a socially acceptable way (Bickel, Nord, Price, Hamilton, & Cook, 2000). Research suggests that Latina/o households have a higher prevalence of food insecurity (28.4%) than White/European Americans (17.3%) (Furness, Simon, Wold, & Asarian-Anderson, 2004). Finally, as a precursor to homelessness, *housing instability* is defined as the inability to pay rent, spending more than 50% of one's income on housing, or frequently moving (The Urban Institute, 2002). Prevalence of housing instability is limited; however, it is likely that Latina/o families experience housing instability because of their high poverty rates.

The second social determinant of health is education. Education includes a number of factors, such as high school graduation, enrollment in higher education, language and literacy, and early childhood education and development. See Chapter 1 for specifics on Latina/o educational profiles. Collectively, Latina/os do not fare well on any of these metrics. Education levels are much lower on average for Latina/os than for their White/European American counterparts. Fewer Latina/os acquire a high school diploma, with a dropout rate of 12% among Latina/os, as compared with 7% for African American students, 5% for White/European American students, and 1% for Asian American students (Krogstad, 2016). While not addressed in Chapter 1 but important to mention here is that fewer Latina/o children participate in early childhood education and development opportunities as compared with White/European American children (U.S. Department of Education—National Center for Educational Statistics, 2000).

The third social determinant of health is social and community context. Factors that influence social and community context include social cohesion, civic participation, discrimination, and incarceration. Unfortunately, there is limited research regarding social cohesion and civic participation in Latina/o communities. However, as addressed in Chapter 1, Latina/os frequently experience discrimination, especially if they are not proficient in English. Finally, Latina/os are incarcerated at nearly double the rate of White/European Americans (Mauer & King, 2007).

The last two social determinants of health are health and health care and neighborhood and built environment. Health and health care includes access to health care, access to primary care, and health literacy. As discussed in Chapter 1, access to health care is traditionally lower for Latina/os than for White/European Americans and African Americans. Estimates based on NHIS data suggest that 19.4% of Latina/os lack health insurance, as compared with 6.2% of White/European American and 9.9% of African

American adults in 2015 (Centers for Disease Control and Prevention, 2015a). Additionally, in 2015 more White/European American adults had a regular medical care provider, as compared with Latina/os (88.8% vs. 82.6%). After adjusting the data for both age and gender differences, 5.4% of Latina/os and 5.8% of African American adults failed to obtain needed medical care because of cost during the past 12 months. However, only 4.1% of White/European American adults failed to obtain needed medical care because of cost (Centers for Disease Control and Prevention, 2015a). We address these health care disparities present between Latina/os and White/European Americans in greater detail in Chapter 3. The neighborhood and built environment includes factors such as access to foods that support healthy eating patterns, quality of housing, crime and violence, and environmental conditions. Some evidence suggests that Latina/os also experience poor conditions in each of these areas (Lopez-Class & Hosler, 2010).

Given Latina/os' status in each of the social determinants of health, we would theoretically expect higher morbidity and mortality rates than for White/European Americans. In other words, since their high-risk profile is evident, we should conclude that Latina/os have poorer health indicators. However, this relationship is more complex and has led to discussions regarding *the Latina/o paradox*.

The Latina/o Paradox

Latina/os are surprisingly healthy in terms of their physical health, despite their high-risk profile, which includes less education, being medically underserved, and having lower income levels. This paradoxical relationship is often termed the "Hispanic or Latina/o paradox" (Markides & Coreil, 1986). While Latina/os exhibit high-risk profiles based on the aforementioned demographic characteristics, their average life expectancy at age 65 is 86.7, two years more than among non-Latina females, whose life expectancy is 84.7 (Hummer & Hayward, 2015). However, Latinas over the age of 65 also experience greater disability as compared with White/European American females (Hummer & Hayward, 2015).

Certain research supports the Latina/o paradox. For example, Dominguez and colleagues (2015) examined vital statistics data among Latina/os aged 18 to 64 to examine the relationship between demographic data and health profiles. Although Latina/os are younger, less likely to have a high school diploma, twice as likely to live below the poverty line, and over 20 times as likely to not speak English as proficiently as their White/European American counterparts, the all-cause mortality rate is 24% lower among Latina/os as compared with White/European Americans. Moreover, the cancer mortality rate is 28% lower and heart disease is 25% lower among

Latina/os as compared with White/European Americans. In contrast, morality rates are higher for Latina/os as compared with White/European Americans for diabetes (51% higher), chronic liver disease (48% higher), and homicide (96% higher).

The Latina/o paradox is challenged by competing theories. These alternative theories explain the paradox in terms of the health of the migrating population (the healthy migrant hypothesis; Abraído-Lanza, Dohrenwend, Ng-Mak, & Turner, 1999) or in terms of elder immigrants returning to their country of origin (the salmon bias hypothesis; Medina-Inojosa, Jean, Cortes-Bergoderi, & Lopez-Jimenez, 2014). The *healthy migrant hypothesis* posits that because of the physical and psychological challenges associated with the immigration process, Latina/os who successfully immigrate to the United States are healthier, younger, and more resilient as compared with Latina/os who remain in their home country and as compared with their U.S.-born counterparts. Therefore, Latina/o immigrants' better health profile existed before their move to the United States, and this theory partially explains why the advantages of Latina/os diminish as their generational statuses increase (Balcazar, Grineski, & Collins, 2015; Giuntella, 2016). However, research testing this theory compared the health profiles of Mexicans who immigrated to the United States and those who continued to reside in Mexico. Outcome data do not indicate a health advantage for Mexicans who immigrated to the United States as compared with their Mexican counterparts. In fact, Mexican immigrants are not as healthy as their counterparts who reside in Mexico (Bostean, 2013).

The *salmon bias hypothesis* suggests that older Latina/os travel back to their home country. Their deaths are recorded in their home country and thus bias U.S. mortality rates. For example, Abraído-Lanza et al. (1999) investigated the salmon bias using data from the National Longitudinal Mortality study. Respondents' self-reported national or cultural group determined their Latina/o heritage group—Mexican or Mexican American, Puerto Rican, Cuban, and Central or South American or other. They controlled for SES, age, and gender in their analysis and also analyzed mortality status over time. However, Abraído-Lanza et al. (1999) concluded that there is insufficient evidence to support the salmon bias hypothesis.

The Latina/o paradox may not exist across all Latina/o heritage groups when compared with White/European Americans (Markides & Eschbach, 2005). For example, research suggests that smoking prevalence is lower among Latina/os despite their high-risk profiles; however, when the data are disaggregated by Latina/o heritage groups, Puerto Ricans have a 66% higher prevalence of smoking as compared with Latina/os of Mexican descent (Dominguez et al., 2015). Physical and psychiatric comorbidity is lower among Mexican and other Latina women as compared with White/

European American women; however, it is higher among island-born Puerto Rican men as compared with White/European Americans (Erving, 2017). These factors suggest further research is needed to understand contributors of the Latina/o paradox, which may explain why the paradox exists for some Latina/o heritage groups and not others.

The Latina/o paradox is partially informed by nativity status and is typically identified as the "immigrant paradox" when applied in this scenario. Research suggests that U.S.-born Latina/os have a higher prevalence of obesity, hypertension, smoking, heart disease, and cancer as compared with foreign-born Latina/os (Dominguez et al., 2015). Given the relatively lower incomes, education levels, and access to resources of newly immigrated Latina/os as compared with their U.S.-born counterparts, it is surprising foreign-born Latina/os exhibit better health outcomes. Evidence for the immigrant paradox not only includes the initial superior health of immigrants, but research also demonstrates that as generational statuses increase, the mortality advantage and other positive health advantages exhibited by Latina/os also decrease. For example, despite the initial advantage of Latinas in birth outcomes as compared with their non-Latina counterparts (Acevedo-Garcia, Soobader, & Berkman, 2007), findings suggest that as their generational statuses increase, their advantages also decrease (Giuntella, 2016). By the third generation, collectively Latina birth advantages diminish for all Latina heritage groups except Mexicans (Giuntella, 2016). Additionally, Latina/o advantages in child health outcomes (e.g., bronchitis, allergies, and asthma) are lost after 2.5 generations of residence in the United States (Balcazar et al., 2015). Researchers speculate that this diminishing health advantage might parallel the lessening of cultural protective factors as Latina/o immigrants acculturate.

An emerging area of research seeks to elucidate the Latina/o paradox by examining the mortality advantage across regions. As discussed in Chapter 1, Latina/os demonstrate divergent relocation patterns in new destination state areas. Brazil (2017) examined the spatial variation in the Latina/o paradox and combined geographic analysis with vital statistics to examine whether the paradox existed in both established and new Latina/o destinations. Using data from 1999 and 2010, Brazil standardized mortality rates and compared age-adjusted mortality rates between Latina/os and White/European Americans. Data suggest that the mortality advantage lessens in established Latina/o communities. Moreover, recent immigrants have a higher mortality advantage but living in an area with a higher number of recent immigrants increases this advantage for recent Latina/o immigrants.

Although further research is needed to understand the underlying mechanism of the relationship between years of U.S. residence and associated health outcomes (Abraído-Lanza, Echeverria, & Florez, 2016), associations can be seen between nativity and risk for disease and life expectancy. Foreign-born Latinas have an average life expectancy at age 65 that is three years longer than White/European American females (23.32 vs. 20.29 remaining years) (Lariscy, Hummer, & Hayward, 2015). However, this advantage is less pronounced when comparing U.S.-born Latinas with their White/European American counterparts (20.04 vs. 20.29 remaining years). Life expectancy varies by Latina/o heritage groups as well, with more favorable patterns for Latinas from Cuba, Mexico, and Central and South America but worse life expectancies for Latinas from Puerto Rico (Hummer & Hayward, 2015). Similar trends are observed in male mortality. Foreign-born Latinos have a higher life expectancy at age 65 as compared with U.S.-born Latinos and White/European American men (19.74, 17.55, and 16.75 remaining years, respectively).

Some researchers believe the Latina/o paradox exists because despite their high-risk profiles Latina/os have protective factors, such as cultural values, that help buffer the potential negative impact of their conditions. Potential protective factors against chronic disease include lower acculturation levels, *familismo*, living in homogeneous neighborhoods, social support, and marriage. Acculturation is the process by which individuals adapt to a new living environment and potentially adopt the norms, values, and practices of their new host society (Abraído-Lanza, Armbrister, Flórez, & Aguirre, 2006). Lower acculturation is also identified as a risk factor in some cases, but lower acculturation also functions as a protective factor against disease risk among Latina/os (Abraído-Lanza et al., 2016). Abraído-Lanza and colleagues (2016) suggest that inconsistencies in associations between acculturation and health are due to differences in the operationalization of acculturation, inconsistent measurement, and conceptual differences. In Chapter 10, we discuss acculturation in greater detail, including research limitations and possible future directions for protecting Latina/os against negative outcomes associated with acculturation, and we provide recommendations for moving this area of research forward. However, it is important to understand that as generational status or years of U.S. residence increase, health outcomes appear to become less than optimal (Abraído-Lanza et al., 2016). This is perhaps due to the assimilation to mainstream U.S. culture and lessening of cultural values that protected previous generations of Latina/os.

As discussed in Chapter 1, *familismo* can serve as a protective factor against various risky health behaviors and negative health outcomes. For example, one study investigated the association between *familismo* and adolescent substance abuse among 117 Latino males (Lopez-Tamayo, Seda, & Jason, 2016). Most participants were descendants of Mexicans, Puerto

Ricans, or Southern American countries, and they all resided in Chicago. *Familismo* serves as a protective factor against substance abuse, as Latinos with higher *familismo* report fewer years of substance abuse than their more assimilated counterparts. Although *familismo* is often investigated in relationship to mental health outcomes, we later explore its relationship to physical health behaviors and outcomes.

Homogeneous neighborhoods can also serve as a protective factor in reducing the risk of stroke and cancer among older Mexican American adults (Eschbach et al., 2004). When Latina/os largely reside in Latina/o neighborhoods in the United States, these enclaves act as a buffer to alleviate the impact of acculturative stress, perceived discrimination, and isolation. Some research suggests these homogeneous neighborhoods can also provide channels for social support, allowing for stronger development of interpersonal networks, which complements preferred communication styles among Latina/os who prefer close relationships (Elder, Ayala, Parra-Medina, & Talavera, 2009). Finally, marriage is also associated with better health outcomes among Latina/os, particularly a decreased risk for cardiovascular diseases (Gallo et al., 2015).

HEALTH ISSUES FACING LATINA/O COMMUNITIES

Cancer among Latina/os

All cancers combined are the leading causes of death for Latina/os. In particular, they demonstrate lower rates of common cancers such as breast, colorectal, lung, and prostate cancer as compared with White/European Americans; however, they have higher rates of stomach and liver cancers (American Cancer Society, 2015). Latina/os experience higher incidence rates for cervical, gallbladder, liver, and gastric cancer, with the largest relative difference observed for gallbladder cancer (Haile et al., 2012). More alarming, in the United States, cervical cancer incidence is higher among Latina/os than among any other major racial/ethnic group (Haile et al., 2012). Latinas also have the highest incidence of gallbladder cancer in the United States. For example, in 2007, the incidence rate was 2 to 2.5 times higher for Latinas than for White/European American, African American, or Asian American/Pacific Islander women (Hayat, Howlader, Reichman, & Edwards, 2007). While not quite as substantial, the rate of gallbladder cancer was about 1.7 times higher for Latina/os as compared with White/European American men.

Breast cancer is the most prevalent form of cancer among Latinas and is projected to impact 29% of Latinas, contributing to 16% of cancer-related deaths among Latinas (Siegel et al., 2015). However, Latinas experience lower incidence rates of breast cancer as compared with White/European

American females (91.9 vs. 128.1 per 100,000) (Siegel et al., 2015). Additionally, mortality rates are lower among Latinas (14.5 per 100,000) as compared with White/European American females (21.9 per 100,000). Breast cancer incidence between 1992 and 2012 increased at twice the rate of the incidence for cancers of the lungs and bronchus, uterine cervix, thyroid, or liver among Latinas (Siegel et al., 2015).

Research using data from the HCHS/SOL examined differences among Latina/o heritage groups in self-reported cancer prevalence and incidence. Cubans and Puerto Ricans demonstrate significantly higher overall reported cancer prevalence rates and higher incidence rates as compared with all other Latina/o heritage groups (Penedo et al., 2016; Pinheiro et al., 2009). Mexicans have the lowest cancer incidence rates (Pinheiro et al., 2009). Among Latina/os, survival rates for most cancers are similar to those for White/European Americans, with the exception of melanoma. Both Latinos and Latinas exhibit lower survival rates for melanoma as compared with White/European Americans (Siegel, Naishadham, & Jemal, 2012). More worrisome, age-adjusted mortality rates are higher among Latina/os as compared with White/European Americans for gastric, liver, and cervical cancers and for all cancers combined (Haile et al., 2012).

Limited data exist to provide information regarding breast cancer risk among various Latina/o heritage groups. One study, however, provides risk estimates for both five-year and lifetime breast cancer risk (Banegas, Leng, Graubard, & Morales, 2013). Although Latinas demonstrate lower risk for breast cancer as compared with their White/European American counterparts, Banegas et al. analyzed data from the 2000 and 2005 NHIS Cancer Control Modules. They used self-reported data on race and country of origin and ancestry to categorize women as White/European American or by Latina heritage group—Mexicans/Mexican Americans, Cubans/Cuban Americans, Puerto Ricans, Dominicans, Central or South Americans, and Other. Risk profiles informed estimates of five-year and lifetime breast cancer risk. They also assessed risk while controlling for key sociodemographic variables. Collectively, Latinas exhibit a lower risk for developing invasive breast cancer over the next five years as compared with White/European American females (0.64% vs. 1.24%). Additionally, Latinas also exhibit lower lifetime risk, as compared with White/European American females (5.88% vs. 8.63%). Among Latina heritage groups, Cuban/Cuban American women have a greater five-year risk of developing invasive breast cancer, but Dominican women have a greater lifetime risk of developing invasive breast cancer. Mexicans/Mexican Americans and Dominicans demonstrate the lowest five-year risk and Cuban/Cuban Americans have the lowest lifetime risk.

Significant variation exists for specific cancer rates among Latiña/os by geographic region and country of origin. Geographically, Latinas from who reside along the U.S.-Mexico border experience higher incidence rates of cervical cancer compared with Latinas who reside elsewhere (Coughlin et al., 2008). Regarding country of origin, Puerto Rican men exhibit the highest incidence of liver cancer (19.2 per 100,000), followed by a much lower incidence among Mexican (10.8 per 100,000) and Cuban men (10.1 per 100,000) (Pinheiro et al., 2009). Latina/os from Mexico and Puerto Rico have a higher incidence (2.2 and 3.6 times, respectively) of gastric cancer rates than White/European Americans. Rates are even less favorable for South or Central American Latina/os, who have rates 4.3 to 5.1 times higher than their White/European American counterparts, whereas rates among Cubans are comparable to rates for White/European Americans (Jemal et al., 2008).

To examine cancer risk factors among Latina/o heritage groups, Cokkinides and colleagues (2012) used two national data sources. The study combined data from the NHIS and NHANES to provide estimates of cancer prevalence and associated risk factor prevalence among Latina/os. Combined, these data sets provide valuable information on several of the risk factors described below. One advantage of the NHIS is the inclusion of data regarding country of origin among Latina/os, allowing for separate analysis among Mexican, Puerto Rican, Cuban, Central/South American, and Dominican heritage groups (Cokkinides, Bandi, Siegel, & Jemal, 2012). Major cancer risk factors among Latina/o adults include age, gender, lack of health insurance, smoking, obesity, poor nutrition, lack of physical activity, alcohol consumption, infectious agents, and lack of screening behaviors (Cokkinides et al., 2012; Penedo et al., 2016; Siegel et al., 2015). Similar risk factors are also observed among children.

Age is positively associated with cancer, and each 10-year increase in age is associated with higher odds of reported diagnosis (Penedo et al., 2016). Gender is also associated with cancer diagnosis, although findings are mixed. Whereas one study identified that males have lower odds of being diagnosed with cancer (Penedo et al., 2016), another study identified that females have lower odds of diagnosis (Hayat et al., 2007). One potential reason for these mixed findings is the data source. For instance, Penedo et al. (2016) used self-reported data while Hayat et al. (2017) used hospital records. Latina/os with health insurance, not surprisingly, have higher odds of being diagnosed with cancer as compared with Latina/os without health insurance (Penedo et al., 2016).

The prevalence of cancer risk factors also differs by Latina/o heritage group. Smoking is overall lower for Latina/o adults combined (11.2%) as compared with White/European Americans (18.3%) (Siegel et al., 2015). However, when comparing smoking behaviors across Latina/o heritage groups, variations are present. Smoking is more common in Cubans (20.7% of men and 15.1% of women) and Puerto Ricans (19.0% in men and 16.6%

in women) as compared with Mexican Americans (Cokkinides et al., 2012). Obesity prevalence among Mexican women in 2011 and 2012 was 45% as compared with White/European American women (33%) and among Mexican men (41%) as compared with 33% among White/European American men (Siegel et al., 2015). South Americans exhibit the lowest prevalence of obesity (27% in men and 31% in women), whereas Puerto Ricans have the highest prevalence of obesity (41% in men and 51% in women) (Daviglus et al., 2012).

Leisure time physical activity among adults in 2009 through 2010 was lower among all Latina/o heritage groups as compared with their White/European American counterparts (Cokkinides et al., 2012). Moreover, Dominican males and females report less leisure time physical activity than the other Latina/o subgroups. Studies using NHIS data suggest that fewer Latina/os report frequent alcohol consumption (three or more drinks per week) than White/European Americans. However, this is in contrast to other studies that suggest that the prevalence of binge drinking (five or more drinks per occasion) in Latino males is higher than for White/European American males (Naimi et al., 2010). Cuban (21%) and Mexican (22%) men exhibit higher rates of alcohol consumption, whereas Dominican men have the lowest rates of alcohol consumption (11.6%) (Cokkinides et al., 2012).

Despite the lower prevalence of common cancers among Latina/os, cancer cases associated with infectious agents are higher among Latina/os than among White/European Americans (Cokkinides et al., 2012). An established risk factor for stomach cancer is *Helicobacter pylori* (Brenner, Rothenbacher, & Arndt, 2009). The seroprevalence of *H. pylori* infection is higher in Latina/os of Mexican descent (64%) as compared with African Americans (52%) and White/European Americans (21%) (Grad, Lipsitch, & Aiello, 2012). *H. pylori* prevalence is also higher among foreign-born Latina/os as compared with their U.S.-born counterparts (Haile et al., 2012). Human papillomavirus infections are associated with nearly all cervical and anal cancers and are sexually transmitted. Latinas of Mexican descent and White/European American women exhibit similar infection rates for human papillomavirus (24.3% vs. 24.2%) (Giuliano, Papenfuss, Schneider, Nour, & Hatch, 1999).

Cardiovascular Diseases among Latina/os

Epidemiological data on cardiovascular disease (CVD) risk among Latina/os is limited (Balfour, Ruiz, Talavera, Allison, & Rodriguez, 2016). Only two major population-based studies directly target Latina/os—the MESA and the HCHS/SOL. However, based on these limited data, it is possible to identify trends in the prevalence of cardiovascular diseases among

Latina/os. Prevalence and mortality associated with CVDs are lower for Latina/os as compared with White/European American and African American adults. When examining coronary heart disease specifically among men, prevalence is lower among Latino men than for African American (6.7% vs. 7.2%) and White/European American men (7.8%). However, among women, Latinas have higher rates (5.9%) as compared with White/ European American women (4.6%) but they demonstrate lower rates as compared with African American women (7%) (Balfour et al., 2016).

CVD risk factors in Latina/os include higher rates of obesity-elevated blood pressure, elevated triglyceride levels, dyslipidemia, and diabetes (Clair et al., 2013). Coronary artery calcium is also present in lesser amounts in Latina/os. For instance, an analysis of CVD risk factors among U.S. Latina/o heritage groups was completed using data from the MESA (Allison et al., 2008). Data from Latina/o heritage groups (Cuban, Dominican, Mexican, Puerto Rican, and other Latina/o Americans) were included in the analysis to determine Latina/o heritage group-specific levels of CVD risk factors and measures of subclinical CVD, as well as the magnitude and significance of associations between these risk factors and subclinical CVD within each Latina/o heritage group. Significant differences are identified in the distributions of CVD risk factors, prevalence, and mean risk values in subclinical CVD. Significant differences in the associations of the risk factors, and subclinical disease by Latina/o heritage groups are also observed. For example, Mexican Americans have the highest prevalence of thoracic aortic calcium, whereas Puerto Rican Americans have the highest prevalence of an ankle-brachial index less than 1.0.

Researchers used data from the Hispanic Community Health Study to further examine differences in CVD risk factors by Latino subgroup (Daviglus et al., 2012). Researchers defined major CVD risk factors using current national guidelines. Based on these criteria, the majority of participants exhibited at least one risk factor for CVD. The study found high levels of at least one CVD risk factor among 80% of Latino men and 71% of Latina women. When examining the data by Latina/o subgroup, Puerto Rican males and females were most likely to have at least three CVD risk factors compared to the other subgroups (Daviglus, Pirzada, & Talavera, 2014). Age-standardized prevalence of CVD risk factors varied by Latino subgroup and sex. For example, Central American males had the highest rate of hypercholesterolemia (54.9%), followed by Mexican men (53.9%), and Cuban men (53.7%). For females, the highest rate of hypercholesterolemia is among Puerto Rican females (41%), followed by Central American (39.4%), and Cuban females (37.5%). Self-reported coronary heart disease and stroke prevalence are low across the sample. Hypertension and smoking are directly associated with coronary heart disease in both men and women. Stroke risk is also associated with hypertension and smoking in women and hypertension and diabetes in men (Daviglus et al., 2012).

Emerging research suggests higher psychological distress among Latina/os as compared with their White/European American counterparts, but research also indicates that psychological distress may increase the possibility of certain CVD risk factors (Castañeda et al., 2016). In women, psychological distress is associated with smoking and obesity. In men, psychological distress is also associated with smoking but instead of obesity, it is associated with diabetes. More research on how psychological distress and acculturative stress are associated with physical health outcomes, such as cardiovascular disease in Latina/os, is needed.

Diabetes among Latina/os

Diabetes is a disease in which the body is either insufficiently producing insulin or unable to use its own insulin (Centers for Disease Control and Prevention, 2016). Diabetes, if uncontrolled, can lead to serious health complications, including but not limited to heart disease, retinopathy, kidney failure, and amputations. Diabetes is typically classified into one of three categories—type 1 diabetes, type 2 diabetes, and gestational diabetes. Type 1 diabetes was previously regarded as "juvenile-onset diabetes" and accounts for approximately 5% of all diagnosed cases of diabetes (American Diabetes Association, 2017). Type 2 diabetes was formerly identified as "adult-onset diabetes," given its emergence later in the life course. However, in more recent years, type 2 diabetes has become increasingly common among younger adults and prevalence among adolescents and children also increased. Type 2 diabetes accounts for 90–95% of diagnosed diabetes cases. Gestational diabetes has its onset during pregnancy. This type of diabetes occurs in approximately 2–10% of all pregnancies and often disappears after pregnancy. Because it constitutes most of the cases of diabetes, the remainder of this discussion will focus on type 2 diabetes.

The prevalence of type 2 diabetes between 2007 and 2009 was almost twice as high for Latina/o adults age 20 or older as compared with White/European American adults (11.8% vs. 7.1%). Research based on data from HCHS/SOL suggests that diabetes rates vary by country of origin (Schneiderman et al., 2014). The prevalence of diabetes is highest among Dominican (18.1%) and Central American (17.7%) adults, whereas the prevalence is lowest among Cuban (13.4%) and South American (10.2%) adults. When examining women alone, prevalence is highest among Puerto Rican women (19.5%) and lowest among South American women (9.8%). Among men, the prevalence is highest among mixed/other men (19.6%) and lowest among South American men (10.6%).

Prediabetes also varies by Latina/o heritage group; Daviglus and colleagues (2016) examined fasting plasma glucose and hemoglobin A1c to assess diabetes risk at baseline in the HCHS/SOL cohort study. They then examined how many Latina/o participants met criteria for prediabetes—a fasting plasma glucose less than 100 mg/dl and hemoglobin A1c of less than 5.7%—and reported not taking medication for diabetes mellitus and having no history of diabetes mellitus. The number of women who met the criteria differed significantly by country of origin. The highest prevalence of prediabetes was among Mexican women (43.5%) and the lowest was among Cuban (32.7%) and South American (33.3%) women. For men, the highest prevalence of diabetes was among Mexican men (53.3%) and the lowest was among South American (43.2%) and Cuban (47.8%) men.

Risk factors for diabetes among Latina/os include poor nutrition, low levels of physical activity, low health literacy levels, and low use of screening. Data from NHANES show that Latina/o adults born in Mexico are more likely to eat lower levels of total fat, saturated fat, fiber, and potassium and consume adequate intakes of vitamin C, vitamin B_6, folate, calcium, and magnesium as compared with U.S.-born Latina/o adults (Dixon, Sundquist, & Winkleby, 2000). This beneficial diet seems to decrease the longer adults reside in the United States, but findings are inconclusive regarding the role of acculturation, if any, in these dietary changes (Perez-Escamilla, 2011). Leisure time physical activity is most associated with reducing diabetes risk. All Latina/o heritage groups report lower levels of leisure-time physical activity as compared with their White/European American counterparts (Cokkinides et al., 2012). Dominican males and females report even less leisure time physical activity as compared with other Latina/o heritage groups.

Diabetes awareness is typically low among Latina/os. Only 58.7% of participants who meet objective criteria for diabetes report receiving a diagnosis for diabetes, and 42.4% report that they have health insurance (Schneiderman et al., 2014). Acculturation is positively associated with an increased risk of diabetes and likelihood of engaging in behavioral risk factors. For example, one study suggests that Latina/o adults who reside in the United States for fewer than five years resemble those born in the United States in terms of diabetes prevalence. However, Latina/os who reside in the United States for 10 years or more have a higher prevalence of diabetes than Latina/os born in the United States (Schneiderman et al., 2014).

Injuries among Latina/os

Injury is a leading cause of death in the United States (Centers for Disease Control and Prevention, 2015b). Latina/o populations are further disproportionately burdened by injury. Unintentional injuries include motor vehicle injuries and interpersonal violence, among others. For motor vehicle injuries, though Latina/o children have a lower rate of deaths per billion vehicle-miles than African American children (8 vs. 14), they outnumber White/European American children, who have a rate of five per billion vehicle-miles (Baker, Braver, & Chen, 1998). Interpersonal violence is also higher among Latina/os. For example, in 2001, homicide was the second leading cause of death among Latina/os aged 15 to 24 years and the rate was over 2.5 times over the U.S. average homicide rate for this age group (Anderson & Smith, 2003).

Occupational injuries are increasing especially among Latina/o workers. Mekkodathil and colleagues (2016) conducted a review to identify occupational injuries between 1984 and 2014. The rate of fatal injuries of Latina/o workers in the United States during 2006–2008 was 4.8 per 100,000 full-time-equivalent employees, as compared with only 4 per 100,000 such employees among the general workforce. Additionally, foreign-born Latina/os incurred 66% of occupational injuries, as compared with 54% incurred by U.S.-born Latina/os. The types of occupations held by foreign-born versus U.S.-born Latina/os partially accounts for these differences.

Human Immunodeficiency Virus (HIV) among Latina/os

The human immunodeficiency virus (HIV) is a transmittable virus spread through certain body fluids (Centers for Disease Control and Prevention, 2017). HIV attacks the body's immune system by reducing the number of CD4 cells (T cells) in the body, weakening the immune system. HIV, if left untreated over time, can disable the body's ability to protect itself from infections and disease, thereby leaving the person with HIV susceptible to a range of serious diseases, such as cancers.

While HIV does not impact Latina/os as much as African Americans or White/European Americans, the rates remain high enough to threaten Latina/o health and warrant discussion. Latina/os constitute almost 24% of all new diagnoses of HIV in the United States and dependent areas of American Samoa, Guam, the Northern Mariana Islands, Puerto Rico, the Republic of Palau, and the U.S. Virgin Islands (Centers for Disease Control and Prevention, 2017). Although HIV diagnoses declined among Latinas from 2005 to 2014, HIV rates increased among Latino gay and bisexual men in the same period (Centers for Disease Control and Prevention, 2017).

An area of interest in HIV research involves examining the risk factors for HIV among men who have sex with men. Research suggests that among Latino men who have sex with men, differences in HIV risk factors might exist between foreign-born and U.S.-born Latinos. A cross-sectional analysis of risky behaviors, such as illicit drug use and binge drinking, did not indicate significant differences between men who have sex with men by place of birth—U.S.-born versus foreign-born (Mizuno et al., 2015). However, other studies suggest that these risky behaviors are more prevalent in U.S.-born Latina/os than in their foreign-born counterparts (Kopak, 2013; Ojeda, Patterson, & Strathdee, 2008).

Latina/o Children's Health

Data from the NHIS indicate that fewer Latina/o than White /European American children (ages 5–18 years old) rate their health as excellent (53.4% vs. 64.6%) (Centers for Disease Control and Prevention, 2014a). Despite this lower perceived health, fewer Latina/o children (11.6%) report missing six or more days of school due to illness or injury compared to White/ European Americans (13.1%) (Centers for Disease Control and Prevention, 2014b).

Obesity is more prevalent among Latina/o children than among White/ European American children (Kuczmarski et al., 2002). *Obesity* is defined as meeting or exceeding the 95th percentile for age and gender. Latino boys have higher rates of obesity (22.7%), as do Latino boys of Mexican descent (22.8%), as compared with their White/European American counterparts (18.7%). This relationship is also true for Latina girls of Mexican descent, who have a 24.2% prevalence of obesity, followed by Latina girls from other countries of origin, with 22.8%, and White/European American girls with 20.4%. These trends mirror data seen among adults and are troublesome given the number of chronic conditions associated with obesity and the increased likelihood of developing adult obesity for obese children (Dietz, 1998).

An ancillary study for adolescents was conducted alongside the HCHS/ SOL study—the SOL Youth study. SOL Youth enrolled a subset of the offspring of SOL study participants. Alike SOL, researchers recruited participants from the four U.S. communities—the Bronx, Chicago, Miami, and San Diego. The subset included 1,466 youth between 8 and 16 years old. While findings are still being published, one study provides initial information on the health of Latina/o youth. Overall, the prevalence of obesity is 28.4% among Latino boys and 24.6% among Latina girls (Isasi et al., 2016). This finding supports prior other studies regarding higher obesity rates among Latina/o children (Kuczmarski et al., 2002). Additionally, the prevalence of prediabetes is 20.9% among Latino boys and 11.8% among Latina girls.

Obesity trends begin fairly early in Latina/o children. In particular, Mexican American preschool children are disproportionately burdened by obesity (16.7%) and its associated consequences as compared with their

White/European American counterparts (10.7%) (Ogden, Carroll, Kit, & Flegal, 2014). Children develop attitudes and behaviors related to diet and physical activity that tend to influence subsequent health behaviors and outcomes later in life (Ogden et al., 2014). Cultural barriers to obesity prevention among Mexican American families include skepticism of clinical standards for childhood obesity, interdependence with extended family members to promote health, emotional distress associated with child feeding, and the acculturation process (Sosa, 2012; Sosa, McKyer, Goodson, & Castillo, 2014). More research is needed in this area to identify opportunities to intervene in meaningful and impactful ways among this high-risk group.

As with adults, the percentage of uninsured Latina/o children is also problematic. In 1997, 13% of children under the age of 18 were uninsured (Centers for Disease Control and Prevention, 2015c). However, in recent years, the number of uninsured Latina/o children has decreased. The rate of uninsured Latina/o children in 2005 was 8.9% and it further decreased to 4.5% in 2015. Possible changes to or the repeal of the Affordable Care Act will likely impact their health insurance coverage in the future.

CONCLUSION

Research on Latina/o health demonstrates the development of a paradigm shift. As seen by the trend data reviewed, there is great variation in the health conditions that impact Latina/o heritage groups as compared to non-Latina/os. Moreover, health conditions vary by country of origin, language, nativity, and immigration status. The prevalence of risk factors also varies among Latina/o heritage groups, highlighting the heterogeneity of Latina/os and their health profiles. These trends support the need to examine Latina/o health with special attention to Latina/o heritage groups and the creation of tailored approaches for these groups. Thus, it is important to remember that Latina/os are not a homogeneous group, and overgeneralized approaches to examine their health is problematic, as doing so results in decreased opportunities to advance the field. A paradigm shift must occur throughout research and practice to shift to informed approaches. New models can inform the study of Latina/o health, particularly as preexisting models typically reference non-Latina/o populations as the norm. Researchers should also continue to examine how immigration and acculturation impact health behaviors and outcomes among Latina/o heritage groups and the unique factors that impact their health.

Chapter 3

Health Care Access and Delivery among Latina/o Populations

There are wide differences between racial and ethnic groups in access to health care and the availability of health insurance. Minorities, especially Hispanic and African-American families, are less likely than whites to have private health insurance.

—Institute of Medicine, 2002

Latina/os are the nation's largest and fastest-growing minority group. They currently comprise approximately 15% of the U.S. population and are expected to nearly double to 29% by 2040 (Colby & Ortman, 2015). Their rapid increase and anticipated growth in the United States warrants providing not only reactionary but also proactive care to this segment of the population. Ensuring improved health outcomes for this underserved ethnic minority group will increase the likelihood of improving our nation's overall health.

Despite the large number of Latina/os in the United States, they are less likely than White/European Americans to access health care services. More than one-fourth of Latina/o adults in the United States lack a usual care provider (Livingston, Minushkin, & Cohn, 2008). Moreover, Latina/os are twice as likely as African Americans and three times as likely as White/European Americans to lack a usual provider (Pleis & Lethbridge-Çejku, 2006). These differences are further impacted by their country of origin and by immigration status—noncitizen versus U.S. citizen. Understanding these trends is critical for researchers, as this information will enable practitioners to better serve Latina/os. This chapter explores health care access among Latina/os and then specifically by Latina/o heritage groups. We examine barriers to accessing health care among Latina/os, including differences in access by nativity status and language barriers. Additionally, this chapter includes a brief discussion of how health care is accessed and utilized among higher-risk individuals, such as Latina/os with one or more chronic diseases. We also address two chronic diseases that impact Latina/os—diabetes and human immunodeficiency virus (HIV) infection. These two diseases are briefly reviewed and their relationship with health care access discussed. The chapter concludes with recommendations for addressing barriers to care and improving access to health care among Latina/os.

HEALTH CARE ACCESS AMONG LATINA/OS

Health care access is a critical aspect of preventive health. Access to health care includes an individual's ability to access health services when needed (see Tables 3.1 and 3.2). Health care access is associated with many health outcomes, and accessing preventive services and other health care services can lead to a reduced likelihood of disease and secondary and tertiary prevention, further reducing complications of diseases and illnesses. Beyond the contribution to reducing health risks, health care access is linked with higher quality of life (Ransford, Carrillo, & Rivera, 2010). However, there are complex associations among health care access, risk reduction, and quality of life. For instance, research indicates that individuals with access

Table 3.1 Age-Adjusted Percentage Distributions (with Standard Errors) of Type of Health Insurance Coverage of Latina/os as Compared with Other Racial/Ethnic Groups, 2015—Under Age 65

	Private	Medicaid	Other	Uninsured
Total	64.9 (.42)	20.7 (0.34)	3.7 (0.16)	10.8 (0.19)
Hispanic or Latino	45.1 (0.73)	30.7 (0.60)	2.4 (0.19)	21.9 (0.52)
Mexican or Mexican American	42.8 (0.93)	30.5 (0.76)	2.1 (0.19)	24.7 (0.70)
White	67.4 (0.47)	18.2 (0.37)	3.5 (0.18)	10.8 (0.23)
Black or African American	50.6 (0.86)	33.4 (0.74)	4.6 (0.32)	11.5 (0.43)

Source: Adapted from U.S. Department of Health & Human Services. (2015). Summary health statistics: National Health Interview Survey.

Table 3.2 Age-Adjusted Percentage Distributions (with Standard Errors) of Type of Health Insurance Coverage of Latina/os, as Compared with Other Racial/ Ethnic Groups, 2015—Age 65 and Over

	Private	Dual Eligible	Medicare Advantage	Medicare Only	Other	Uninsured
Total	41.5	7.3	24.3	18.4	8.0	0.6
	(0.74)	(0.30)	(0.60)	(0.55)	(0.37)	(0.07)
Hispanic or	18.0	24.8	28.0	19.3	6.8	3.1
Latino	(1.37)	(1.44)	(1.64)	(1.41)	(0.75)	(0.46)
Mexican or	16.7	23.3	28.4	19.8	7.6	4.2
Mexican American	(1.93)	(1.97)	(2.35)	(2.08)	(1.21)	(0.78)
White	43.8	6.1	24.2	17.7	7.8	0.6
	(0.83)	(0.31)	(0.67)	(0.61)	(0.41)	(0.07)

Source: Adapted from U.S. Department of Health & Human Services. (2015). Summary health statistics: National Health Interview Survey.

to health care tend to report greater quality of life, after controlling for disease state and other demographic characteristics (Villagran et al., 2012). Moreover, research suggests that health care access is more predictive of health care utilization than cognitive psychological factors, such as perceived benefits of using health care (De Jesus & Xiao, 2014).

Collectively, Latina/os tend to demonstrate lower health care access than their non-Latina/o counterparts. However, similar to research on Latina/o health issues, most research regarding access to health care examines Latina/os collectively, assuming that Latina/os are a homogeneous ethnic minority group. This research is also limited by the sole focus on one Latina/o heritage group, such as Mexican Americans. These aggregate analytical strategies not only limit researchers' ability to compare rates across Latina/o heritage groups but also limits their capability to understand the heterogeneous nature of Latina/os and how or why they access health care. Researchers are unable to identify unique factors by Latina/o heritage group that may explain lower health care access. However, if research across Latina/o heritage groups is conducted regularly, this information will enable practitioners and policymakers to use evidence-based strategies and thus increase health care access among each Latina/o heritage group. The few studies that have examined access by Latina/o heritage groups indicate significant within group differences in access and use of health care (Bustamante, Fang, Rizzo, & Ortega, 2009a; Shah & Carrasquillo, 2006).

HEALTH CARE ACCESS AMONG LATINA/O HERITAGE GROUPS

Researchers are increasingly investigating differences in health care access across Latina/o heritage groups. For example, one study examined health care access and use among Latina/o heritage groups and attempted to characterize the underlying mechanisms that contribute to differences in health care access (Bustamante et al., 2009b). Using National Health Interview Survey (NHIS) data from 1999 to 2007, Bustamante et al. (2009b) examined health care access and use across six Latina/o heritage groups— Mexican, Puerto Rican, Cuban, Dominican, Central/South American, and Other. Because they hypothesized that U.S. Latina/os of Mexican ancestry differ in their access in relation to other Latina/os, they compared Latina/os of Mexican ancestry with all other Latina/o heritage groups combined.

Bustamante and colleagues (2009b) used the decomposition model to examine both observed and unobserved contributors to disparities. Observed variables included the structural composition of the groups, whereas unobserved variables included cultural differences, discrimination, and other factors not accounted for. Latina/os of Mexican ancestry demonstrate a lower probability (68.7%) of having a regular health care facility when ill as compared with all other Latina/o heritage groups combined (79.6%). They are also less likely to have health insurance and also to experience delays in obtaining health care. Regarding the decomposition model, Latina/os of Mexican ancestry have worse access and utilization measures as compared with the combined group. This comparison holds true even after excluding Puerto Ricans and Cubans.

Alcalá and colleagues (2017) used NHIS data to examine differences in health care access and utilization among Latina/o heritage groups after the implementation of the Affordable Care Act. In contrast to Bustamante et al. (2009b), they compared across heritage groups of U.S. Latina/os from Mexico, Cuba, Central America, Puerto Rico, and other countries of origin. They assessed health care access and utilization by insurance status, delayed medical care, forgoing medical care, emergency department visits, and physician visits. Data included the 2011 to 2015 waves to examine the impact of the Affordable Care Act. The study analyzed data from 20,764 Latina/o adults aged 18–64, including 1,995 Puerto Ricans, 12,983 Mexicans, 871 Cubans, 3,592 Central Americans, and 1,323 Other Latinos. Alcalá et al. (2017) estimated logistic regression models for each health care outcome. The Affordable Care Act is associated with improvements in health care access and utilization among most Latina/o heritage groups; however, improvements appear to decrease the following year for certain Latina/o heritage groups. For example, Mexicans and Cubans forgo care a year after the implementation of the Affordable Care Act. Mexicans and Central Americans exhibit lower odds of being insured relative to White/European Americans, whereas Central Americans also have higher odds of forgoing care relative to White/European Americans. Puerto Ricans also have higher odds of visiting an emergency department, while Mexicans have lower odds of visiting a physician as compared with White/European Americans.

BARRIERS TO HEALTH CARE UTILIZATION AMONG LATINOS

Lack of Health Insurance

As indicated in Chapter 1, Latina/os comprise the highest percentage of uninsured persons in the United States (23.7%) and surpass the percentage of the total uninsured population (12.0%; Stepler & Brown, 2016). The role of employer-covered health insurance partially contributes to observed trends in the increasing number of uninsured Latina/os because they tend to be employed in professions that fail to provide health insurance coverage compared to their White/European American counterparts (Kaiser, 2008). Although 70% of Latina/o households have at least one employed person, 40% of employed Latinos are uninsured (Kaiser, 2008).

Some longitudinal data suggest that there are significant differences in insurance trends among Latina/o heritage groups (Shah & Carrasquillo, 2006). A study using the Current Population Survey data from 1993 to 2004 examined 12-year trends among Latina/o heritage groups and by immigration status. The Current Population Survey used an in-person household survey and oversampled for Latina/o households. The number of uninsured Latina/os increased significantly, from 8.4 million in 1993 to 13.7 million in 2004. Among Latina/o heritage groups, Mexicans demonstrate increased uninsured rates, rising from 67% in 1993 to 72% in 2004. In contrast, Dominicans and Cuban demonstrate decreased uninsured rates. While the number of uninsured U.S.-born Latina/os increased between 1993 and 1998, this number decreased between 2000 and 2004. The number of uninsured noncitizen Latina/os increased throughout the 1993–2004 era. White/European Americans demonstrate limited changes in the percentage of uninsured persons between 1993 and 1998; however, the number of uninsured Latina/os appears to increase by nearly 4%.

Using data from the NHIS from 1999–2007, Bustamante and colleagues (2009a) compared insurance status between Latina/os of Mexican ancestry and U.S. non-Mexican Latina/os. As hypothesized, Latina/os of Mexican ancestry are less likely to have health insurance than non-Mexican Latina/os. Approximately 65% of these disparities are attributed to differences in observed characteristics among Latina/os of Mexican ancestry, such as their age, gender, income, employment status, education, citizenship, language, and health condition. Bustamante et al. (2009a) indicate that other significant determinants, such as risk aversion and cultural differences, may also help explain differences in insurance status between Latina/os of Mexican ancestry and non-Mexican Latina/os.

Among Latina/os with chronic conditions, such as diabetes, access to health care is critical. For instance, Hu and colleagues (2014) examined predictors of access to health care among patients with diabetes using the Diabetes Care Survey of the 2010 Medical Expenditure Panel Survey, an annual nationally representative survey conducted by the Agency for Healthcare Research and Quality and the National Center for Health Statistics. The Medical Expenditure Panel Survey includes five rounds of interviews of household respondents, providers, and employers and assesses health care utilization, medical expenditures, access to care, quality of care, and insurance coverage. Findings suggest that Latina/os have lower access to health care. However, after controlling for demographic characteristics such as race/ethnicity and socioeconomic status and health status, insurance remains associated with quality of care.

Lack of Usual Care Provider

Access to a usual health care provider refers to whether individuals have a facility for health care when they are ill or need health advice, excluding a hospital emergency department. Having a usual care provider can facilitate use of health care services. However, according to a survey conducted by the Pew Center and the Robert Wood Johnson Foundation that investigated Latina/os' access to health care, including their use of a usual health care provider, 27% of Latino adults lack a usual health care provider (Livingston, Minushkin, & Cohn, 2008). The lack of a usual health care provider is impacted by, but not completely explained by, whether individuals have health insurance. Approximately 42% of uninsured Latina/os lack a usual health care provider, as compared with 19% of insured Latina/os (Livingston et al., 2008). Despite several underlying factors that contribute to their limited health care access, many of these underlying factors are modifiable and, if addressed, can help reduce health disparities among Latina/os.

Livingston et al. (2008) report that Latina/os who lack a usual health care provider include men (36%), the young (37% of Latina/os between the ages of 18 to 29), and those with lower levels of education (32% lack a high school diploma). However, Latina/os who lack a usual provider indicate that a usual health care provider is unnecessary because they are seldom ill, prefer to treat themselves, and perceive the cost of health care as a barrier (Livingston et al., 2008). The reliance on self-care practices and use of alternative medicine presents its own set of risks, which we address in greater detail in our discussion of nontraditional health practices in Chapter 5. The importance of having a usual care provider cannot be overemphasized, even for preventive services. For example, Latina/os with a regular health care provider (86%) report a prior blood pressure examination, as compared with only 62% of Latina/os without a regular health care provider (Livingston et al., 2008). Access to preventive services is likely to reduce treatment costs subsequently incurred by the health care system and warrant further examination.

Language Barriers

Perceived language barriers and difficulty communicating with a health care provider can greatly impact the likelihood of seeking health care services. Several studies demonstrate how Latina/os forgo their health services if they anticipate communication challenges with their provider (Jacquez, Vaughn, Zhen-Duan, & Graham, 2016; Pearson, Ahluwalia, Ford, & Mokdad, 2008; Pippins, Alegría, & Haas, 2007). Additionally, health care providers are less receptive to patients with limited English proficiency.

Thus, it is critical to examine the relationship between language proficiency and receipt of quality primary care. Pippins et al. (2007) examined language proficiency as a predictor of health care utilization and quality of care received by Latina/os by using data from the National Latina/o and Asian Americans Study (NLAAS). The study solely focused on Latina/os with health insurance ($N = 1,792$). Researchers used data from 2002 to 2003 and included four outcome variables to measure the quality of primary care—not having a regular and continuous source of care, difficulties obtaining an appointment over the telephone, long waits in the waiting room, and difficulties obtaining information or advice by telephone. Participants who lacked continuity or a regular physician were categorized as having low continuity of care; all others were categorized as having adequate continuity. Additionally, data included country of origin to allow for the analysis of Latina/o heritage groups, including Mexican, Puerto Rican, Cuban, or other.

Latina/os with lower English proficiency experience greater negative experiences with health care than their more English-proficient counterparts. Low English proficiency is associated with longer wait times and greater difficulty obtaining information or advice by telephone but is not associated with difficulty obtaining an appointment over the telephone (Pippen et al., 2007). Regression models tested the associations among Latina/o heritage groups. Puerto Ricans experience greater difficulty obtaining an appointment over the telephone as compared with Mexicans. Cubans report greater long waits in waiting rooms as compared with Mexicans. Puerto Ricans, Cubans, and other Latina/os are more likely to report difficulty obtaining information or advice by telephone as compared with Mexicans. Puerto Ricans and other Latina/os are more likely to report no regular source of care as compared with Mexicans.

The issue of language barriers can be exacerbated in areas with smaller Latina/o communities. One example is the new migration area in Greater Cincinnati. Using a community-based approach, Jacquez et al. (2016) examined 516 Latina/o immigrants in Greater Cincinnati to assess their health care experiences in an emerging Latina/o community. Participants were largely from Mexico (51%) but included Latina/os from Guatemala (28%), Honduras (8%), Nicaragua, (5%), and others (10%). Participants were recruited through school events, festivals, grocery stores, and Latin American corner stores. Jacquez et al. also conducted four focus groups to engage community members in order to interpret the data and explore potential access barriers. Barriers to health care include language, limited availability of high-quality interpreters, frustration with wait times to speak with interpreters, and variable quality of interpretation provided. Participants note a significant need for systemic changes to increase their health care access. Many participants express the need for more Spanish-speaking health care providers. Additionally, they identify the need for more Spanish language health education in settings easily accessible to Latinos.

Immigration Status

Assumptions that unauthorized workers abuse health care expenditures are not strongly supported by empirical research (Goldman, Smith, & Sood, 2006; Nandi et al., 2008). In fact, while unauthorized immigrants account for 3.2% of the U.S. population, they solely account for approximately 1.5% of U.S. medical costs (Goldman et al., 2006). This is in part attributed to their lower health care utilization. For instance, only 36.5% of unauthorized Latina/os report access to a regular health care provider (Nandi et al., 2008). These estimates are larger in certain border areas. For example, in Southern California, it is estimated that approximately 68–84% of unauthorized Latina/os are uninsured (Kaiser, 2008). Data from the 2003 California Health Interview Survey of 42,044 participants indicate that unauthorized Mexicans report lower use of health care services and poorer experiences in their health care encounters as compared with their U.S.-born counterparts. This relationship remains after adjusting for confounding variables, such as education and income (Ortega et al., 2007). Unauthorized Latinas are perhaps less likely to enter the health care system in these border areas because of fear of deportation.

Analysis of insurance trends suggests that unauthorized Latina/os experienced a continuous increase in the proportion of uninsured persons (Shah, Zhu, Wu, & Potter, 2006). Unauthorized immigrants are typically ineligible for many government programs. Additionally, they tend to work in nontraditional jobs that do not provide employee benefits, such as health insurance. One study compared health care use between unauthorized Latina/os and other Latina/os (Rodriguez, Bustamante, & Ang, 2009). Using data from the Pew Hispanic Center/Robert Wood Johnson Foundation Hispanic Healthcare Survey, a telephone survey of over 3,847 Latina/o adults, researchers examined nativity/immigration status and whether participants had a usual source of health care, health insurance, and prior screening behaviors. Their analysis controlled for sociodemographic variables such as age, marital status, gender, and education. Fewer unauthorized Latina/os as compared with U.S.-born Latina/os have a usual source of health care (58% vs. 79%), insurance coverage (37% vs. 66%), blood pressure examinations within the past two years (67% vs. 81%), and cholesterol screenings within the past five years (56% vs. 79%). Unauthorized Latina/os have lower odds of undergoing cholesterol screenings and worse perceived health care quality than U.S.-born Latina/os. They also report significant financial and linguistic constraints to access health care.

Additional Barriers

Qualitative research is helpful in unraveling complex barriers to health care access among Latina/os. For example, a qualitative study conducted by Ransford and colleagues (2010) examined barriers among 12 hometown association leaders from Mexico, El Salvador, and Guatemala as well as with 96 community respondents who reside in the Pico-Union area of Los Angeles. Barriers include long waits, rude behavior, being hurried through the health care system without sufficient medical explanations, and costs. Most participants (65%) cite long waits as a barrier to using health care and report waiting between 6 and 12 hours to receive medical attention. Participants who lose a full day's pay to seek medical care find the long waits especially burdensome. Participants also identify financial constraints (51%), rude behavior and communication problems once they meet with their provider, as they also feel hurried through their visit and consequently fail to receive proper medical information (35%).

Perceptions regarding quality of health care received among Latina/os are generally positive. For example, in a survey of Latina/os who received medical care in the past year, only 23% report poor-quality treatment (Livingston et al., 2008). More educated Latinos and those with access to the medical system tend to have positive evaluations regarding the quality of their medical care. For instance, having health insurance or a usual health care provider is associated with positive perceptions of quality of care, as Latina/os who receive their medical care in a physician's office rather than a medical clinic report positive perceptions. More worrisome is that among Latina/os who perceive poor-quality treatment, many perceive that their poor treatment is due to their poverty status (31%), ethnicity (29%), or accent (23%) (Livingston et al., 2008).

Unfortunately, these findings underscore the importance of addressing how perceived discrimination among Latina/os influence their perceptions of inequality in the heath care system. Moreover, there is ample research indicating that discrimination is also a health barrier among Latina/os. For example, in a study of racial bias (Johnson, Saha, Arbelaez, Beach, & Cooper, 2004), Latina/os report that their physicians fail to listen to them and perceive that their physicians do not actively involve them with decision making about their treatment. They also report that the medical staff unfairly judge them or treat them with disrespect because of their ethnicity (Johnson et al., 2004).

In addition to the aforementioned barriers, low health competence can also create barriers to accessing health care among Latina/os. A cross-sectional study of 330 foreign-born Latina/o adults in Baltimore, MD, suggests that low health competence can create barriers to accessing health care (Fonseca-Becker et al., 2010). Health competence includes knowledge, attitudes, skills, and resources that are necessary to improve and maintain health. For example, health competence appears to predict health care–seeking behaviors among foreign-born Latina/os. Moreover, increased education also appears to increase their knowledge of existing barriers for accessing care as a Latina/o immigrant. These findings have implications for practice and can inform interventions aimed at increasing health care utilization via increasing health care competence.

HEALTH CARE ACCESS AND UTILIZATION AMONG CHILDREN AND YOUTH

Latina/o children tend to have lower access to health care as compared with White/European American children (Perez-Escamilla, Garcia, & Song, 2010). Factors that contribute to Latina/o children's lack of insurance include poverty, immigration status, unfavorable labor policies, language barriers, discrimination, and acculturation status, among others (Perez-Escamilla et al., 2010). Children at highest risk are children of migrant farm workers. A multiethnic cross-sectional study examined health insurance among 900 unauthorized and other Latina/o parents of children 18 years and younger (Flores, Abreu, & Tomany-Korman, 2006). Findings suggest that many Latina/o children lack health insurance. Moreover, among Latina/o children without health insurance, 55.1% have one working parent and an additional 33.1% of children who lack health insurance have parents employed in jobs that do not provide health insurance and employee benefits. Parents report barriers such as difficulties scheduling an appointment, lack of health insurance, long wait periods, high costs, inconvenient office hours, language barriers, and health care staff with a limited understanding of Latina/o culture.

Along the U.S.-Mexico border, similar trends exist. One study examined the health choices of Latina/o farmworkers who reside along the U.S.-Mexico border (Seid et al., 2003). The study includes children from Head Start centers in California. Among the children of migrant farmers who reside along the U.S./Mexico border, over half receive their health care in Mexico, even if they possess health insurance. Parents of children who largely receive their health care in Mexico report greater accessibility and receive coordinated primary care in Mexico.

Similar to adults, health care access and utilization among children also varies by Latina/o heritage group. Another study examined youth health care access and utilization across Latina/o heritage groups (Perez et al., 2009). Researchers used data from the 1998 to 2006 NHIS to assess health insurance, child demographics, parent demographics, parent ratings of the child's health status, and access to health care, such as a usual source of care. The sample included 56,007 children aged 1 to 17 years. Mexican children demonstrate the lowest access to health care as compared with White/European American children and other Latina/o heritage groups. Additionally, when controlling for predisposing (i.e., age, gender, parental education, interview language, citizenship and nativity status, and survey year), enabling (i.e., predisposing factors and family income below poverty level, health insurance, and U.S. regions), and need (i.e., predisposing, enabling factors, and health status) factors, Mexican children are the only group to demonstrate lower rates of access and utilization as compared with White/European American children. The NHIS does not collect data regarding parent citizenship status, so the influence of fear related to legal authorization is not assessed. However, the authors posit that fear related to legal authorization may also contribute to lower health care access among Latina/o children.

Latina/o children who live in Limited English Proficiency (LEP) households are less likely to have access to enter and navigate the health care system (Avila & Bramlett, 2013). Polk, Carter-Pokras, Dover, and Cheng (2013) outline five recommendations for improving access among Latina/o children with limited health literacy—comprehensive efforts to increase community engagement, interpreter availability, workforce diversity, health care access, and inclusiveness in research efforts. Polk et al. (2013)

first recommend that clinicians, health care delivery systems, and policy-makers engage Latina/o community members within the design, implementation, and evaluation of health information and services. This is particularly critical for families with LEP. Second, Polk et al. argue for the universal availability of interpreter services in clinical settings. Trained professional interpreters can help provide appropriate linguistic services, that are associated with improved patient satisfaction, fewer errors in communication, better adherence to medication regimens, and improved clinical outcomes (Flores et al., 2002).

Third, a culturally competent and more inclusive workforce is needed to speed health care improvements. In addition to increasing diversity in the workforce, all health care training must include lessons in cultural competence and cultural humility. Fourth, it is necessary to create a more accessible health care system. Outreach services may be required to enroll individuals in medical care, as well as health insurance coverage. Finally, health research must better reflect the U.S. population, including Latina/o families, LEP individuals, and their children. Health research should aim to include more diverse samples that include Latina/o families and must also engage in the increased development and testing of Spanish language instruments.

Furthermore, children of immigrants are at especially high risk to lack access to health care. Children of immigrants are less likely to have a usual source of care (Kaiser Family Foundation, 2004), lower immunization completion rates (Findley, Irigoyen, & Schulman, 1999), and lower access to dental care (Isong & Weintraub, 2005) as compared with their U.S.-born counterparts. Moreover, parental legal status is associated with better social well-being.

HEALTH CARE ACCESS FOR LATINA/OS WITH CHRONIC DISEASE

Diabetes

Given the disproportionate burden diabetes on Latina/os, it is increasingly important to understand their unique barriers and how Latina/os with diabetes navigate the health care system. As mentioned in Chapter 2, diabetes is a condition in which the body is either unable to produce insulin or unable to properly use its insulin. If left untreated and poorly managed, diabetes can lead to several other complications. Given the chronic nature of diabetes, ongoing access to health care is extremely important. Patients with diabetes require ongoing medical care and assistance with self-management and preventive care.

Data from the MESA suggest that Latina/os with shorter U.S. residence or Latina/os who speak Spanish at home have diabetes and less metabolic control over their conditions than their more acculturated counterparts (Eamranond et al., 2009). Additionally, other research suggests that Latina/o adults with diabetes and with a usual health care facility have higher diabetes knowledge than Latina/o adults with diabetes but without a usual health care facility (Livingston et al., 2008).

Additional research suggests that differences in health-related beliefs exist among Latina/o heritage groups. A qualitative study examined diabetes-related beliefs of 24 Latina/os—6 Mexicans, 6 Guatemalans, 5 Colombians, and 7 Puerto Ricans—with diabetes or a diabetic family member or friend (Long et al., 2012). Focus group data suggest that not all Latina/o heritage groups perceive diabetes as an inevitable disease. For instance, Puerto Ricans are more likely to indentify that the development of diabetes is inevitable, while others indicate that diabetes is caused by unhealthy living or due to spiritual elements. Interestingly, Mayans perceive that diabetes is preventable by increasing one's spiritual connections with the environment and by also maintaining healthy communication with family members. Despite the study's small sample, these qualitative findings suggest the need for culturally tailored outreach for Latina/os with diabetes to examine heritage group differences in cultural beliefs and how those beliefs might impact diabetes care and diabetes prevention.

HIV/AIDS

Rates of HIV infection disproportionately burden Latina/os. Rates of HIV infection are twice as high among Latino men as among White/European American men and four times higher among Latina women as among White/European American women (Hall et al., 2008). See Chapter 2 for information on the prevalence of HIV in Latina/o communities. A needs assessment for HIV/acquired immunodeficiency syndrome (AIDS) prevention among Latina/os was conducted among Latinos who were HIV-positive and at risk for HIV infection across 14 U.S. cities (Rios-Ellis et al., 2008). Community-based organizations and participants were recruited to take part in interviews and focus groups. Latina/o participants, demonstrate limited awareness of HIV risk factors and findings also illustrate the need for culturally and linguistically appropriate programming. Cultural gender roles, such as *machismo*, also appear to play a role in promoting risky sexual behaviors.

Programs targeting Latina/o heritage groups that exhibit higher rates of HIV infection might also show promise for addressing HIV-related disparities. A study based on 2000 NHIS data compared HIV testing by Latina/o heritage group. Mexicans (odds ratio [OR] = 1.59) and Mexican Americans (OR = 1.61) are more likely to report that they are not tested for HIV as compared with their Puerto Rican counterparts (Lopez-Quintero, Shtark-shall, & Neumark, 2005).

STRATEGIES FOR ADDRESSING BARRIERS IN ACCESS TO HEALTH CARE AMONG LATINA/OS

Many of the strategies below are informed by a literature review of 77 studies on health care access barriers (Perez-Escamilla, 2009). The review includes key studies and authoritative reviews based upon a Medline search. Additionally, the review includes studies and reviews recommended by experts in the field. Studies include both convenience sampling techniques and representative sampling techniques; however, Perez-Escamilla (2009) prioritize studies that either use representative sampling or are comprehensive systematic literature reviews. The results of the review indicate many similar barriers among the studies and systematic reviews. Perez-Escamilla (2009) identifies many of the same barriers as discussed throughout this chapter—lack of health insurance, lack of a usual care provider, language barriers, and unauthorized status. Perez-Escamilla (2009) recommends addressing these barriers by increasing access to insurance, improving cultural competency, using patient navigators, and several policy recommendations. Additionally, because of the significant impact of language barriers on accessing health care, we provide a specific discussion regarding the need for increased access to trained and high-quality interpreters.

Health Insurance

Increasing access to health care through increasing health insurance has great promise. Health insurance from employers is limited, as Latina/o workers are more likely to be uninsured as compared with other employed groups (McCollister et al., 2010). From 1997 to 2007, data from the NHIS suggest that Latina/os have a sharper decline in health insurance coverage than White/European Americans or African Americans (McCollister et al., 2010). This number is most pronounced among Latina/o blue-collar workers, who experience the largest drop in the number of insured individuals.

With the potential repeal and replacement of the Affordable Care Act, there is an urgent need to advocate for policies aimed to increase access to health insurance for extremely vulnerable groups, such as Latina/os. Additionally, access to health insurance for unauthorized workers is imperative. A pathway to citizenship is certainly a long-term solution. In the short-term, decreasing barriers to accessing care among the uninsured is also critical.

Improving Cultural Competency among Health Care Providers

Cultural competency among health care professionals is necessary to provide responsible care to Latina/o patients. Cultural competence is generally defined as the condition when a set of congruent behaviors, attitudes, and policies come together in a system, agency, or among professionals to enable effective cross-cultural work (Cross, 1989). Without cultural competence, health care providers neglect the needs of patients from cultures that differ from their own since they fail to provide informed and appropriate care to groups with the greatest need (Perez-Escamilla, 2009). Increasing cultural competence can involve several approaches. Cultural competence and recommendations are described in greater detail in Chapter 10. However, we present two approaches to increase cultural competence in the short term—increasing the pipeline of culturally competent individuals and providing training to health care providers.

Increasing the pipeline of individuals with cultural competency and an interest in health-related careers can be a long-term solution to decrease the cultural gap in health care services. Increasing the diversity of health professionals by including underrepresented groups can aid in the elimination of health disparities. For example, bilingual and bicultural Latina/os who are familiar with Latina/o cultural values and who also possess the skills to effectively communicate with Latina/o patients can inform efforts to increase cultural competence. Adequate training and support (e.g., mentorship opportunities) to address potential barriers in pursuing professional training can minimize obstacles and increase the likelihood of success for these professionals.

It is paramount to provide cultural competency training to all health care providers (Polk et al., 2013). Their initial training can incorporate cultural competency to provide health care providers with a greater understanding of their patient's cultural beliefs, particularly those of their Latina/o patients. This can help improve patient–provider communication and decrease current barriers. Although these two approaches alone are insufficient to establish cultural competence, they are feasible approaches to prioritize in the short term while larger systemic changes are pursued.

Increasing Access to Trained Interpreters

While Title VI of the Civil Rights Act of 1964 requires organizations with federal support to ensure that patients with Limited English Proficiency (LEP) have access to interpreter services. However, implementation of the mandate is inconsistent and inadequate (Polk et al., 2013; Wu, Ridgely, Escarce, & Morales, 2007). Nonetheless, creative models can be used to provide language access services for patients with LEP. *Hablamos Juntos* is a $10-million multiyear demonstration project funded through the Robert Wood Johnson Foundation (Wu et al., 2007). The demonstration provided funding to 10 organizations and tasked them to: (1) plan and implement activities to recruit, assess, train, and place medical interpreters throughout the health care system; (2) develop a supportive environment for interpretation; and (3) beta test an assessment of language proficiency and develop training program for interpreters.

Researchers estimated the annual operating costs at approximately $666,000 per site. They learned that providers needed convincing regarding the quality rationale to increase their buy-in. Many physicians did not easily recognize the benefit of using professional interpreter services and relied upon their prior use of bilingual housekeeping staff or patient's family members. The prerequisite implementation strategies required consistency, as staff members failed to frequently utilize the interpreter services because of their limited time. In these instances, staff members relied on their previous sources of translation, such as patient's family members. Additionally, there are limited interpreter proficiency standards and a need for comprehensive training programs for medical interpreters. Moreover, health professions will benefit from the requirement of minimal standards to serve as an interpreter. This effort will increase the quality of translation services provided to patients.

Patient Navigators/Community Health Workers/Health Educators

To bridge the gap between health professionals and patients, several other professionals and para-professionals can be employed. For instance, these individuals can serve a critical role, such as patient navigators, community health workers/*promotoras*, and health educators. Patient navigators are trained community health workers who help patients overcome access to health care barriers and help patients navigate the health care system to obtain timely health care (Freeman, 2004). Navigators help connect patients with resources and also help patients understand the health care system. *Promotoras* (the Spanish term for female community health workers), are lay community members who provide health education and social support to Latina/o community members (Balcazar et al., 2006). Patient navigators and *promotoras* can provide support to patients and help them overcome traditional barriers to the complex health care system.

One reason *promotoras* are effective and well accepted among Latina/os is that they fit a natural model of communication in the Latina/o community. Latina/os value and prefer interpersonal communication and close relationships (Elder, Ayala, Parra-Medina, & Talavera, 2009). Additionally, Latina/os are open to receiving health information through informal health communication sources (Katz, Ang, & Suro, 2012). *Promotoras* are able to assist in health promotion efforts by increasing access to health information, implementing health programming, and providing ongoing social support (Balcazar et al., 2000). For more information on *promotora* approaches to health, see Chapter 4. A diversified health information communication network can help increase awareness of health issues among Latina/os and become more proactive in maintaining their health.

Another group that is beneficial in providing services despite limited resources is *health educators*. Health educators are trained educators who also have earned a Bachelor's degree in Health. Clinics can employ health educators to bridge the care that otherwise might not be provided because of limited time and resources. The national certification provides a standard for health educators to meet to become certified health education specialists. These trained health educators can assess individual needs, provide education to meet specific goals, and advocate for patient needs. Because of the lower education requirements for health educators as compared with other health professionals, a health educator position might provide an avenue for engaging culturally competent individuals in the health care system. This fills the immediate but urgent need for cultural competence among health professionals. This can complement efforts to increase the number of culturally competent physicians and other health care providers.

Programmatic Efforts

Programmatic efforts can help bridge the gap between health care and community member's needs. For example, to address the barrier to accessing health insurance, a four-year study evaluated the success of the Los Angeles Healthy Kids Program (Hill et al., 2008). The program aimed to improve health care access for 40,000 children, a majority of whom were immigrant Latina/o children. The program was funded through Proposition 10 funds (revenues from a 50-cent tax on cigarettes) and provided health insurance to low-income children who were age five or younger and ineligible for Medicaid or Healthy Families coverage. The program successfully increased health insurance, with 86% of new enrollees living below the poverty line and 91% noncitizens. However, the program's expansion is problematic and sustainability is dependent on comprehensive health care reform.

As we consider ways to become more inclusive of Latina/os, the following recommendations may help health care professionals prepare to work with them:

- Increase programmatic efforts for Latina/o workers who may lack health insurance.
  - Engage nontraditional worksites in health promotion efforts, since these sites are more likely to be places of employment for Latina/os.
  - Examples of programmatic efforts may include mobile health screenings and other outreach efforts.
- Incorporate telephone interventions to reach Latina/o communities since telephone communication is convenient, less expensive than face-to-face interventions, circumvents transportation issues and child care needs, reduces time commitment, and can be provided in English and Spanish (Elder et al., 2009).
- Partner with Latina/os to help inform practice. Engage members of the target population at all stages to identify the most pressing needs, opportunities for addressing the needs of the Latina/o community despite access limitations, potential activities, evaluation, and sustainability.

Assess Latina/o cultural competence prior to engaging in Latino/o communities. Practitioners and researchers can assess their Latina/o cultural competence and that of their teams using a self-assessment tool that asks questions about their familiarity with aspects of the Latina/o community such as Latina/o beliefs, custom norms, and values; Latina/o understanding of disease and illness; Latina/o strengths; Latina/o history in the geographic area; and the role of family in decision making and language preferences. The lack of knowledge in any of these areas can be addressed prior to engaging with the Latina/o community to increase inclusivity and receptiveness among Latina/os.

CONCLUSION

There are a large number of barriers that prevent access to health care services for Latina/os. Efforts to reduce these barriers are greatly needed if we are to serve this fast-growing segment of the population in meaningful ways. Barriers such as the rapidly increasing number of Latina/os who do not have insurance, especially among Latina/os of Mexican heritage; language barriers; immigration status and other cultural factors need to be addressed to reduce health disparities experienced among this group.

Chapter 4

Community Efforts for Health Promotion in Latina/o Communities

Much of the task of developing successful community programs can be pared down to the use of clear and effective communication with entire communities, their organizations, and the families and individuals who reside in them.
—Elder, Ayala, Parra-Medina, and Talavera, 2009

Given the number of Latina/os who experience difficulty accessing the health care system, finding alternative routes for delivering health promotion and disease prevention services is critical. Within Latina/o communities, language, family, and religion are often paramount. Accordingly, these elements are potential points of entry and support for health promotion delivery in the Latina/o community. By capitalizing on natural help systems that exist in the Latina/o community, practitioners can use culturally appropriate approaches such as *promotora*/community health workers and family-based interventions. Additionally, alternative sites that are frequented by Latina/os, such as churches and schools, can serve as channels for delivering health promotion and screening to Latina/os. Understanding these delivery channels and forming collaborations with these entities can enable increased evidence-based approaches and culturally tailored resources to better serve the Latina/o community.

This chapter explores nontraditional settings for community health promotion and health care efforts for Latina/os. More importantly, we present a sample of culturally tailored programs for Latina/os and discuss their ability to engage Latina/os in health promotion efforts. We also highlight collaborations across various channels and highlight processes to successfully recruit and engage Latina/o-serving entities and provide health-related resources for Latina/os. Additionally, this chapter explores programmatic efforts to address key health issues in Latina/o communities, such as obesity, cancers, diabetes, and human immunodeficiency virus (HIV) infection. Given the rapid increase in the number of culturally tailored programs for Latina/os, we discuss current frameworks for developing culturally appropriate programs. We also provide recommendations for new programs and how to reach traditionally underserved Latina/o communities, and we identify important considerations for community-based participatory research and other research efforts to inform future programming.

MOVING OUTSIDE TRADITIONAL HEALTH SETTINGS

Now is the time for collaborative efforts to address complex health-related issues that impact Latina/o communities. Collaborative efforts have several advantages, including but not limited to, sharing of resources, increased buy-in among community members and increased program sustainability (Mattesich & Monsey, 1992). Moreover, when diverse partners are able to share their own perspectives on complex health issues, they can identify comprehensive solutions that are informed by diverse insights (Zuckerman, Kaluzny, & Ricketts, 1994).

Complex health issues are impacted not only by health care access but also by the living and working conditions of everyday life. Accordingly, multiple partners across sectors are necessary to address multifactorial health issues. Beyond health issues, collaborative partnerships can address social issues and other issues that impact Latina/o communities.

Religion

Religion plays a central role in Latina/o culture and is associated with better health outcomes across a number of indicators (Lujan & Campbell, 2006). Theoretically, religiosity serves as a coping mechanism during the acculturation process (Lujan & Campbell, 2006), and Latina/os view churches as trustworthy sources of social support and resources (Schwingel & Gálvez, 2016). Religion may play an important role among immigrant Latina/os. For example, Ransford, Carrillo, and Rivera (2010) examined the role of religiosity in health among 96 Latina/o immigrants. They interviewed Latina/o immigrants in Los Angeles who resided in a Latina/o ethnic enclave of primarily Mexican and Central American unauthorized immigrants. They observed that prayer is essential to the health of Latina/o immigrants and plays a key role in their survival process. Latina/o immigrants perceive that prayer is a method that assists with this process but is insufficient by itself for, disease prevention.

FAITH-BASED PROGRAMS FOR LATINA/O HEALTH PROMOTION

Given the central role of religion among Latina/os, the rise of faith-placed and faith-based programs for Latina/o health is not surprising. Faith-based organizations have a natural fit with public health efforts. The intersection of faith-based and public health sectors contains long-standing partnerships as well as newer initiatives (Levin, 2014). Faith-based organizations serve their congregations and are a potential partner to increase health education, screening behaviors, and access to health-related services. Additionally, a needs assessment among Latina/o faith leaders indicates that most leaders recognize the need to address health issues, such as diabetes and obesity, and believe that the church can play a key role in addressing those issues (He et al., 2013).

Faith-based programs include those that incorporate health programming and messaging into the activities of faith-based organizations. For example, a church might include several ministries, one of which is a church health ministry that oversees the program and leads implementation efforts. The faith-based organization should be an active partner in all program activities. In contrast, faith-placed programs simply house programs and services at the physical location of a faith-based organization.

Faith-based programs can improve health outcomes, but additional research regarding their effectiveness is needed (DeHaven et al., 2004). A review of 106 articles indicates that the majority of faith-based health programs focus on primary prevention and few focus on secondary and tertiary prevention. Program topics largely include chronic disease prevention but also address general health maintenance. Most studies do not clearly communicate outcome measures associated with their faith-based programs. However, among studies that report outcome measures, faith-based programs are associated with increased knowledge of the disease, improved screening behaviors and readiness to change, and reduced disease risk (DeHaven et al., 2004).

Faith-Based Interventions for Cancer Prevention

One area of interest for faith-based programs is increased screening behaviors among Latina/o adults (Allen, Leyva, et al., 2014; Kaplan et al., 2009; Sauaia et al., 2007). Faith-based interventions often aim to promote screening behaviors for various types of cancers, such as breast cancer

(Sauaia et al., 2007). Although evaluation outcomes are limited for various studies in this area, evidence suggests that cancer prevention studies as faith-based interventions can have high buy-in from the congregation, acceptability in the church setting, and greater retention (Allen et al., 2014).

One faith-based program that demonstrates some success is the *Tepeyac Project* in Colorado (Sauaia et al., 2007). The project was created to increase breast cancer screenings among Latinas in Colorado. Two interventions were specifically developed to address breast cancer screenings—a printed material intervention, in which congregants receive culturally tailored breast-health promotion packages through their Catholic church, and a *promotora* intervention, in which a *promotora* delivers the health promotion message on an individual basis. Catholic churches serve as an instrument in distributing the printed material, make announcements, display printed materials, and publish messages in the bulletin. While the printed-material intervention demonstrates minimal success, the *promotora* intervention in the faith-based program is associated with increased breast cancer screening among Latinas with health insurance, as measured through insurance claims.

Faith-Based Interventions for HIV

Faith-based interventions often provide a less stigmatized method for Latina/os to access screening and prevention related to stigmatized diseases, such as HIV infection. Despite scant research in this area, there is evidence for reduced HIV stigma among Latina/os (Bogart et al., 2015; Derose et al., 2016) and increased HIV screening through faith-based interventions (Bogart et al., 2015; Williams et al., 2016). The familiarity of faith-based organizations may provide a safe place for high-risk communities to access these services.

The stigma associated with HIV and screening behaviors for HIV presents a significant barrier to secondary prevention of HIV. One church-based intervention with six churches, including a large Latina/o Roman Catholic Church and a pair of small Latina/o Pentecostal churches, aims to reduce stigma and promote HIV testing among Latina/os and African Americans (Derose et al., 2016). The intervention includes HIV education workshops to increase HIV awareness and knowledge, peer leader workshops for participants to develop skills for discussion stigma with others through role-play, an HIV sermon/imagined contact scenario where a priest or pastor deliver a sermon, and a congregation-based HIV testing event where rapid oral fluid testing is provided through a mobile clinic. Surveys are collected at baseline and six-month follow up to collect data on HIV stigma (e.g., discomfort, shame, blame and rejection), HIV-related mistrust, HIV testing during the study, and demographic data. Findings indicate significant reductions in HIV stigma and HIV mistrust within the Latina/o Catholic intervention church and Latina/o Pentecostal intervention church from baseline to follow-up. The Latina/o Pentecostal intervention church demonstrates higher HIV testing during follow-up as compared with the Latina/o Pentecostal control church. Although statistically significant reductions exist within the Latina/o intervention churches, these same findings are not observed in the African American intervention churches. Derose et al. (2016) note that they are underpowered to detect significant differences and significant differences in the Latina/o churches are surprising.

Faith-Based Interventions for Cardiovascular Disease

Despite the disproportionate burden of cardiovascular disease (CVD) on Latina/os, there are relatively few faith-based interventions targeting CVD among Latina/o populations. Most faith-based initiatives that target CVD prevention often focus on African American communities (Lancaster et al., 2014). However, one of the few programs that targets Latina/os, is the American Heart Association (AHA) *Search Your Heart Program* (Kalenderian et al., 2009). The program includes a network of ambassadors for Latina/o churches that serve as liaisons to educate congregants about cardiovascular diseases and stroke. After receiving training through the AHA, ambassadors educate their congregation on topics related to cardiovascular disease. Ambassadors also administer a survey to their congregations to collect data on CVD knowledge, stroke risk factors, self-efficacy and behavior, diet, physical activity, tobacco use, and physician visits. After the intervention, 78% of participants recognize all five warning signs of stroke; however, less than half speak with their physicians about heart disease and stroke risk factors. These findings are similar to those of another study among Latinas that uses a four-month community-based bilingual preventive cardiovascular education program (Altman, Nunez de Ybarra, & Villablanca, 2014). Upon the completion of the intervention, participants report significant improvements in symptom knowledge and risk factors for CVD and engagement in heart healthy behaviors.

Faith-Based Interventions for Diabetes

Diabetes prevention and self-management are two concerns among Latina/os. Faith-based interventions in Latina/o churches can help to prevent diabetes (Gutierrez et al., 2014; He et al., 2013) and promote diabetes self-management (Baig et al., 2014). The Fine, Fit and Fabulous program is a 12-week faith-based diabetes prevention program that aims to increase nutrition knowledge and increase physical activity among African American and Latina/o congregants in New York City (Gutierrez et al., 2014). Gutierrez and colleagues originally developed the curriculum for African American churches but subsequently made cultural and linguistic adaptations to the curriculum for use with Latina/o churches. The curriculum includes dietary information, cooking classes, and an emphasis on the association between spirituality and health behaviors. Interestingly, there are stark differences in health insurance coverage among participants, as only 28% of Latina/o participants have health insurance, as compared with 80% of African American participants.

Over the 12 weeks, participants lost an average of four pounds or 2% of their body weight. Most Latina/os are motivated by a desire to become healthy and feel better (98.5%), followed by religious or spiritual beliefs about healthy living (92.4%). Latina/o participants significantly increased their knowledge about their daily dietary intake and how to judge portion sizes. Significantly more Latina/os report exercising in the past 30 days, eating fruit daily, drinking plenty of water, and reading food labels when shopping, from baseline to follow-up (Gutierrez et al., 2014).

SCHOOL HEALTH SERVICES FOR LATINA/OS

Schools provide a wealth of resources and are geographically located within the neighborhoods they serve. For these reasons, school-based programs can circumvent common barriers among Latina/o parents who participate in these programs (Garcia-Dominic et al., 2010). Schools can also take advantage of having a captive audience of students and the potential to engage parents in health promotion. School-based programs that are culturally tailored and provided in the child and family's preferred language demonstrate greater efficacy than programs without these cultural and linguistic considerations (Kreuter et al., 2003).

School-Based Health Centers

While school-based health centers are not unique to the Latina/o community, their emergence can significantly help improve access to health services among Latina/os, including primary and secondary prevention services. School-based health centers can provide basic services, such as primary medical care, dental/oral health care, health education and promotion, and nutrition education (U.S. Department of Health & Human Services, 2011a). These services are often provided as a partnership between schools and community health care centers. Over 2,000 school-based health centers currently exist and can help eliminate disparities in access to health care among Latina/o children and their families.

Research suggests that school-based health centers can reach students who might otherwise not have access to health care. Additionally, they can reduce health disparities between Latina/o and White/European American students. For instance, a study of 414 adolescent school-based health center users suggests that students who do not have health insurance are more likely to report that the school-based health center is their only usual source of care (Parasuraman & Shi, 2015). Additionally, overweight adolescents are 2.34 times more likely to identify the school-based health center as their only usual source of care and are almost twice as likely to report that the school-based health center is their usual source for sick care.

Evaluations of school-based health centers are not without their limitations. For example, there are challenges evaluating the impact of school-based health because of selection bias, maturational and historical effects, and clustering effects (Bersamin et al., 2016). Students who utilize school-based health centers can significantly differ from their peers who do not utilize school-based health centers. Maturation and historical effects are not traditionally controlled in observational studies that examine the impact of school-based health centers on health outcomes. Finally, clustering effects potentially impact results, as students are enrolled in schools by geographic boundaries and most likely share traits that are tangentially related to their geographic location, socioeconomic status, etc.

School-Based Health Centers and HPV

One area in which school-based health centers can positively impact health behaviors is immunization delivery. For example, completion of immunization against human papillomavirus (HPV) is lower among Latina/os as compared with their White/European American counterparts. In a study of retrospective immunization delivery among adolescents, Federico et al. (2010) examined immunization registries through either a school-based health center or a community health center. Both centers serve a large urban population that is primarily Latina/o and many patients do not speak English. Findings indicate that completion rates are significantly higher for adolescents who use school-based health centers across a number of immunizations, including hepatitis B and HPV. These findings highlight important implications for increased access and immunization delivery for Latina/o adolescents. For example, school-based health centers help decrease access barriers in the delivery of immunizations, as they deliver free immunizations in a safe setting and target medically underserved youth (Federico et al., 2010).

School-Based Health and Obesity

Several school-based health programs attempt to address the prevalent issue of childhood obesity among Latina/o children. A review of school-based studies that focuses on obesity prevention in schools with at least 50% Latina/o participants demonstrates mixed findings and the need for increased evaluative rigor (Holub et al., 2014). The review aims to examine the effects of evidence-based research of obesity-related interventions on Latina/o children in U.S. schools. Holub et al. (2014) indicate that of the 15 U.S. studies, 13 solely focus on children whereas two focus on both parents and children. Five of the studies include both a school-based and a community-based component. Out of the 15 studies, 11 focus on prevention and 13 focus on both physical activity and nutrition, while the other two studies exclusively focus on physical activity. These studies demonstrate mixed results regarding their impact on obesity outcomes. Only three studies report statistically significant reductions in obesity-related outcomes compared to control groups. Effect sizes also range considerably but are seldom reported in most studies, and consequently make it difficult to compare results across studies. While these interventions include large Latina/o enrollments and in many cases specifically target Latina/os, only four studies include some aspect of cultural tailoring.

FAMILY-BASED INTERVENTIONS FOR LATINA/O HEALTH

The importance of family in Latina/o culture provides another unique opportunity for health promotion through the family unit. In recent years, several culturally tailored family-based studies have emerged for the Latina/o community. Families are often the main source of social support, especially among Latina/os and new immigrants who may not have established other social ties (Elder et al., 2009). This makes family-based studies ideal for addressing health disparities among Latina/o populations.

Parent engagement is an important factor when considering any early childhood intervention. A systematic review of interventions for obesity prevention in early care and education settings examined studies published between 2010 and 2015 (Ward et al., 2016). The authors conclude that components of parent engagement add to the effectiveness of the reviewed early care and education interventions. At least one significant anthropometric measure is correlated with interventions when parent engagement is included. Parent engagement is not correlated with obesity prevention outcomes when simultaneously examining all anthropometric measures. However, Ward et al. (2016) hypothesize that these studies are not adequately powered to detect changes across multiple outcomes. One important consideration from this review is that of the 43 interventions included in the review, only 9 are identified as strong quality, 14 are moderate, and 20 are weak based on the study's selection, design, potential for bias, and analytic methods. This once again underscores the need for more rigorous evaluations.

Family-Based Interventions for Obesity Prevention

One intervention, *Active and Healthy Families*, is a randomized controlled trial targeting obesity among Latina/o children through group medical appointments. The intervention lasts 10 weeks and targets parent–child dyads (Falbe et al., 2015). Primary care physicians from two federally qualified health centers refer parents and children to the program. *Promotoras* follow up with parents by telephone to assess interest and prescreen interested candidates. The program includes five 2-hour group medical appointments every other week for 10 weeks in the families' medical home. A registered dietitian, physician, and *promotora* lead all sessions. The content focuses on expert recommendations to promote healthy growth and reduce obesogenic behaviors, such as the consumption of sugar-sweetened beverages and excessive screen time. The program successfully reduces body mass index over a 10-week period among children who participate in the *Active and Healthy Families* intervention (Falbe et al., 2015).

Another successful family-based intervention worth noting is the *Entre Familia—Reflejos de Salud* study. This intervention combines a unique entertainment-education component with a *promotora* model to improve the dietary behaviors of families of predominantly Mexican origin. The family-based intervention includes a nine-part, Spanish-language, sitcom-style DVD series. The series includes 12-minute storyline episodes that follow a Mexican family who seeks to improve their eating habits. Families are also provided with a manual to supplement the DVDs. The manual includes homework in the form of goal setting and self-monitoring forms. Finally, an interpersonal intervention includes *promotora* home visits and telephone calls. The intervention has high attendance and low attrition.

Family-based approaches are efficacious when disseminated through Head Start centers. For instance, *The ¡Miranos! Program* family-based component is part of a larger quasi-experimental study that includes both center- and family-based activities (Yin et al., 2012). Family-based activities include parent education sessions, bilingual newsletters, and take-home bags. Parent peer educators, recruited through centers, offered biweekly parent education sessions. The parent education sessions circumvent traditional issues for parents who attend educational sessions (e.g., transportation, child care) by offering the sessions at the conclusion of the school day when parents arrive to pick up their children. Teachers volunteer to watch children in their classrooms until parents complete their short session. Head Start centers provide bilingual newsletters to parents that include information on healthy growth promotion for their children. Finally, when parents attend an educational session, they receive a take-home bag for their children. The bag includes an age-appropriate activity that promotes a shared physical activity for parents and their children. The take-home bag also includes a children's book that reinforces lessons about nutrition and physical activity. The parent educational sessions have high attendance, with approximately 80% of parents attending. Parents in the family-based intervention recall more key messages regarding healthy growth for their children than parents in the control group. Finally, children in the centers with the family-based intervention have better gross motor development than children in centers with only center-based activities.

PROMOTORA INTERVENTIONS FOR LATINA/O HEALTH

Promotores de salud (community health workers) who work within the Latina/o community can include both Latina/o men and women. Female community health workers are commonly known as *promotoras*, while male community health workers are commonly known *promotores*. However, in Spanish *promotores* also connotes mixed gender or plural community health workers (Ayala et al., 2010). Because most work in this area uses the term *promotora*, we also use this term to describe these community health workers. *Promotora* projects use a train-the-trainer approach, whereby interventionists train *promotoras* to disseminate information and skill sets to the community. *Promotoras* help improve clinical outcomes and cost savings (WestRasmus, Pineda-Reyes, Tamez, & Westfall, 2012). For example, *promotoras* motivate families to increase their heart-healthy behaviors and reduce their CVD risk behaviors (Balcazar et al., 2006). *Promotoras* also deliver diabetes education programs to significantly reduce A1C levels among Mexican Americans with diabetes (Lujan, Ostwald, & Ortiz, 2007).

The success of *promotoras* is attributed to their personal credibility as community members since they reside within the same communities where researchers and interventionists hope to work. *Promotoras* also share the same language, culture, and values of program participants and are also experts on their local community (WestRasmus et al., 2012). Their expertise can assist program developers ensure that interventions are informed and tailored to the needs of the local community. Their impact has been recognized such that the task force on the Health and Human Services Action Plan to Reduce Racial and Ethnic Health Disparities recommends the increased use of *promotores* to promote participation in health education, behavioral health education, prevention, health insurance programs, and to reduce disparities among racial and ethnic minority groups (U.S. Department of Health & Human Services, 2011b).

Despite the potential benefits of *promotora* models, there are limitations within this body of research. First, there is considerable heterogeneity in the manner in which *promotora* programs are implemented. Some programs employ *promotoras* to recruit participants and deliver diabetes intervention programs (McCloskey, 2009), whereas others task *promotoras* to link community members with other health care providers or provide direct services such as immunizations; well child and woman care; and blood pressure, diabetes, and cholesterol screening and management (WestRasmus et al., 2012). Second, and perhaps more problematic, is the lack of information and detail provided in many studies regarding the specific role of *promotoras* in their interventions (Swider, 2002). This is critical because the educator-only role differs from the educator-bridge role, as the latter requires the provision of direct health information, as well as emotional and instrumental support. Moreover, these distinct roles potentially differ in their efficacy in reaching health outcomes (Ayala et al., 2010). Third, the types of *promotora* roles appear to differ geographically, as a larger number of *promotoras* serve as bridges to health care in Northeastern regions. Finally, a review of *promotora* studies suggests that only 5 of the 61 studies reviewed appear to target a Latina/o heritage group other than those of Mexican descent (Ayala et al., 2010).

Promotora Interventions for Nutrition

To address the issue of poor nutrition, de Heer and colleagues (2015) developed an intervention based on the Centers for Disease Control and Prevention's best practices. The four-month intervention is facilitated by *promotoras* who assist with the use of parks and recreational facilities and lead cooking classes, grocery store tours, and coffee talks for Latina/os (Mexican Americans) who reside along the U.S.-Mexico border to promote heart-healthy nutrition practices. Each weekly session includes four to five structured activities and at least one activity specifically focuses on nutrition.

Intervention evaluations include clinical measurements that are taken at baseline and postintervention, including height, weight, waist and hip circumference, and blood pressure (de Heer et al., 2015). Spanish and English questionnaires also collect data on health habits. Results suggest that participants significantly improve their health behaviors from baseline to postintervention. For example, whereas only 33.3% consume at least five daily servings of fruits and vegetables at baseline, 67.4% of participants consume this recommended amount after the intervention ($p<0.001$). There are also improvements in weight, waist and hip circumference, and CVD risk scores. Findings also indicate that greater attendance of program activities is key to the intervention's success (de Heer et al., 2015).

Promotora Interventions to Address Cardiovascular Disease and Hypertension

Given the sociocultural roles of risk factors related to cardiovascular diseases, a culturally relevant and tailored approach, such as the *promotora* model is warranted for the Latina/o community (Rodriguez et al., 2014). One such program that utilizes the *promotora* approach to address control of risk factors associated with hypertension is the *Promotoras de Salud Contra La Hipertension* Program (Balcazar et al., 2009). The program is based on the *Salud Para Su Corazon* promotora program, an effective community outreach model implemented in the U.S.-Mexico border (Balcazar et al., 2006). A community-based participatory research approach also informs the project. The participatory research includes holding community forums, collaboratively developing a community plan with the *promotoras*, conducting focus groups, implementing a community survey, pilot testing the curriculum, implementing a train-the trainer approach, and implementing a pilot program.

Promotoras de Salud Contra La Hipertension includes a nine-week *promotora*-led intervention (Balcazar et al., 2009). All intervention materials are available in Spanish. *Promotoras* are instrumental throughout the project, as they help develop the community plan, and evaluate the survey. During implementation, *promotoras* work in pairs to deliver the intervention. Sessions last approximately two hours. A total of 98 participants enrolled in the study—50 are assigned to the intervention group and 48 are assigned to the control group. Results suggest significantly greater reduced intake of sodium, cholesterol and fat from baseline to follow up among the intervention group compared to the control groups. In addition, perceived benefits significantly differ between the intervention and control group from baseline to follow-up. However, no clinical variables significantly differ between the intervention and control groups after controlling for confounding variables. The authors attribute the lack of significant differences in clinical outcomes to the study's short duration.

Promotora Interventions for Diabetes

Several *promotora* interventions focus on diabetes prevention among Latina/os (Babamoto et al., 2009; Prezio et al., 2013; Spencer et al., 2011).

One example of a *promotora*-led program is the *Promotora-Led Diabetes Prevention Program* (PL-DPP) (O'Brien et al., 2015). The program is a culturally tailored translation of the Diabetes Prevention Program (DPP), the gold standard for evidence-based interventions targeting type 2 diabetes. The DPP is a clinical trial that uses an intensive lifestyle intervention to target an increase in moderate physical activity and modest weight loss to reduce the development of type 2 diabetes among individuals with prediabetes by 58%. This surpasses the effectiveness of a comparison group that uses metformin. Given the potential impact of *promotoras* to improve health outcomes among Latina/o populations, O'Brien et al. (2015) culturally adapted the DPP lifestyle program and delivered PL-DPP through *promotoras*. The pilot trial includes one intervention arm. Measurements are collected before the intervention and after 12 months. Latina/o-serving nonprofit organizations recruit interested Latinas who are asked to complete the American Diabetes Association's 7-item Diabetes Risk Assessment Questionnaire. Latinas with scores of 5 or greater are asked to take part in fasting lab work. To be eligible for participation, Latinas must be fluent in Spanish, at least 20 years of age, and have a body mass index of 25 (calculated as the weight in kilograms divided by the square of the height in meters) or higher.

The participants' two main goals include weight reduction (7%) from baseline to postintervention and performing 150 minutes per week of moderate physical activity. The program lasts for one year and begins with weekly sessions for the first 12 weeks, then 10 sessions are offered biweekly, and final sessions are offered monthly. The PL-DPP program is culturally adapted for Latina/os and offers all materials in Spanish, incorporates Latina/o family context into messages, adds two additional sessions to better explain dietary recommendations and self-management, and uses culturally appropriate tools for dietary self-monitoring. All sessions are delivered in Spanish. From baseline to 12 months, participants lost an average of 10.8 pounds. A total of 42% achieved their 7% weight loss goal and approximately 58% achieved at least a 5% weight loss. Participants also report reduced waist circumference, diastolic blood pressure, low-density lipoprotein (LDL) cholesterol, and fasting insulin levels. However, while outcomes do not surpass the original DPP study, the delivery by *promotoras* increases the potential sustainability and scalability of the program.

COMMUNITY-BASED PARTICIPATORY APPROACHES FOR LATINA/O COMMUNITIES

Many research studies that target Latina/os, regardless of setting, use a community-based participatory research approach. Community-based participatory research is highly accepted as a method to address health disparities in underserved communities (Minkler, Blackwell, Thompson, & Tamir, 2003). Community-based participatory research engages the community as an active partner in the research process to identify health needs, develop solutions, and evaluate outcomes. Among certain studies, this involves partnering with *promotoras* to garner community expertise, whereas in other studies church leaders provide the expertise (Allen et al., 2014).

One example of a community-based participatory approach to address health disparities using a faith-based initiative is the *Bronx Health REACH faith-based initiative* (Kaplan et al., 2009). The community-based approach began with the formation of a community advisory group and community research committee from within the group. Members of the community research committee included members of the community who were previously involved in the larger REACH coalition. Members who no longer resided in the community had the opportunity to continue their participation. The community research committee began by reflecting on the importance of evaluation and research to ensure that committee members perceived their evaluative role as meaningful and important. The community research committee hosted five large focus groups with church members to assess program effectiveness and replication. During the focus groups, researchers gained increased insight regarding important issues. For example, their initial enrollment of predominantly Latina/o churches was low. They learned during the focus groups that the low participation of Latina/o churches in part was due to language barriers. At one large church, only the coordinator felt comfortable to attend a meeting in English; when he was no longer able to attend, the church discontinued its participation. Focus groups also assessed the acceptability of the program's key messages. Finally, the community research committee helped develop and administer a survey to the congregation members.

CULTURAL TAILORING FOR LATINA/O COMMUNITIES

There has been a push in recent years to culturally tailor programs for their intended communities. This push is partly due to the increased recognition that culturally tailored programs are effective for target communities as compared with programs that are not culturally tailored (Resnicow, Baranowski, Ahluwalia, & Braithwaite, 1998). Whereas many studies include a statement that the program is culturally tailored to the Latina/o community or to a specific Latina/o heritage group (e.g., Mexican), these studies rarely provide a specific description that outlines their process for cultural tailoring. Kreuter and colleagues (2003), however, outline five common strategies used for enhancing cultural appropriateness—peripheral, evidential, linguistic, constituent-involving, and sociocultural. Many programs use more than one of these strategies, and they are not necessarily exclusive of each other. Next, we describe each strategy and highlight a few aforementioned studies that align with this strategic approach.

Peripheral strategies are characterized by program materials that use colors, images, fonts, pictures of group members or titles indicating that they are designed for the target group (Kreuter et al., 2003). These types of strategies are peripheral because they do not actually reflect a change in the content delivered but instead reflect surface-level changes that make the target group more receptive and accepting of the information. Studies that utilize these types of strategies include many of the aforementioned studies that use Spanish words in their program title (Balcazar et al., 2006; de Heer et al., 2015; Lujan et al., 2007; Sosa et al., 2016). Although this may resemble a linguistic strategy, which we later discuss, the use of Spanish titles clearly illustrate how target groups include Spanish-speaking communities or individuals descended from Spanish-speaking countries.

Evidential strategies provide evidence of the health problems' relevance to the target group through the use of epidemiological data or some other form of evidence (Kreuter et al., 2003). For example, a study focusing on cardiovascular health might present data on how Latina/os are at higher risk for cardiovascular diseases. These types of strategies help the target population to identify with the information. Most studies insufficiently describe their intervention content to discern whether this strategy is utilized within their interventions.

Linguistic strategies provide the information in the target group's language (Kreuter et al., 2003). Almost all studies that culturally tailored their approaches for the Latina/o community provide information in Spanish or in both English and Spanish. One study that includes a large number of Latina/os but does not use a linguistic strategy is the *Bronx Health REACH faith-based initiative* (Kaplan et al., 2009). The authors identify the lack of available Spanish materials and resources as a major limitation in their success with Latina/o churches. Although linguistic strategies are common in culturally tailored programs for Latina/o communities, their sole use is insufficient. Also, program developers should consider maintenance of the meaning of the message rather than simply direct translation.

Constituent-involving strategies include those that recruit members of the target community as active participants in the research process (U.S. Department of Health & Human Services, 2011b). These strategies are most commonly observed within *promotora* projects (Ayala et al., 2010; Elder et al., 2009; Nuno, Martinez, Harris, & Garcia, 2011; Prezio et al., 2013; Spencer et al., 2011). When *promotoras* are actively involved in the research process, they can inform all research aspects. As previously mentioned, the level of involvement of *promotoras* varies across studies (Ayala et al., 2010). However, there is evidence that *promotoras* appreciate learning and understanding the research process, and future training programs should incorporate a research training aspect (Otiniano, Carroll-Scott, Toy, & Wallace, 2012).

Sociocultural strategies present health-related information within broader social and cultural values (Lujan et al., 2007). These types of programs are designed within the context of the target group's shared beliefs and values. Several culturally tailored programs appear to focus on the value of religiosity (Allen et al., 2012, 2014; DeHaven et al., 2004; He et al., 2013; Sauaia et al., 2007). These faith-based programs do not simply present the information within their faith-based organization settings. These programs incorporate health messages into a religious context and identify values that are central to both the religion and desired health behaviors.

Before offering a program to the Latina/o community, program developers should consider the use of these questions to assess additional opportunities to ensure their programs are culturally tailored:

- Are there additional ways to incorporate peripheral strategies?
  - Do program materials contain pictures of Latina/os?
  - Do these pictures reflect the diversity of Latina/os (i.e., various countries of origin)?
  - Is it possible to provide a Spanish title or otherwise connect with Latina/o cultures (e.g., program's name reflects familiar characteristics)?
  - Are the colors that are associated with Latina/o culture used throughout?
- Are there additional ways to incorporate evidential strategies?
  - Are the messages about health risk specific to the Latina/o community?
  - Is the information provided about Latina/os and their health risks specific to their heritage group (e.g., Cuban American, Mexican American)?
  - Is the information provided about Latina/o health placed in context of other race/ethnic groups so it is apparent if Latina/os are at higher risk for the health outcome?
- Are there additional opportunities to incorporate linguistic strategies?
  - Are all materials available in English and Spanish?
  - When both English and Spanish are used, are materials provided in large fonts to ensure their legibility?
  - Are all materials field tested and checked with members of local communities to ensure the terminology and phrasing is appropriate and understood as intended for the Latina/o target community?
- Are there additional opportunities to incorporate constituent-involving strategies?
  - Are constituents involved in all aspects of program development, implementation and evaluation? If not, is it possible to involve these constituents?

- Is it possible to increase engagement among constituents (e.g., increase opportunities for feedback prior to implementing changes, leadership roles, and increased cross-training)?
- Are there additional opportunities to incorporate sociocultural strategies?
  - Is there a way to clearly connect program goals with Latina/o values?
  - Are there other issues important to Latina/os that can be incorporated into the program?

CONCLUSION

Multiple partners across sectors are necessary to address the multifactorial health issues of Latina/os. Beyond health issues, collaborative partnerships can address social issues and other issues that impact Latina/o communities. A number of programs and community efforts have emerged to address the needs of Latina/o communities. However, there are significant gaps within the existing literature. For example, there are a limited number of programs that target Latina/o heritage groups other than those of Mexican descent. Additional research is needed to translate programs for use with other Latina/o heritage groups and assess program effectiveness in varied settings. Translation of programs can help identify and address the unique barriers, values, and needs of each Latina/o heritage group. Secondly, current interventions are not extensively evaluated. Evaluation research is limited especially for newer intervention types that aim to use innovative approaches to address Latina/o health. As rigorous evaluations are conducted, including longer follow-up assessments, a stronger body of research can support the effectiveness of Latina/o-focused interventions. Finally, there is a significant need for assessment measures that are developed and validated for use with Latina/o populations. One should not assume that assessments that provide reliable and valid data in White/European Americans populations are appropriate for Latina/os. Program developers and researchers are tasked to develop psychometrically sound assessments for use with Latina/os. Spanish materials that are direct translations from English are often inappropriate, as they lack linguistic and cultural relevance.

Chapter 5

Nontraditional Health Practices

Latina/o communities exhibit higher rates of obesity, diabetes, human immunodeficiency virus (HIV) infection, and some cancers, yet they experience lower access to health care (see Chapter 3). However, many Latina/os access treatments and care outside of the traditional health care system. It is important to understand the worldviews and health practices of Latina/os, as they also shape their receptivity to traditional health practices. Although the health practices of Latina/os are not uniform, many are accustomed to nontraditional health practices and demonstrate greater dissatisfaction with the bureaucratic and costly American health care system. The loss of confidence in physicians (Martinez, 2009) and the need for cultural empathy (Lopez, 2005) may lead to the increased use of complementary and alternative medicine. Thus, when health practitioners understand the roles that nontraditional health practices play in Latina/o health and subsequently demonstrate respect for these practices, they can increase their communication with Latina/o patients, develop trust, and increase the likelihood that their Latina/o patients will self-disclose their use of nontraditional practices. Doing so will increase the likelihood that health providers will provide culturally competent assessments, diagnoses, and medical treatments.

A common theme throughout Latina/o cultures is a holistic perspective on health, where spirituality and physical and mental/emotional health are equally important and intertwined (Avila & Parker, 2000). Illness may result from natural and emotional causes, as well as spiritual or supernatural causes. This is in contrast to Western medicine, which separates physical health from mental and emotional health, and this inconsistency in perceptions is a barrier to care among some Latina/os (Morales, Lara, Kington, Valdez, & Escarce, 2002). Additionally, Western medicine does not address many folk illnesses commonly recognized among Latina/o communities. These folk illnesses, also known as culture-bound syndromes or idioms of distress, include *ataque de nervios* (nervous attack), *susto* (fright), *mal de ojo* (evil eye), *mal aire* (bad air), *embrujo* or *mal puesto* (supernatural hex), *espanto* (extreme fright), *caída de mollera* (sunken fontanelle in infants), *empacho* (blocked intestine), *envidia* (envy), *hechizo/bilongo* (Hex or spell), *bilis* (anger/rage), *matris caida* (fallen womb), *aire del oido* (air in the ear), *pasmo* (frozen face) and *fatiga* (fatigue; Bauer & Guerra, 2014; Jones & Hernandez, 2009; Lopez, 2005; Murguía, Peterson, & Zea, 2003; Titus, 2014). For example, *caída de mollera* occurs among infants because of inefficient sucking and quickly removing an infant from the nipple during breastfeeding. Symptoms may include vomiting, colic, diarrhea, failure to suck, and/or sunken eyes. Although treatment may vary, the overall goal is to restore the infant's fontanelle. It is noteworthy that Western practitioners often treat *caída de mollera* with rehydration methods, while *curandera/os* may apply warm and soapy water over the fontanel and press the infant's palate with their finger (Titus, 2014, p. 197).

Unfortunately, health practitioners do not always demonstrate positive attitudes toward healing systems that help their Latina/o patients address physical, spiritual, or mental ailments (Muñoz, Servin, Kozo, Lam, & Zuñiga, 2013). These systems can include the use of indigenous healers such as *espiritistas, curandera/os, santera/os, yierbera/os,* and *partera/os* (see Chapter 9), religious or spiritual practices, *remedios* (herbal remedies) that include various types of herbs/plants that are ingested in various ways, such as tablets, capsules, as well as raw or cooked herbs and plants (Amirehsani & Wallace, 2013). Drinks can also include *tés* (teas), *licuados* (smoothie-like mixture of natural products), *aguas frescas* (cold drinks that are often prepared with an herb; Amirehsani & Wallace, 2013), or *botellas* (bottled plant mixtures; Vandebroek et al., 2010).

Therefore, it is vital for health practitioners to become knowledgeable about the nontraditional practices of their Latina/o patients and to also demonstrate respect for their diverse worldviews. Unfortunately, research indicates that Latina/o patients seldom disclose their use of herbal remedies to health care providers (Amirehsani & Wallace, 2013; Murguía et al., 2003). Failure to demonstrate respect will most likely result in the lack of self-disclosure regarding nontraditional practices as well as concealment of contraband medications, as Latina/os may fear ridicule from their heath practitioners (Lopez, 2005; Murguía et al., 2003; Titus, 2014). Furthermore, disrespect and disinterest among health providers may contribute to poor patient compliance and poor use of community medical services (Murguía et al., 2003).

This chapter will explore the various nontraditional health practices utilized by Latina/os. Although there is scant research regarding nontraditional health practices among Latina/o heritage groups, when available, these data are presented. We provide a brief history of common nontraditional health practices, such as complementary and alternative medicines and the use of indigenous healers, such as *curandera/os* and *sobadores*. Finally, we present implications for practice among health professionals who seek to work with the Latina/o community.

NONTRADITIONAL MEDICINES (COMPLEMENTARY AND ALTERNATIVE MEDICINES)

Complementary and alternative medicine (CAM) use among Latina/o populations is relatively common. The National Center for Complementary and Integrative Health (2011) defines complementary medicine as a group of diverse medical health care systems, practices, and products that are not presently considered a part of Western medicine, such as natural products (e.g., vitamins, minerals, herbs) and mind and body practices (e.g., deep breathing, meditation, acupuncture, yoga). Research suggests at least 25% of Latina/os use some form of traditional, complementary, or alternative medicine (Ortiz, Shields, Clauson, & Clay, 2007). For example, data from the National Health Interview Survey indicate that Latina/os are the second largest ethnic group, following Black/African Americans, to report CAM use, with a prevalence of 24% (Barnes et al., 2004). However, a smaller study that oversampled ethnic minority groups indicates that CAM use is equally prevalent among all ethnic groups with a prevalence of 41% among Latina/os (Mackenzie et al., 2003). CAM use varies by region among Latina/os. For example, as many as 77% of Mexican Americans living along the Mexico-Texas border report CAM use within the past year (Rivera et al., 2002) compared with 55% of primarily Mexican American participants in St. Louis (Grafford, Nieto, & Santanello, 2016).

Understanding the types of CAM methods is also important to address the needs of the Latina/o community. A cross-sectional study conducted in California surveyed Latina/o patients from a local family health center and their CAM use and treatments prescribed by their doctors (Ho et al., 2015). Of the 150 patients, 63% of patients report using at least one CAM method in the past year, and their CAM use is often for weight loss. The most frequent CAM practices include the use of vitamins/supplements (32%), followed by herbal medicine (29%), dietary/nutritional therapy (26%), and massage (24%). Fewer patients appear to use yoga (11%), acupuncture (11%), and energy healing (3%). Latina/o patients also express an interest in other specialized CAM therapies that are associated with diet and lifestyle improvements, including massage, mind–body relaxation techniques, and acupuncture.

Most research regarding CAM use among Latina/os largely focuses on Mexicans or Mexican Americans. However, data from the 2007 National Health Interview Survey suggest that 23.7% of Latina/os use CAM and that there are differences in CAM use among Latina/o heritage groups (Barnes, Bloom, & Nahin, 2008). For instance, Puerto Ricans (29.7%), Dominicans (28.2%), Mexican Americans (27.4%), and Central and South Americans (23.4%) report greater CAM use than their Cuban or Cuban American (22.9%) and Mexican (18.2%) counterparts. Findings also indicate differences in type of modality, as Latina/os report greater use of biologically based therapies (11.8%), and mind–body therapies (10.8%), as well as lower use of manipulative and body-based therapies (6.7%) and alternative medical systems (3%). Latina/o heritage groups also differ in their use of modality type; Dominicans (18.5%) and Puerto Ricans (16.8%) report greater use of mind–body therapies, while Puerto Ricans (14.2%) and Mexicans (14.0%) report greater use of biologically based therapies. However, Cubans (8.5%) and Mexican Americans (7.9%) report greater use of manipulative and body-based therapies (Barnes et al., 2008)

A descriptive study of ethnomedical approaches (i.e., spiritual and folk healers, and home remedies) and illness among Central American immigrants from a community clinic in the District of Columbia (Murguía et al., 2003) suggests that 83% use remedies and 46% use a combination of folk and spiritual healers and remedies. Interestingly, 23% use a combination of folk and spiritual healers, and physicians for medical conditions. Central American immigrants also use folk remedies more frequently than attending medical visits with their health care providers to treat medical conditions such as arthritis, asthma, migraines, and ulcers.

It is also common for parents to use CAM for their children. The underlying factors that contribute to CAM use among parents for their children appear to differ by ethnicity and language. Whereas some research suggests non-Latina/o White adults use CAM more than do Latina/o adults (43% vs. 24%; Barnes et al., 2008), less is known regarding trends in CAM use among parents of different ethnicities. Nonetheless, Fortier et al. (2014) examined the independent and collective role of ethnicity and language on mothers' CAM use for their children. Participants self-identified as either Spanish-speaking Latinas, English-speaking Latinas, or English-speaking non-Latina White mothers (Fortier et al., 2014). They examined 27 different methods of CAM use, such as acupressure, deep breathing exercises, diet-based therapies, and homoeopathy. Additionally, participants completed the Holistic and Complementary and Alternative Medicine Questionnaire to report their holistic health beliefs and beliefs regarding the benefits, safety, and risks of using complementary and alternative medicines.

Fortier et al. (2014) found that of the 206 participants, all mothers reported high CAM use regardless of ethnicity and language, as 98% of English-speaking White mothers, 92% of English-speaking Latina mothers, and 75% of Spanish-speaking Latina mothers use at least one form of CAM. Spanish-speaking Latina mothers use massage, deep breathing, herbology, chiropractic techniques, relaxation, aromatherapy, meditation, yoga, guided imagery, and megavitamins significantly less often than English-speaking White mothers. English-speaking Latina mothers report greater use of exercise and prayer than English-speaking White and Spanish-speaking Latina mothers.

Acute conditions in children may also increase their use of CAM. In a literature review, Evans, Tsao, and Zelter (2008) examined parental use of CAM to address acute pain in children, including studies that address CAM and studies without Latina/o participants. Although systematic literature review procedures are followed, the review provides some insights into contexts in which parents currently use CAM. Interventions studies report varying evidence of effectiveness for different methods such as hypnosis, music therapy, acupuncture, massage, and humor therapy. The effects of hypnosis differ by ailment and age group, with less effective results with younger children. Music therapy demonstrates some evidence of effectiveness, but further research is needed, particularly with randomized controlled trials. Intervention studies that are based on other methods—acupuncture, massage, and humor therapy—appear to show extremely limited evidence of effectiveness.

Complementary and Alternative Medicine Use among Latina/os with HIV

CAM use is also observed among HIV Latina/os who reside along the US-Mexico border. This research indicates that Latina/os frequently access clinical care and medication within the United States and Mexico (Muñoz et al., 2013; Shedlin et al., 2013) and they seldom report their CAM use to their health providers. For example, Rivera et al. (2005) examined CAM use among 35 HIV-positive and 439 non-HIV-positive Mexican American patients from El Paso, Texas and Las Cruces, New Mexico. Seventy-one percent use herbal products, primarily *manzanilla* (chamomile), *flor de Jamaica* (hibiscus), as well as the use of *ajo* (garlic). While most Latina/os without HIV purchase their herbal products in the United States, most

HIV-positive Latina/os (56%) cross the border and purchase products in Mexico. Also, friends and relatives are the most common source of advice regarding CAM treatments (Rivera et al., 2005). Lamentably, most Latina/os do not disclose their CAM use to their health providers because they fear being judged and their providers seldom inquire about their CAM use. However, these herbal products cause potential clinical interactions with their ARV treatment and necessitate that providers establish a positive relationship with their patients and encourage open discussions regarding their CAM use, particularly their use of herbs and over the counter products.

Shedlin et al. (2013) also examined CAM use among 113 HIV-positive Latina/os who also reside in El Paso, Texas. Their qualitative findings indicate that Latina/os report CAM use to support general health and their immune systems and to address symptoms of HIV-related diseases and antiretroviral (ARV) side effects. However, while CAM appears to complement ARV treatment, their CAM use is seldom reported to health care providers due to concerns regarding disapproval and loss of care privileges. While they regard their health care providers and biomedicine as legitimate resources, Latina/os may relinquish their physician's warnings regarding specific practices or remedies if they perceive that a particular herb works in a certain manner.

Shedlin et al.'s (2013) findings underscore how HIV-positive Latina/os do not disclose their use of CAM to their health providers. In a binational comparison of 19 HIV providers from the San Diego, CA region, Muñoz et al. (2013) indicate that providers from both San Diego, and Tijuana, Mexico report that their patients seldom disclose their CAM use and almost half do not routinely ask about CAM practices. However, at least one-third of their Latina/o patients cross the border to purchase their medications or CAM. Providers demonstrate both positive and negative views regarding CAM. While most providers lack information about CAM, they are primarily concerned about potential CAM-ART interactions and the effect of CAM on treatment compliance.

Complementary and Alternative Medicine Use among Latina/os with Diabetes

One concern when addressing diabetes among Latina/os is their potential use of herbal self-care remedies. The use of herbal self-care remedies becomes problematic when addressing diabetes because of the potential for drug interactions with commonly used diabetes medications (Rivera et al., 2002). Research suggests that Latina/o immigrants with type 2 diabetes use a variety of herbal self-care remedies (Amirehsani & Wallace, 2013). For example, in their mixed-methods study, Amirehsani and Wallace (2013) examined 75 Latina/o adults from North Carolina with type 2 diabetes (8.37 average A1c level). Seventy percent reported the use of herbal remedies to manage their diabetes, including 49 herbal remedies. They described simultaneously using between one and nine different remedies. These remedies included a variety of vegetable food products, teas, herbs, and commercially packaged products. However, their most frequently reported natural products include a blend of Mexican herbs, horsetail, oats, and chamomile tea. Common products include *nopale* (prickly pear cactus leaves), *sábila* (aloe vera), *apio* (celery), and *chayote* (vegetable pear). Participants also report various types of herbal remedy preparation, such as *licuados* (smoothie-like mixture of natural products), with 20 differing herbal products that are blended with juice, milk, or other vegetables. *Tés* (teas) are also commonly used with 19 herbal remedies, as well as *aguas frescas* (cold drinks that are often prepared with an herb), and raw or cooked herbs and plants (Amirehsani & Wallace, 2013).

Amirehsani and Wallace also indicate that Latina/os report various reasons for using their remedies, such as "lower sugar," "for diabetes," "for triglycerides or cholesterol," "for my kidneys," and "to feel better." Most remedies are purchased locally but some are purchased in their home country. Most participants perceive that their herbal remedies are beneficial but also describe experiencing side effects associated with their herbal remedies, such as bitterness (6 of 75). Forty-five percent (34 of 75) also report that they trust a combination of herbal remedies and prescription diabetes medications and the majority (39 of 75) consider prescription diabetes medications safe. However, 77% do not disclose the use of their remedies to their health care providers.

Howell and colleagues (2006) suggest that Latina/o patients may withhold information about their use of herbal remedies and CAM because of the fear that their physicians will disapprove of this use. In addition, few physicians inquire about their patients' use of herbs. For example, in their sample of 640 Latina/o patients from Indiana, 80.3% reported the use of herbal remedies but only 17.4% of their physicians inquired about their use of herbal remedies (Howell et al., 2006). Black et al. (2016) also report that despite the high prevalence of CAM use among Latina/os with cancer, 76.3% do not discuss their CAM use with their health care providers. Their lack of disclosure is attributed to the following: uncertainty if they should disclose their CAM use (25.6%); health care providers do not ask about these practices (24.1%); insufficient time during their office visit (12.3%); and perceptions that their health care provider is unfamiliar with the topic (9.4%).

Complementary and Alternative Medicine Use among Latina/os with Cancer

Among the 12 million persons with a cancer diagnosis, 40–80% use CAM (Horneber et al., 2012). Most CAM research with Latina/o cancer patients focuses on breast cancer. However, one study examined Latina/o colorectal cancer patients' use of CAM (Black et al., 2016). For example, Black et al. interviewed 631 Latina/o patients diagnosed with colorectal cancer and found that 40.1% report CAM use and that most use herbal products/dietary supplements (35.3%), followed by body work (16.5%), mind–body practices (7.8%), and homeopathy (6.7%). Approximately 60% use CAM to address their specific health conditions. Women report significantly higher use of CAM than do men (45.1% vs. 35.9%). However, there are no significant differences in CAM use by clinical stage, time since diagnosis, or preferred language.

In a related study, Gonzalez-Mercado, Williams, Williams, Pedro, and Colon (2017) examined the alleviation practices of Puerto Rican children undergoing cancer treatment in a pediatric hospital in San Juan, Puerto Rico, as reported by their mothers ($N=65$). Puerto Rican mothers report greater alleviation strategies for their children's symptoms of irritability, nausea, loss of appetite, hair loss, and depression. Although they use biological treatments significantly less often than mind–body control strategies or other methods for their children, mothers use vitamins and herbal remedies, such as drinking aloe vera juice. They also apply honey in their child's mouth, and provide a massage with arnica ointment and eucalyptus. Puerto Rican mothers also report the use of spiritual alleviation methods, such as religious family rituals, including praying and reading the Bible with their children. Gonzalez-Mercado et al. (2017) suggest that the limited use of CAM among Puerto Rican mothers is perhaps due to Puerto Rican pediatric physicians who may not allow mothers to use home remedies, such as herbal plants, to manage their children's symptoms.

Religious Practices

The examination of religious beliefs and their impact on health behaviors among Latina/os demonstrates mixed results. Whereas some studies suggest that Latina/os perceive that God causes disease and disability and therefore demonstrate a sense of fatalism, other studies indicate more positive implications. For example, research suggests that religiosity is associated with coping and overall well-being among patients with arthritis (Abraído-Lanza, Vásquez, & Echeverría, 2004). Similarly, Latina breast cancer survivors who report high levels of spirituality also report greater health-related quality of life (Wildes, Miller, San Miguel de Majors, & Ramirez, 2009). Glover and Blankenship (2007) examined religiosity and perceptions of fatality among 160 Latina/os who reside along the Texas-Mexico border. Most participants (68.1%) do not perceive that disabilities are due to punishment from God. In fact, they perceive that God rewards people who care for others with disabilities, thus increasing caregiving behaviors (Glover & Blankenship, 2007).

For many Latina/os spirituality and religiosity are interwoven and function as a source of strength when coping with challenges, such as chronic illness (Campesino & Schwartz, 2006). Spirituality also appears to support adaptation and resilience and improves quality of life among Latina/os with cancer and other chronic illnesses (Hunter-Hernández, Costas-Muñiz, & Gany, 2015). For instance, Nedjat-Haiem, Lorenz, Ell, Hamilton, and Palinkas (2012) indicate that although Latinas with advanced cancer experience depression, they do not demonstrate psychological distress but instead demonstrate a fighting spirit. Nedjat-Haiem et al. also note that Latinas are not fatalistic about their disease or treatment and accept their illness as God's will. They report that through faith, prayer, and acceptance they can alter the outcome of their illness. Latinas are also active participants in their healing process and follow their providers' instructions for care.

Researchers have also examined the role of religiosity to predict CAM use. A cross-sectional study examined traditional (herbal therapies, home remedies, *sobador*, *espiritualista*, *vidente media* (psychic), and *curandera/o*) and mainstream CAM among 306 Latina/o adults (Heathcote, West, Cougar Hall, & Trinidad, 2011). Common forms of CAM therapies include traditional CAM, such as home therapies (64%), herbal therapies (35%), and *sobador* (24%), as well as mainstream CAM, such as megavitamins (20%) and chiropractic care (20%). These findings also indicate demographic differences in CAM use. For instance, South Americans report significantly higher mainstream CAM than do Mexicans and Central Americans. Females are significantly more likely to use traditional CAM than men, and Latina/os between the age of 30 and 69 also report greater traditional CAM use. Lastly, Latina/os who report higher levels of religiosity also report greater traditional and mainstream CAM use, after controlling for age, gender, and income.

Using data from the first wave of the Hispanic Established Population for the Epidemiological Study of the Elderly (EPESE), Loera, Reyes-Ortiz, and Kuo (2007) examined predictors of CAM among 3,050 non-institutionalized older Mexican Americans. Thirty-two percent report the use of at least one CAM therapy within the past year, and common therapies include herbal medicine (27.9%), followed by massage therapy (2.7%), chiropractic (2.4%), relaxation techniques (1.3%), and spiritual healing

(0.4%). Independent predictors of CAM include female gender, being on Medicaid, frequent church attendance, and a higher number of medical conditions. Interestingly, frequent church attendance increases the likelihood among 46% of the overall sample and by 59% of elderly Mexican-born Latina/os.

The role of religiosity and perceptions of medical encounters among Latina/os has gained recent attention. Research using data from Wave 1 of the Pew Hispanic Center/Robert Wood Johnson Foundation Latina/o Health Survey examined religiosity and medical perceptions among 4,013 randomly selected U.S. Latina/o adults (Reyes-Ortiz, Rodriguez, & Markides, 2009). In particular, they examined the association between *curandera/o* use and feelings (confusion, frustration) regarding information provided during the medical encounter or perceptions of quality of medical care. For Latina/os, feeling confused by the information received during a medical visit is significantly associated with consulting a *curandera/o*, praying for healing, asking others to pray for healing, and considering spiritual healing very important, even after controlling for language concordance between patient and provider. The use of a *curandera/o* or increased use of spiritual therapy is also associated with dissatisfaction with medical care (Reyes-Ortiz et al., 2009).

Self-Prescription Practices

There is limited research regarding self-prescription practices among Latina/os. Self-prescription includes using restricted medications without medical advice or a prescription from a health care provider. Despite the lack of research in this area, extant research suggests that Latina/os' use of medicines obtained outside of formal medical care is common (Larson, Dilone, Garcia, & Smolowitz, 2006). Small Latina/o markets known as *bodegas* or *tiendas* are common places where Latina/os can obtain prescription medications while navigating the medical health care system (Coffman, Shobe, & O'Connell, 2008). Benefits to obtaining prescription medications through Latina/o markets include convenience and familiarity (Kiefer, Bradbury, & Tellez-Giron, 2014). Familiarity with the products sold in Latina/o markets and their ability to speak Spanish in the market, allows Latina/os to ask questions about complex health issues without the typical language barriers encountered in the Western medical system (Coffman et al., 2008). Additionally, Latina/o markets provide access to a variety of medications without a prescription, and Latina/os can bypass U.S. physicians, who may hesitate to dispense antibiotics (Coffman et al., 2008).

Unfortunately, there are several disadvantages and risks associated with the purchase of medications from Latina/o markets. One major issue pertains to the lack of safety regulations for medications that are secretly imported from outside the United States because they are not subjected to the same strict regulations and high standards as medications manufactured in the United States. Without these required safety regulations, medications in Latina/o markets risk being mislabeled, expired, or pose a significant health risk to the consumer (Nolen, Ball, Pinon, & Shepherd, 2002). Workers who sell these medicines lack formal health-related training and are poorly equipped to provide appropriate consultations regarding these medicines. Additionally, drug enforcement officials estimate that 25% of all Mexican medications are counterfeit or substandard (Nolen et al., 2002).

Recent Latina/o immigrants may engage in self-prescription practices for various reasons. For example, in their qualitative study, Coffman et al. (2008) examined self-prescription practices among 19 recent Latina/o immigrants without health insurance. Recent Latina/o immigrants use self-prescriptions practices for various reasons and the practice of obtaining prescription medications without a prescription is widespread. Common reasons include difficulty accessing health care, cultural norms, self-care, and self-prescription. Latina/o immigrants also perceive that medications from their country of origin are stronger and more effective than medications from the United States. In addition, self-diagnosis is common and Latina/os rely on past experiences and advice from family and friends to treat various conditions.

Latina/o immigrants also receive medications via courier, mail, and proxy. For example, they may contact family members in Mexico and request medications by mail, or receive medications from Mexico via courier service. Coffman et al. (2008) indicate that Latina/o immigrants frequent Latina/o markets to access their desired medications. These medicines are kept behind the counter and dispensed solely upon request. When pills are sold separately and without packaging, participants must attempt to quickly examine the box to verify the product and expiration dates. For example, when Latina/os are unfamiliar with the name of their medicine, they often rely upon the color of the box. Cashiers at the Latina/o markets are often asked for advice regarding the medication. Despite their limited background in health care or pharmaceuticals they also provide recommendations for medications.

The popularity and accessibility of *botánicas* (stores that sell folk or alternative medicine) or specialty markets also appeal to Latina/os. An ethnographic study of *botánicas* in the Los Angeles area investigated the presence of *botánicas* and their products; in their examination of 26 traditional healers, Jones and Hernandez (2009) suggested that healers treat a variety of conditions, including physical, emotional, and other ailments. Physical illnesses include headaches and chronic diseases. Folk healers also treat *susto* (fright), *empacho* (intestinal problems), *mal de ojo* (evil eye), and *mal aire* (bad air). They utilize more than 300 different herbs and medicines; however, approximately 40–50 plants are commonly grown for medicinal or spiritual use.

Curanderismo as a Source for Latina/o Health

Curanderismo is a term that comes from the Spanish word *curar*, meaning "to heal" and is a complex folk-healing system used in Latina/o cultures (Hendrickson, 2014; Trotter & Chavira, 2011). *Curandera/os* are healers who use aspects of the *curanderismo* healing system to help their patients address physical, spiritual, or mental ailments. A variety of specialties exist for *curandera/os*, such as being an herbalist or midwife or specializing in massages or psychic communications (Avila & Parker, 1999). Additionally, *curandera/os* differ in their source of power. Whereas some believe their healing capabilities are from a higher power, others complete apprenticeships to acquire their skills, which results in varying degrees of expertise among *curandera/os* (Tovar, 2017).

The origins of *curanderismo* predate the Spanish conquest. When the Spanish conquistadors arrived in the New World, the merging of Spanish medical practices and indigenous healing processes resulted in *curanderismo*. Spanish medical knowledge at the time was largely influenced by Greek Hippocratic humoral theory (Tovar, 2017). *Curanderismo* is common among Latina/o heritage groups; however, it is most common among Mexican and Mexican American populations. The overlap of *curanderismo* and humanistic frameworks commonly used in health research provides an opportunity to merge *curanderismo* with modern medical intervention (Chávez, 2016).

Curanderismo is based on a holistic concept of health and focuses on addressing underlying causes of disease, such as imbalances of the body's humors, fractures in the soul caused by fright or trauma, and curses (Trotter, 2001). The resulting treatments align with these potential causes of disease. For example, imbalances in the body's humors are addressed using hot and cold treatments and herbal remedies. The four humors (i.e., blood, phlegm, yellow bile, and black bile) are bodily fluids that when kept in balance, result in a balance of hot and cold and overall wellness (Tovar, 2017). The Spanish believed that a deficiency or excess in any one of the humors resulted in illness. Treatments often involved reducing the amount of fluid in the human (e.g., bloodletting) or balancing the excess temperature with an opposite (e.g., using a warm remedy to balance excessive coldness). Additionally, the Spanish believed in a holistic approach to well-being. Factures in the soul and curses are addressed using spiritual practices. *Curandera/os* are believed to have a gift from God or a higher power to heal their patients. Accordingly, often their work areas include religious figurines and statues to assist in the healing process.

Curanderismo differs from Western medicine in one more important aspect—it uses a collectivistic focus to address health issues. The individual is not the focus of treatment, as in modern Western medicine. Instead, *curanderismo* includes a comprehensive examination of factors that likely impact patients' health, including their family, community, and society and include all of those individuals as part of the healing process (Tovar, 2017). *Curanderismo* includes three overlapping domains of healing knowledge and practice: the spiritual, mental, and material (Cavender, Gladson, Cummings, & Hammet, 2011). The spiritual aspect of *curanderismo* includes contact with spirit beings and spirit currents by *curandera/os* who serve as mediums. The mental aspect of *curanderismo* focuses on the abilities of *curandera/os* to manipulate their own mental energy to heal others. Finally, the material aspect of *curanderismo* includes the *curandera/o*'s use of objects and rituals to diagnose or treat illness (Trotter, 2001). While *curanderismo* is used to address issues related to mental illness (see Chapter 9), this chapter focuses solely on its application to physical health.

The prevalence of *curandera/os* varies throughout the United States. One study examined *curandera/o* use among 3,623 Mexican Americans from the Southwestern United States (Higginbotham, Trevino, & Ray, 1990) based on data from the Hispanic Health and Nutrition Examination Survey, the first national study of Latina/o health from 1982 to 1984. Approximately 4.2% of the participants report consulting a *curandera/o* in the past 12 months. Similar studies suggest a prevalence rate of 5% (Feldmann, Wiemann, Sever, & Hergenroeder, 2008). However, other studies indicate divergent lifetime prevalence rates. For example, among Latina/os who use a public hospital, one-third have visited a *curandera/o* during their lifetime (Padilla, Gomez, Biggerstaff, & Mehler, 2001).

REASONS LATINA/OS SEEK OUT *CURANDERA/OS*

Because Latina/os utilize *curandera/os*, it is important to understand why they seek out their services in conjunction with or in lieu of modern Western medicine. A review examining why Latina/os seek and utilize *curandera/os* throughout the United States (Titus, 2014) examined English-language journals between 2000 and 2012. While 30 research studies examine *curandera/o* use among Latina/os; only 9 studies address why Latina/os seek and utilize *curandera/os*. Nonetheless, these studies suggest that Latina/os seek *curandera/os* because of their affordability and Spanish literacy. Less common reasons include immigration status, cultural appropriateness, spiritual healing, acculturation, and dissatisfaction with the current Western medical system. In addition, these studies suggest that Latina/os utilize *curandera/os* for a range of illnesses, including folk illnesses and treatments that are unfamiliar to health care practitioners.

Chapter 3 discussed issues that contribute to lower access of health care services among Latina/os. These barriers are not present when accessing a *curandera/o* for many Latina/os. Previous research suggests that many Latina/os seek out *curandera/os* because they cannot afford to access Western medical health care (Iniguez & Palinkas, 2003). Moreover, *curandera/os* do not typically charge for their services, and patients determine an appropriate fee for their treatment (Trotter, 2001). This aspect of free or low-cost treatment is a reason why *curandera/os* are sought out by lower-income populations.

One characteristic of *curandera/os* that makes them especially appealing is their similar social and cultural background, meaning that there are fewer barriers between *curandera/os* and their patients (Trotter & Chavira, 2011). In addition to similarities in their social and cultural background, *curandera/os* can speak Spanish. *Curandera/os* can lessen the confusion that is often present when Latina/os need to communicate in English about complex medical terminology (Reyes-Ortiz et al., 2009). Latina/os also express an appreciation for the use of practices that are deemed culturally appropriate and aligned with their cultural traditions (Titus, 2014).

Acculturation is also associated with the likelihood to seek out and utilize the services of *curandera/os*. Research suggests that *curandera/os* can assist with the acculturation process (Trotter & Chavira, 2011). As Latina/os become accustomed to their new home in the United States, they might seek out a *curandera/o* to help ease their transition and provide a sense of familiarity with their country of origin (Rogers, 2010). However, additional research on these relationships is needed.

Dissatisfaction with the Western health care system also contributes to seeking out *curandera/os*. A study of Latina/os and their perceptions regarding medical encounters reveals that many Latina/os experience confusion after a medical encounter or after receiving unsatisfactory treatment with Western medicine (Titus, 2014). This confusion is associated with language issues. However, the overall ability of *curandera/os* to spend time with their patients also contributes to Latina/os' preferred use of *curandera/os*.

One ethnographic study examined six *sobadores* in North Carolina to understand their practices (Quandt et al., 2016). All *sobadores* informally receive their training from family members who are also lay practitioners. They treat a variety of symptoms and ailments, including musculoskeletal pain. Pain is typically a result of a sports injury or overexertion. Additionally, *sobadores* treat twisted nerves, muscles, or tendons and also make referrals to health providers. Another appealing element of sobadores is their ability to validate the pain of their clients. For example, his study of *sobadores* in South Texas, Hinojosa (2008) found that pain sufferers seek *sobadores* because their medical providers and assessments fail to seriously consider their pain reports. Their limited pain validation discourages Mexican Americans from relying on formal care and prompts them to seek folk alternatives, such as *sobadores*.

Curandera/os and Childhood Obesity

Research on how *curandera/os* can partner with researchers to address childhood obesity is limited despite the significant impact of childhood obesity on Latina/o children. As part of a preliminary study, Clark, Bunik, and Johnson (2010) interviewed seven *curandera/os* to assess their perceptions of childhood obesity, prevention, and potential role in working with families to reduce childhood obesity. Findings suggest that *curandera/os* believe health is aligned with a "natural world." They also perceive that the shift from eating natural foods from the earth and consuming processed foods significantly contributes to childhood obesity. They also perceive that breastfeeding is a protective measure because breast milk is more natural than formula. *Curandera/os* also identify feeding strategies that are potentially harmful to children, such as using food to show affection and to bribe children. *Curandera/os* also report that parents feel sorry for their overweight or obese children because of social stigma. Moreover, *curandera/os* indicate that without addressing the issue of poverty and hopelessness among Latina/o families, childhood obesity interventions alone are ineffective. Finally, *curandera/os* highlight that childhood obesity interventions are solely efficacious if they are culturally tailored. They suggest the use of storytelling to communicate messages because storytelling is a culturally acceptable mode of communicating information.

NONTRADITIONAL HEALTH PRACTICES FOR CHILDREN

Folk healing and biomedicine are used among Latina/o families, although the extent of their use is uncertain. For example, a study examined the choices of Mexican American adults regarding folk healing and biomedicine for their children with gastrointestinal problems (Andrews, Ybarra, & Matthews, 2013). Participants include 36 families from the state of Washington with children younger than 2 years of age. Among the parents interviewed, 21 either use traditional healing alone for their children's condition or use traditional and biomedicine. *Sobadores*, folk-healing specialists who use massage and bone manipulation, are often used by families for stomach problems associated with *empacho, susto, caída de la mollera*, and *mal de ojo. Curandera/os* are also sought out depending upon the child's age. Teas are commonly used among families—including *manzanilla* (chamomile) tea and rice water, followed by *yerbabuena* (mint tea) and *atole* (corn- or rice-based drink). Parents who use both traditional and biomedicine first utilize traditional treatments and if they perceive that their children are not improving they use biomedicine.

Andrews et al. (2013) also examined the perceived use of folk healing and biomedicine among 12 biomedical health care staff, including eight care providers and four support staff. Most health care staff members perceive that their Latina/o clients use some form of folk healing. Providers believe they can comprehensively provide for their clients if they learn their practices and incorporate their Latina/o patient's current biomedical treatments. They perceive that doing so will help increase their client's receptivity to their prescribed medical treatments. However, providers indicate that one limitation of this approach is their limited time with their patients, as time constraints often prevent a deeper level of communication to occur.

Implications for Practice

Research suggests that physicians' knowledge and communication about their Latina/o patients' CAM use is quite limited (Bauer & Guerra, 2014). For example, in their exploratory study, Bauer and Guerra (2014) examined 10 physicians from Oakland, CA who typically treat large Latina/o populations. Only 6 of the 10 physicians received information about the cultural health beliefs and practices of Latina/os during an orientation at their current institute. Five physicians received extensive cultural competency training during their medical residency or fellowships at their academic institutions. All physicians report that they always ask their patients about over-the-counter medications; however, only four report that they always ask their Latina/o patients about herbal remedies, supplements, traditional healers, alternative practitioners, or spiritual practices. This finding is particularly problematic because when Latina/o patients are not directly asked about their CAM use, they are unlikely to volunteer this information. In fact, other studies report high rates of Latina/os who do not discuss their CAM use with their physicians, often because they fear disapproval or perceive their providers are unfamiliar with their nontraditional practices (Black et al., 2016; Howell et al., 2006; Mikhail, Wali, & Ziment, 2004). However, when Latina/os communicate with their physicians, they regard them as respectful, open-minded, and willing to listen (Howell et al., 2006).

Howell et al. (2006) note that regardless of whether patients self-disclose their CAM use, the "onus is on health practitioners" to inquire about their CAM use. However, health practitioners must first understand the roles that nontraditional health practices play in Latina/o health and subsequently demonstrate respect for these practices. Thus, it is essential that health practitioners continually educate themselves regarding the specific CAM practices of their patients to provide effective and culturally sensitive care (Ortiz, 2007). Health practitioners should be mindful that the healing traditions of Latina/os provide cultural stability and continuity (Trotter & Chavira, 1997). Their healing traditions reflect the cultural perspectives and worldviews of Latina/os regarding their conceptualizations of health and illness (Holliday, 2008). Therefore, health providers must recognize that Latina/os may conceptualize their illness or medical concerns from a non-Western, non-medical perspective and may discuss their illness in a different manner (Amirehsani & Wallace, 2013).

Furthermore, there are numerous benefits of addressing spirituality and religiosity, particularly as Latina/os often favor integrative, holistic, and syncretic healing approaches (Comas-Díaz, 2012c). Respect for worldviews and practices can increase their communication with Latina/o patients and gain their trust to discuss their CAM use in an open and nonjudgmental manner (Howell et al., 2006). Doing so will increase the likelihood that increase the likelihood that their Latina/o patients will self-disclose their use of nontraditional practices and increase their treatment compliance (Ortiz et al., 2007). Effective provider-patient communication will also aid in the provision of culturally competent assessments, diagnosis, and medical treatments.

CONCLUSION

Implications for practitioners in the medical care industry include the necessity to increase communication regarding CAM use. Greater communication regarding the use of CAM can help to screen for potentially dangerous drug interactions and prevent harmful herb use among Latina/os. Additionally, training regarding CAM is needed for health care professionals who work with Latina/os, including seasoned and novice medical providers. Also, greater knowledge of *curanderismo* and other nontraditional health care practices can enable practitioners to become better informed to discuss these practices with their patients and increase patient trust and comfort to disclose their use of nontraditional practices.

Chapter 6

Prevalence of Mental Health Disorders

There can be no mental health where there is powerlessness, because powerlessness breeds despair; there can be no mental health where there is poverty, because poverty breeds hopelessness; there can be no mental health where there is inequality, because inequality breeds anger and resentment; there can be no mental health where there is racism, because racism breeds low self-esteem and self-denigration.

—Marsella and Yamada, 2007, p. 812

Despite the increased visibility of Latina/os, there are limited national data to document the prevalence of their mental health disorders, unmet needs, and the factors that are associated with their mental illness (Alegría et al., 2004). It is also important to understand how social, cultural, and contextual factors influence the well-being of Latina/os. Their increased risk for mental health disorders is attributed to discrimination, family conflict, immigration challenges, language barriers, poverty, and other factors. However, the culture-based assets and strengths of Latina/os, such as social support, religious involvement, racial/ethnic identity, and biculturalism also play an important role in their mental health and help buffer against the development of mental illness. Understanding factors that protect and exacerbate mental illness are crucial, as they may function differently depending on gender, immigrant status, Latina/o heritage group, and other salient variables. This understanding will help inform interventions and research targeted toward Latina/os who are at risk for mental health disorders (Scott, Wallander, & Cameron, 2015). Further, an understanding of the prevalence of mental health disorders among Latina/o heritage groups indicates the need to avoid aggregating Latina/os into a single, homogeneous group, as this masks the significant variability within their lifetime and current risk of psychological disorders (Alegría, Chatterji et al., 2008b).

The present chapter presents a brief overview of the protective and risk factors that impact the mental health of Latina/os. We also review epidemiological studies that are largely based on the National Latina/o and Asian American Study (NLAAS; Alegría et al., 2004). While we recognize that the NLAAS and related studies are not based on the current *Diagnostic and Statistical Manual of Mental Disorders* (5th ed.; DSM-5; American Psychiatric Association, 2013), the current chapter focuses largely on epidemiological studies from the NLAAS because of the focus on immigrant status, gender, sexual orientation, and other key variables that impact the mental health of Latina/os. Similarly, epidemiological studies from the comprehensive report from the Centers for Disease Control and Prevention (CDC) *Mental Health Surveillance among Children—United States, 2005–2011* (Perou et al., 2013) are reviewed largely to identify the prevalence of mental health disorders among Latina/o children and adolescents. However, alike epidemiological studies that focus on Latina/o adults, studies that focus on Latina/o children and adolescents are also reviewed to address important cultural and psychosocial variables.

It is equally important to understand prominent idioms of distress among Latina/os. For example, idioms of distress are culturally sanctioned constructions of physical, psychosocial, or psychospiritual distress (Guarnaccia, Lewis-Fernández, & Marano, 2003; Salgado de Snyder, Diaz-Perez, & Ojeda, 2000). More specifically, they are culturally accepted illnesses that signal distress through a variety of somatic and physical symptoms among Latina/os. Scholars often focus upon *susto* (fright), *nervios* (nerves), and *ataque de nervios* (attack of nerves) because of their associations with depression, anxiety, and panic disorder (Durà-Vilà & Hodes, 2012; Guarnaccia et al., 2003; Salgado de Snyder et al., 2000; Weller, Baer, Garcia de Alba Garcia, & Rocha, 2008). Thus, these idioms of distress are discussed.

EARLY PSYCHIATRIC EPIDEMIOLOGICAL STUDIES OF LATINA/O ADULTS

Prior to the 1980s, few large population-based epidemiological studies examined the mental health of Latina/os within the U.S. mainland and Puerto Rico. However, researchers conducted several important studies within the past four decades. These studies include the following:

- *Los Angeles Epidemiologic Catchment Area Study* (LAECA; Burnam, Hough, Karno, Escobar, & Telles, 1987)
- *Puerto Rican Epidemiologic Catchment Area Study* (PR-ECA; Canino et al., 1987)
- *Hispanic Health and Nutrition Examination Survey* (HHANES; National Center for Health Statistics, 1985)
- *Mexican American Prevalence and Services Survey* (MAPSS; Vega et al., 1998)
- *National Comorbidity Survey* (NCS; Kessler et al., 1994)
- *National Comorbidity Survey Replication* (NCS-R; Kessler & Merikangas, 2004)
- *National Epidemiological Survey on Alcohol and Related Conditions* (NESARC; Grant, 1996)

An in-depth review of these studies by Canino and Alegría (2009) indicates that while these studies find support for the immigrant paradox (i.e., lower prevalence of mental health disorders among Latina/o immigrants as compared with their U.S.-born counterparts) among Latina/os born outside the United States, these initial studies largely focus on Latina/os of Mexican heritage and fail to focus upon other Latina/o heritage groups (for a review of the Latina/o paradox, see Chapter 2). However, in their analysis of mental health disorders among Puerto Ricans and Cubans based on NESARC data, Alegría, Canino, Stinson, and Grant (2006) found that the immigrant paradox does not generalize to all Latina/o heritage groups or all mental health disorders. In particular, nativity is solely protective of substance abuse disorders and not depressive or anxiety disorders.

NATIONAL LATINA/O AND ASIAN AMERICAN STUDY (NLAAS)

National epidemiological studies are instrumental in examining the lifetime prevalence of mental health disorders among diverse Latina/os, such as the NLAAS (Alegría et al., 2004). The NLAAS examines mental health disorders, including lifetime and last year DSM-5 diagnoses as measured by the Composite International Diagnostic Interview (CIDI) schedule. In particular, the NLAAS examines mental health disorders between immigrant and U.S.-born adults (18 and older), and among Latina/os from diverse heritage groups, to identify protective factors of mental health disorders. Conducted between May 2002 and December 2003, the NLAAS is a national household survey (75.5% overall response rate) of English and Spanish adults who reside in the conterminous United States, and includes both Latina/os ($N=2,554$) and Asian American ($N=1,097$). More specifically, Latina/o participants include Mexican ($N=868$), Cuban ($N=577$), Puerto Rican ($N=495$), and Other Latina/os ($N=614$) (Alegría et al., 2008b). Another contribution of the NLAAS is the comparison of lifetime rates of psychological disorders with non-Latina/o Whites from the

NCS-R since similar measures and methods are utilized within both studies (Alegría et al., 2008b). For example, after adjusting for age and gender, Latina/os, demonstrate significantly lower rates for all disorder categories as compared with non-Latina/o Whites (Alegría et al., 2008b), including any depressive disorder (15.4% vs. 22.3%), any anxiety disorder (15.7% vs. 25.7%), and any substance disorder (11.2% vs. 17.7%).

In addition to the examination of protective factors, another contribution of the NLAAS is the examination of dual minority status arising from both sexual orientation and race/ethnicity. There is accumulating evidence indicating that compared to their heterosexual counterparts, individuals who self-identify as LGBTQIA face increased risk for psychological and substance use disorders. For example, Cochran, Mays, Alegría, Ortega, and Takeuchi (2007) examined the substance use and mental health of LGBTQIA Latina/os and Asian Americans. Approximately 4.8% identified as lesbian, gay, or bisexual and/or report recent same-gender experiences. Despite few sexual orientation–related differences, gay/bisexual men report greater one-year suicide attempts (2.4%) than heterosexual men (0.3%). Lesbian/bisexual women report greater lifetime (24.7% vs. 17.2%) and one-year histories (16.0% vs. 9.2%) of depressive disorders than heterosexual women, as well as greater one-year histories of drug use disorders (2.9% vs. 0.2%).

CORRELATES OF LIFETIME MENTAL HEALTH DISORDERS AMONG LATINA/OS

Large-scale epidemiological studies are helpful to identify correlates of lifetime mental health disorders among Latina/o heritage groups. For example, after adjusting for age and gender, Alegría et al. (2008b) found significant differences among Latina/o heritage groups indicating that Puerto Ricans report the greatest prevalence of any lifetime mental health disorder (38.98%), followed by Mexicans (28.42%), Cubans (28.38%), and Other Latina/os (27.29%). Canino and Alegría (2009) also report that while rates for any lifetime depressive disorder do not significantly differ among these groups, lifetime prevalence rates for any lifetime anxiety disorder differ statistically—21.7% among Puerto Ricans, 15.5% among Mexicans, 14.4% among Cubans, and 14.1% among Other Latina/os. Similarly, prevalence rates for any lifetime substance disorders also differ among Puerto Ricans (13.8%), Mexicans (11.8%), Other Latina/os (9.8%), and Cubans (6.6%).

There are demographic differences in the prevalence of lifetime mental health disorders (Alegría et al., 2007b). Prevalence rates are slightly higher among Latinas (30%) than Latinos (28%). In terms of age, Latina/os between the ages of 35 and 49 report higher lifetime mental health disorder prevalence rates (32%), as compared with those between the ages of 18 and 34 (27%). Also, Latina/os who immigrate before the age of 13 or after the age of 34 (28%) have the highest lifetime mental health disorder prevalence rates, as compared with those who immigrate at other ages (Alegría et al., 2007a). When adjusting for age, gender, and socioeconomic status, there is support for the immigrant paradox. For example, U.S.-born Latina/os (N=924) report significantly higher risk for any lifetime disorder than their immigrant peers (N=1,630; 37.1% vs. 24.9%), as well as major depressive episodes (18.6% vs.13.4%), any depressive disorder (19.8% vs. 14.8%), any anxiety disorder (18.9% vs. 15.2%), and social phobia (8.5% vs. 6.0%) (Alegría et al., 2008a).

There are similar trends for alcohol and drugs, including any lifetime substance abuse disorder (20.4% vs. 7.0%), alcohol abuse (9.3% vs. 3.5%), alcohol dependence (6.9% vs. 2.8%), drug abuse (6.1% vs. 2.2%), and drug dependence (5.1% vs. 1.7%). Interestingly, despite support for the immigrant paradox (Alegría et al., 2008a), not all Latina/o heritage groups benefit, as Mexican immigrants demonstrate a consistent pattern across mood, anxiety, and substance abuse disorders (see Table 6.1). Among Cubans and Other Latinas/os, foreign nativity is solely protective for substance disorder and there are no significant differences in the risk of any lifetime disorder between migrant and U.S.-born Puerto Ricans (Alegría et al., 2008a). Thus, these findings suggest that the protection against mental health disorders among Latina/o immigrants varies by specific disorders (i.e., mood, anxiety, and substance abuse) and the immigrant paradox applies to certain Latina/o heritage groups, such as Mexicans but not others, such as Puerto Ricans. These findings also suggest that other factors beyond nativity may play a role in the development of mental health disorders (Canino & Alegría, 2009) and also underscore how aggregating Latina/os into a single, homogeneous group masks significant variability within their lifetime risk of psychological disorders (Alegría et al., 2008a).

These findings underscore the need to examine the increased vulnerability of lesbian, gay, bisexual, transgender, queer or questioning, intersex, asexual, and ally (LGBTQIA) Latina/os, such as their risk for substance abuse disorders. For instance, McCabe, Bostwick, Hughes, West, and Boyd (2010) examined associations among multiple types of discrimination—based on race/ethnicity, gender, and sexual orientation and substance abuse disorders—in a national sample of self-identified lesbian, gay, and bisexual women and men (N=577) from Wave 2 of the 2004–2005 NESARC. Approximately 46.0% of lesbian, gay, and bisexual adults who report discrimination based on their race/ethnicity, gender, and sexual orientation meet criteria for any past-year substance use disorders, as compared with 17.2% of their counterparts who do not report discrimination.

Table 6.1 Bayesian Lifetime Prevalence of Mental Health Disorders—Percentage (95% Confidence Intervals) for NLAAS Latina/o by National Origin and Immigrant Status[a]

Disorder	Puerto Rican		Cuban		Mexican		Other	
	U.S.-Born (N=278)	Immigrant (N=217)	U.S.-Born (N=76)	Immigrant (N=501)	U.S.-Born (N=380)	Immigrant (N=488)	U.S.-Born (N=190)	Immigrant (N=424)
Any depressive disorder	21.0 (16.8–25.5)	19.9 (16.1–23.7)	20.3 (13.7–27.2)	19.7 (15.3–24.1)	**20.4 (16.6–24.1)**[b]	**12.9 (9.9–16.0)**[b]	17.3 (13.4–21.7)	15.8 (12.2–19.2)
Dysthymia	4.0 (1.8–6.2)	5.5 (3.0–8.1)	4.2 (1.4–7.6)	4.0 (2.2–5.9)	3.3 (1.8–4.8)	2.8 (1.3–4.5)	3.3 (1.2–5.8)	2.7 (1.4–4.4)
Major depressive episode	20.2 (16.3–24.2)	17.6 (14.1–21.6)	17.9 (11.9–25.1)	18.5 (14.5–22.8)	**19.2 (15.7–22.7)**[b]	**11.8 (9.1–14.5)**[b]	16.2 (12.2–20.1)	14.1 (10.9–17.4)
Any anxiety disorder	21.6 (17.9–25.7)	21.8 (16.9–26.7)	16.7 (10.7–22.6)	14.1 (10.8–17.5)	**20.0 (16.2–23.8)**[b]	**14.2 (11.3–17.1)**[b]	14.1 (10.3–18.8)	16.0 (12.5–19.5)
Agoraphobia without panic dx	4.0 (1.9–6.1)	6.9 (4.1–9.9)	5.1 (1.9–8.7)	3.7 (1.7–6.3)	4.0 (2.2–6.2)	3.4 (1.9–5.0)	2.5 (0.8–4.3)	3.4 (1.8–5.2)
Generalized anxiety disorder	6.9 (4.5–9.4)	7.7 (4.9–10.7)	5.2 (1.9–9.0)	5.1 (3.3–7.0)	3.8 (2.2–5.5)	4.8 (3.2–6.5)	4.2 (1.4–7.2)	3.5 (1.9–5.3)
Panic disorder	4.8 (2.8–7.0)	5.3 (2.7–8.0)	4.5 (1.4–8.2)	3.3 (1.5–5.9)	4.8 (2.8–6.8)	3.4 (1.6–5.1)	3.7 (1.5–5.9)	3.2 (1.6–4.9)

Post-traumatic stress disorder	3.8 (1.9–5.7)	5.4 (2.5–8.7)	3.5 (2.1–5.0)	5.9 (3.8–8.3)	5.0 (2.3–8.2)	7.0 (3.3–11.0)	7.2 (4.2–9.9)	6.5 (4.0–9.1)
Social phobia	7.3 (4.8–10.0)	4.5 (2.1–7.1)	4.7 (2.9–6.6)[b]	10.0 (7.2–12.8)[b]	6.6 (4.3–9.2)	6.1 (2.9–9.9)	10.0 (6.8–13.4)	8.1 (5.5–10.9)
Any substance disorder	5.7 (3.3–8.0)[b]	20.4 (15.6–25.3)[b]	7.0 (4.7–9.5)[b]	21.4 (17.9–25.0)[b]	6.4 (3.4–9.5)[b]	20.9 (13.5–28.1)[b]	11.1 (7.5–14.9)	15.9 (12.4–19.5)
Alcohol abuse	3.2 (1.4–5.0)[b]	10.4 (7.0–13.7)[b]	3.5 (1.9–5.4)[b]	9.4 (6.6–12.1)[b]	3.4 (1.4–5.5)	6.5 (3.1–10.4)	4.6 (2.5–7.1)	7.7 (5.2–10.4)
Alcohol dependence	2.2 (0.9–3.5)[b]	5.3 (2.2–8.4)[b]	2.8 (1.4–4.2)[b]	7.7 (5.5–10.1)[b]	2.2 (25.7–32.0)[b]	8.2 (3.8–12.8)[b]	5.3 (2.5–7.1)	5.6 (3.1–8.3)
Drug abuse	2.1 (0.8–3.5)[b]	8.4[b] (5.0–11.8)[b]	2.0[b] (0.8–3.4)[b]	5.8 (3.7–7.8)[b]	2.2 (0.4–4.2)	3.6 (30.6–42.5)	4.3 (1.8–7.0)	4.6 (2.2–7.0)
Drug dependence	1.0 (0.1–2.1)[b]	5.2 (1.9–8.7)	1.7 (0.5–3.0)	5.3 (3.2–7.4)[b]	1.9 (0.3–3.8)	5.7 (0.7–6.8)	3.6 (1.3–6.3)	4.3 (2.6–6.4)
Any disorder	24.2 (19.9–28.2)[b]	31.4 (25.7–36.5)[b]	23.9 (20.6–27.2)[b]	39.2 (34.7–43.6)[b]	26.2 (21.1–31.1)	32.2 (24.5–39.8)	32.6 (27.0–38.5)	37.2 (32.5–42.2)

Note: [a]Bayesian lifetime prevalence adjusted for age, gender, and socioeconomic status (education and household income). Data were drawn from the NLAAS. Composite diagnostic categories were restricted to any depressive disorder, any anxiety disorder, any substance disorder, and any disorder.
[b]Wald chi-square test.

Source: Alegría et al. (2008a). Prevalence of mental illness in immigrant and non-immigrant U.S. Latino groups, Table 4. *American Journal of Psychiatry, 165,* 359–369.

Factors That Impact the Mental Health of Latina/os

The psychological literature suggests that there are numerous factors that impact the mental health of Latina/os. However, depending on the context, these factors can operate as both protective and risk factors. For example, while biculturalism is a protective factor and buffers Latina/os from negative outcomes, bicultural stress among Latina/o adolescents can accumulate and lead to the development of depressive symptoms and substance use (Romero, Edwards, Bauman, & Ritter, 2014a). Protective factors are characteristics that buffer between a stressor and person's reaction to the stressor (Romero et al., 2014a). Ecological perspectives aid in understanding the resilience and mental health of Latina/os (Kuperminc, Wilkins, Roche, & Alvarez-Jimenez, 2009), as their mental health is best explained in the context of linguistic, sociocultural, political, and socioeconomic stressors (see Figure 6.1).

Bronfenbrenner's Ecological Model (1997) considers the individual as well as the exchanges that occur with his/her environment. Accordingly,

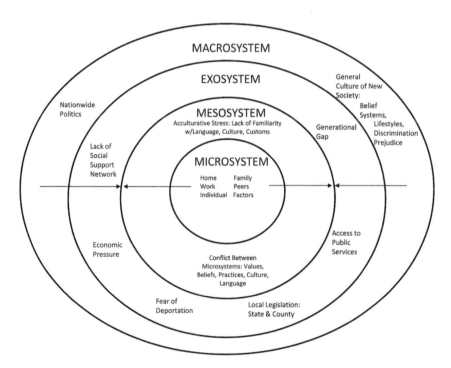

Figure 6.1 Ecological Model.

Source: Pimentel-Narez, D. (2017). The effects of immigrant status, gender and years of U.S. residency on the acculturative stress and psychological symptomatology of Mexican immigrants. Unpublished dissertation. University of La Verne, La Verne, CA.

four main levels of social settings surround individuals—the microsystem, mesosystem, exosystem, and macrosystem. In addition, interactions between the individual and environment are viewed as reciprocal—the individual influences these environments and vice versa. For Latina/os, there are unique interactions with the macrosystem because of the current political climate and punitive immigration policies contribute to their experiences of discrimination, anti-immigrant sentiments, stereotypes, social marginalization, and other forms of oppression (Romero et al., 2014a). However, strong social support at home ameliorates the effects of discrimination and other stressors among immigrant Latina/o adolescents (Potochnick & Perreira, 2010).

Protective and Risk Mental Health Factors

A significant body of research suggests that the culture-based assets and strengths of Latina/os are protective factors (social support, religiosity/spirituality, racial/ethnic identity, and biculturalism) and that these play an important role in their mental health (Ai, Aisenberg, Weiss, & Salazar, 2014; Alegría et al., 2007b; Alegría & Woo, 2009; Mulvaney-Day, Alegría, & Sribney, 2007). For example, the collectivistic nature of Latina/os (see Chapter 1) often plays a role in the multidimensional and complex process of their adaptation in the United States. While individualism dominates in most Western cultures, collectivism is often salient among Latina/os because of the role of *familismo* (Adames & Chavez-Dueñas, 2017; Añez, Silva, Paris, & Bedregal, 2008; Arredondo et al., 2014; Falicov, 2013; Gallardo, 2012; Santiago-Rivera et al., 2002). *Familismo* and strong family ties are protective of the mental health of Latina/os and contribute to their pride, sense of belonging, and obligation (Falicov, 2013). As a natural support system, *familismo* provides physical, emotional, and social support for Latinas/os, and this support may act as a buffer during stressful situations (Dunn & O'Brien, 2009). Data from the NLAAS indicates that support from family and friends, as well as neighborhood social cohesion, is positively associated with positive self-rated physical and mental health (Mulvaney-Day et al., 2007). Among adolescents, *familismo* is also associated with decreased parent–adolescent conflict and mediates the negative association between acculturation conflicts and adolescent aggressive behavior (Smokowski & Bacallao, 2006).

Ethnic identity, often defined as a sense of belonging to one's ethnic group, is also a protective factor among Latina/os (Ai et al., 2014). Ethnic identity is associated with self-esteem (Romero & Roberts, 2003; Umaña-Taylor, Diversi, & Fine, 2002) and coping abilities among Latina/o adolescents (Romero, Edwards, Fryberg, & Orduña, 2014; Romero et al., 2014b), and decreased externalizing and externalizing problems among Mexican and Dominican children (Serrano-Vilvar & Calzada, 2016). As a source of resilience, ethnic identity helps Latina/o adolescents deal with discrimination and prejudice (Romero et al., 2014a,b) and may reduce their risk for drug use, particularly among Latinas (Castro, Stein, & Bentler, 2009). Similarly, a strong ethnic identity helps them cope with their experiences of discrimination and helps buffer against unhealthy behaviors, such as substance use (Molina, Jackson, & Rivera-Olmedo, 2016). Similarly, school support helps to increase their academic achievement and sense of belonging (Kuperminc et al., 2009; Romero et al., 2014b). In addition, teacher support is important for Latina/o youth. For example, Brewster and Bowen (2004) note that social support from teachers is an important factor for the school engagement of at-risk Latina/o middle and high school youth. In particular, teachers exert an important effect on these students' school engagement, beyond the effect of parental support.

Biculturalism is also regarded as a cultural asset for Latina/os, because of associations with better family relations and psychosocial adjustment and the ability to maintain social connections and cultural ties (Mulvaney-Day et al., 2007). Biculturalism is also salutary for children and adolescents (Gonzales, Knight, Morgan-Lopez, Saenz, & Sirolli, 2002), including fewer internalizing problems and higher self-esteem (Smokowski & Bacallao, 2007). Among a community sample of Latina/o adolescents, biculturalism is associated with less depressive symptomatology and greater optimism (Carvajal, Hanson, Romero, & Coyle, 2002). Biculturalism and bilingualism also contribute to the success of adolescents within various social contexts because of the ability to access resources from both Latina/o and U.S. mainstream cultures (Bacallao & Smokowski, 2009).

Church attendance and religiosity enable Latina/o immigrants to cope with their stressors because of the formation of social networks and the establishment of spiritual and social support (Barranco, 2016). Religious beliefs may protect against substance abuse disorders and suicide (Barranco, 2016) because religion discourages deviant behaviors. For example, Robinson, Bolton, Rasic, and Sareen (2012) found that increased church attendance is associated with both decreased suicidal ideation and attempts, as well as decreased anxiety among Latina/os. Among Latina/o college students, religiosity helps moderate relationships between discrimination and anxiety symptoms (Corona et al., 2017). In addition, spirituality also serves as a protective factor and source of strength for Latina/os (Comas-Díaz, 2014). Comas-Díaz (2014) suggests that despite the diverse religious orientations among Latina/os, spirituality is a "vital force" and provides healing, empowerment, and transformation, as well as connections within their communities (p. 217).

Several factors appear to contribute to mental health risk factors of Latina/os, and these factors may explain variation in their risk of mental health disorders, such as discrimination (Ai et al., 2014; Araújo & Borrell, 2006; Chou, Asnaani, & Hofmann, 2012; Cook et al., 2009; Lee & Ahn, 2012). For example, data from the CPES suggests an independent effect of racial discrimination on major depressive disorder, panic disorder, post-traumatic stress disorder, and substance use disorders among Latina/os (Chou et al., 2012). Data from the NLAAS indicate that discrimination is also associated with major depression, general anxiety, suicidal ideation, and smoking (Ai et al., 2014). Discrimination is also a risk factor for a range of internalizing and externalizing problems among Latina/o adolescents, including general externalizing and internalizing problems (Smokowski & Bacallao, 2007; Smokowski, Chapman, & Bacallao, 2007), lower self-esteem (Smokowski & Bacallao, 2007), and social problems (Smokowski et al., 2007).

The experience of discrimination also creates challenges to men's masculinity and well-being. For example, among Latinos with a strong ethnic identity, an awareness of their devalued social position as men of color creates heightened levels of threat, internalization of a devalued status, and greater distress. Latinos engage in harmful behaviors such as substance use to numb their pain from discrimination and threats to their identity (Molina et al., 2016; Negi, 2013). Similarly, Latina/os with darker phenotypic characteristics (see Adames & Chavez-Dueñas, 2017, for a review of colorism) and certain cultural characteristics (e.g., Spanish language use) also experience increased discrimination (Araújo & Borrell, 2006). Similarly, Latinx (Reichard, 2015) experience multiple forms of oppression because of their intersecting identities as ethnic and sexual minorities. For instance, Ibañez and colleagues (2012) found that Latinx with darker skin, greater indigenous features, increased U.S. residence, and low self-esteem report greater racism within both general and gay contexts. In addition, some research suggests that Latinx are vulnerable to poor mental health and that they experience suicidal ideation, anxiety, and depressed mood (Díaz, Ayala, Bein, Henne, & Marín, 2013), as well as severe physical and sexual assault and loss of social support from family and friends (Cerezo, Morales, Quintero, & Rothman, 2014).

The process of acculturation is associated with stressors that increase mental health risk factors, such as acculturative stress. Among Latina/os, *acculturative stress* refers to psychological or social stressors that emerge as a result of dissimilar beliefs, values, and other cultural norms between their country of origin and the United States (Sanchez, Dillon, Ruffin, & De La Rosa, 2012). The process of acculturation also impacts Latina/o youth because of the significant associations between acculturation and internalizing and externalizing problems (Lawton & Gerdes, 2014). Acculturative stress is often linked to financial burden, language problems such as limited English proficiency, perceived cultural incompatibilities, and decreased commitment to culturally prescribed values that contribute to the increased likelihood of cultural conflict and family burden (Alegría et al., 2007b; Alegría & Woo, 2009). Traditional family relationships appear to erode with increasing numbers of years in the United States and are replaced with increased intergenerational conflict, decreased family support, and decreased endorsement of traditional Latino values, such as *familismo*. Differences in the experience of acculturative stress also exist among Latina/o heritage groups. For instance, Mexicans report greater acculturative stress, while Puerto Ricans report lower acculturative stress but also demonstrate greater family cultural conflict (Guarnaccia et al., 2007).

Although biculturalism is a protective factor for Latina/o adolescents, bicultural stress (the stress that may arise among youth due to pressure to navigate values, norms, and languages of two cultures) is a risk factor (Romero & Roberts, 2003; Romero et al., 2014a). For example, bicultural stress among a community sample of Latina/o adolescents is associated with engagement in risky behavior and higher levels of depressive symptoms (Romero, Martinez, & Carvajal, 2007) and with depressive symptoms and hopelessness among adolescents of Mexican descent from a U.S.–Mexico border region (Romero, Piña-Watson, & Toomey, 2017). In addition, a longitudinal study of diverse immigrant Latina/o adolescents from Miami and Los Angeles (Cano et al., 2015) indicates that greater cultural stress (e.g., bicultural stress, perceived discrimination, and perceived negative context of reception), predicts higher odds of cigarette smoking, binge drinking, aggressive behavior, rule breaking, and depressive symptoms.

Unfortunately, Latina/o immigrants often reside in poor and disadvantaged urban areas. Poverty and limited opportunities are associated with negative outcomes for adolescents and their families (Pantin, Schwartz, Sullivan, Coatsworth, & Szapocznik, 2003). Immigrant adolescents who reside in neighborhoods with increased exposure to peer and community drug abuse, crime, violence, and risky behaviors are at risk for the development of mental health disorders (Alegría et al., 2007b; Alegría & Woo, 2009; Canino & Alegría, 2009; Pantin et al., 2003). These experiences may lead to perceptions among adolescents that peer and community drug abuse, crime, and violence are normative, thereby contributing to their increased risky behaviors (Pantin et al., 2003). It is hypothesized that victims of violence may use substances to cope with their exposure to violence (Poquiz & Fite, 2016). For example, community violence is associated with increased risk for lifetime use of illegal substances, tobacco, and marijuana among Latina/o adolescents (Poquiz & Fite, 2016).

The Role of Exposure to U.S. Culture and Mental Health Disorders

Factors beyond nativity—such as acculturation, including changes in language and cultural practices—appear to contribute to the development of mental health disorders among Latina/os. As Latina/os shift their language use, a number of important cultural and social experiences change (Guarnaccia et al., 2007). For instance, socialization into U.S. values and lifestyles, as well as exposure to greater problem behaviors, such as illicit drug use (Vega et al., 2002) contribute to increased mental illness. Exposure to English and U.S. culture may also create intergenerational conflict and distance among family members. Conversely, later-arrival immigrants may share norms and values that are similar to their parents because of their greater identification with Latina/o cultural values.

Alegría et al. (2007c) examined associations among age at arrival, length of residence, and birth cohorts. They observed that the longer Latina/o immigrants remain in their native country, the lower their risk of mental health disorders over their lifetimes. Much of the low risk of Latina/o immigrants in their country of origin is attributed to their protective familial and cultural values (i.e., *familismo*) and Latina/os may lose these protective resources upon their immigration to the United States. NLAAS data indicate that Latina/o immigrants experience similar onset risks as their U.S.-born counterparts of the same age. In particular, shorter U.S. residence is associated with less cumulative risk for the onset of psychopathology, resulting in lower rates of mental health disorders, as cultural and familial factors among Latina/os may erode with longer residence in the United States.

Using NLAAS data to identify factors associated with psychopathology risk, Alegría et al. (2007b) observed differences among Latina/o heritage groups. For example, unadjusted values indicate that more than half of Puerto Ricans are born in the mainland United States and report high levels of family cultural conflict, perceived exposure to discrimination, and good or excellent English language proficiency. In addition, they report low levels of perceived neighborhood safety, increased likelihood of marital disruption, greater prevalence of any 12-month disorder, and greater prevalence of any anxiety disorder as compared with other Latina/o heritage groups. Conversely, Cubans are mostly late-arrival immigrants, arriving in the United States after the age of six. Cubans report high levels of family support, greater Latina/o ethnic identity, and good or excellent Spanish language proficiency, and low levels of family burden or family cultural conflict as compared with Latina/os who self-identify as "Other." Conversely, Mexicans are younger, have lower mean household incomes, are less likely to be divorced, and demonstrate the lowest prevalence of any 12-month disorder. However, while these unadjusted figures highlight the significant variability among Latina/o heritage groups, these differences diminish after adjusting for differences in age, gender, nativity, and age at arrival.

Successful adaptation to U.S. culture is a complex and multidimensional process that includes maintenance of family harmony, integration into advantageous U.S. neighborhoods, and positive perceptions of social standing (Alegría et al., 2007b). In addition, differences in the prevalence of mental health disorders among Latina/o heritage groups are a function of multiple factors beyond nativity. For example, to varying degrees, family burden and family cultural conflict, perceived low neighborhood safety, exposure to discrimination, disrupted marital status, unemployment, and perceived low social standing are all risk factors for the prevalence of 12-month depressive, anxiety, and substance use disorders.

Alegría et al. (2007b) also identify several risk and protective factors that are linked to mental health disorders among Latina/os. For example, cultural conflict and family burden are associated with increased risk for depressive and anxiety disorders. After age and gender adjustments, the risk for anxiety disappears among later-arrival Latina/os as compared with Latina/os who resided in the United States as children. For substance use disorders, family factors do not offset the elevated risk of early exposure to neighborhood disadvantage, but arrival in the United States after the age of 25 does offset such risk. Alegría et al. (2007b) suggest that for substance abuse disorders, arrival in the United States as an adult may protect against exposure to risky social networks linked to drug use, and strong family bonds may offer a protective environment. In addition, religious attendance also facilitates social participation and integration into positive social networks that protect against the negative impact of disadvantageous neighborhoods and substance use disorders.

Correlates of Eating Disorders

In addition to the examination of depressive, anxiety, and substance abuse disorders, the NLAAS also includes the examination of lifetime and 12-month prevalence of DSM-IV eating disorders and their correlates. Alegría et al. (2007d) report elevated rates of binge eating and binge eating disorder among Latina/os but a low prevalence of anorexia nervosa and bulimia nervosa. Foreign nativity is associated with a decreased risk for binge eating, and those who spend more than 70% of their lifetime in the United States report higher rates of lifetime bulimia nervosa. Despite the lack of differences in gender or Latina/o heritage group, there are age cohort differences, as those aged 30 and older are significantly less likely to have bulimia nervosa and any binge eating disorder. Alegría et al. (2007d) suggest that the low prevalence of anorexia nervosa among Latina/os is perhaps attributable to cultural differences in the presentation of eating disorder symptoms, as they are more inclined to exhibit binge eating rather than restricting behaviors. Moreover, criteria for eating disorders are perhaps inappropriate for understanding restricting eating disorders of Latina/os and reflect nosological criteria for Western populations and do not capture illness expressions (Alegría et al., 2007d).

Marques et al. (2011) also pooled data from the National Institute of Mental Health (NIMH) CPES that includes data from three nationally representative U.S. samples—the NLAAS, the National Survey of American Life (NSAL), and the NCS-R—to examine the prevalence and correlates of eating disorders among Latina/os, Asian Americans, African Americans, and non-Latina/o Whites. Findings indicate similar prevalences of anorexia nervosa and binge eating disorder across all groups. However, 12-month and lifetime prevalence of bulimia nervosa are significantly greater among Latina/os and African Americans. Despite the similar prevalence of binge eating disorder among Latina/os, African Americans, and Asian Americans, lifetime prevalence of any binge eating is greater among these ethnic minority groups in comparison to non-Latina/o Whites.

It is also possible that ethnic minority women, including Latinas, experience comparable sociocultural pressure to conform to majority U.S. culture and that the media and Western values promote unrealistic slender standards and create disordered eating among Latinas (Viladrich, Yeh, Bruning, & Weiss, 2009). However, researchers should also examine associations between disordered eating and discrimination, given the multiple oppressions among Latinas. For example, while Velez, Campos, and Moradi (2015) did not find direct and mediated associations of objectification theory constructs and racist discrimination with eating disorder and depressive symptomatology in a sample of diverse Latinas, they nonetheless found that racist discrimination yields significant positive indirect links with both eating disorder symptomatology and depressive symptomatology through the mediating role of body shame. Similarly, using escape theory, Higgins Neyland, and Bardone-Cone (2016) found support that discriminatory stress has a significant effect on increased binge eating. In addition, the effect of discriminatory stress on binge eating is also mediated by negative affect. Thus, these studies highlight the importance of incorporating cultural factors and discrimination into models of binge eating for Latinas (Higgins Neyland & Bardone-Cone, 2016).

Correlates of Suicidal Ideation and Suicide Attempts

Using data from the NLAAS, Fortuna and colleagues (2007) examined the prevalence and correlates of lifetime suicidal ideation and suicide attempts among Latina/o heritage groups. Lifetime prevalence of suicidal ideation and suicide attempts among Latina/os is 10.1% ($N = 263$) and 4.4% ($N = 117$), respectively. Puerto Ricans are more likely to report suicidal ideation as compared with other Latina/o heritage groups, but this difference is eliminated after adjusting for demographic, psychiatric, and sociocultural covariates. Among Puerto Ricans, 62% report that their attempted suicide occurred when they were under the age of 18. Latina/os with any lifetime DSM-IV depressive, anxiety, or substance abuse disorder, including dual diagnoses, are more likely to report lifetime suicidal ideation and suicide attempts than Latina/os without those disorders. Female gender, acculturation, and high levels of family conflict are also independently and positively correlated with suicide attempts, even among those without any mental health disorders. However, church attendance is a significant protective factor among Latina/os without mental health disorders. These findings highlight the importance of understanding the process of acculturation, the role of the family, and the sociocultural context for suicide risk among Latina/os, especially among young Latina/os.

Data from Metropolitan Statistical Areas (MSAs) indicate that after controlling for a number of variables (Wadsworth & Kubrin, 2007), native-born and immigrant Latina/os are similarly affected by assimilation, mobility, and divorce. However, higher levels of White/Latino inequality lead to greater suicide among native-born Latina/os, while greater African American/Latino inequality lead to less suicide among immigrant Latina/os. Interestingly, MSAs with larger concentrations of well-educated, high-income Latina/os demonstrate lower suicide rates. Wadsworth and Kubrin (2007) suggest that cultural assimilation may contribute to suicide among Latina/os by weakening their cultural protective factors. In addition, increased cultural assimilation increases their isolation and alienation from other Latina/os because of diminished belief systems, rituals, and social networks that promote integration into ethnic communities and strengthen group solidarity.

Domestic Violence among Latinas

Domestic violence against Latinas is a serious social problem and Latinas are often underrepresented within national studies of intimate partner violence (IPV). For example, Hass, Dutton, & Orloff (2000) found that physically and/or sexually abused immigrant Latinas experience significant threats from their abusers, including threats to harm her children and other family members, taking her money, contacting Immigration and Naturalization Services (INS), and threats to kill her. Unfortunately, Latina immigrants are reluctant to report IPV because of their distrust of institutions, fear of immigration authorities, cultural and religious family values that focus on family and community cohesion, financial challenges, embarrassment, social isolation, and limited awareness regarding their legal rights and protections (Coffin-Romig, 2015; Flores-Ortiz, 2004; Hass et al., 2000).

Correlates of IPV among Latinas vary according to within-group variables such as country of origin, level of acculturation, socioeconomic status (SES), and cultural and contextual factors such as marital satisfaction and discrimination (Cho et al., 2014). For example, Cho et al. (2014) examined the prevalence of IPV and associated risk factors among Latinas ($N=604$). Using NLAAS data, participants include Cuban ($N=173$), Puerto Rican ($N=137$), and Mexican ($N=294$) married women, since the data on IPV includes only married couples. Foreign-born Mexican women report greater IPV compared to foreign-born Cuban and Puerto Rican women and greater instances of less injurious IPV (e.g., pushing, grabbing, and object throwing from partners) than their U.S.-born counterparts. Cho et al. (2014) suggest that these rates may reflect how social groups, such as family of origin and formal institutions within Mexico, may fail to recognize IPV as a serious social problem.

However, Latinas with higher levels of education and employment report higher levels of IPV across three heritage groups. Their increased self-reports are attributed to their higher levels of education and empowerment to report IPV, particularly since they tend to have greater knowledge of their legal rights and protections. Lastly, findings indicate that greater marital satisfaction and quality of relational partnership are also associated with a lower incidence of IPV, while perceived discrimination and neighborhood safety are associated with a greater risk for IPV (Cho et al., 2014).

Intermittent Explosive Disorder

An area of research that is limited within the psychological literature is intermittent explosive disorder (IED) among Latina/os. However, Ortega, Canino, and Alegría (2008) examined the occurrence, correlates, and psychiatric comorbidities of lifetime and 12-month prevalence of IED based on NLAAS data. Of the entire sample, 5.8% are classified with lifetime IED and 4.1% with 12-month IED. Unemployment, male gender, and not being married are common risk factors for IED. However, protective factors for both lifetime and 12-month IED include nativity, such as nonmainland nativity, and poor/fair English proficiency. Findings indicate within-group differences, in IED, as Cubans, Mexicans, and other Latina/os have lower odds of both lifetime and 12-month IED as compared with Puerto Ricans. However, Puerto Ricans with lifetime IED do not demonstrate worse impairment as compared with other Latina/os with IED.

Ortega et al. (2008) suggest that the observed odds of IED among Puerto Ricans may not reflect disabling psychopathology, but differences in response styles, as they are often more expressive in their responses to mental health questions. However, depressive, anxiety, substance abuse, and conduct disorder are correlated with IED. Latina/os with lifetime IED on average are six times more likely to report lifetime panic disorder and alcohol dependence. These findings underscore the need for continued studies of IED among Latina/os, as they raise questions whether IED is a manifestation of symptoms among vulnerable individuals who face a wide range of challenges and stressors or whether IED is a valid disorder.

PSYCHIATRIC EPIDEMIOLOGICAL STUDIES OF LATINA/O CHILDREN AND ADOLESCENTS

Mental health disorders among children and adolescents are an important public health issue because of their prevalence and early onset. Moreover, the impact of mental health disorders affects not only children, but also their families and communities, with an estimated annual cost of $247 billion among persons younger than the age of 24, including health care costs, use of services such as special education and juvenile justice, and decreased productivity (Perou et al., 2013). Many epidemiological studies of children rely on parental self-reports, since they are frequently the first adults to identify a child's emotional or behavioral problems. The comprehensive report, *Mental Health Surveillance among Children—United States, 2005–2011* from the CDC (Perou et al., 2013), summarizes data from ongoing federal U.S. surveillance systems and provides prevalence estimates of mental disorders and indicators of children's mental health.

Within this report, data from nine federal surveys and surveillance systems that collect data on children's mental disorders include the following:

- *Autism and Developmental Disabilities Monitoring Network (ADDM)*
- *National Health and Nutrition Examination Survey (NHANES)*
- *National Health Interview Survey (NHIS)*
- *National Survey of Children's Health (NSCH)*
- *National Survey on Drug Use and Health (NSDUH)*
- *National Violent Death Reporting System (NVDRS)*
- *National Vital Statistics System (NVSS)*
- *National Youth Behavior Survey (NYBS)*
- *School-Associated Violent Death Study (SAVD)*

Despite the differences in goals and methodologies of these surveillance systems, mental health disorders addressed within this report include the following DSM-IV (Text Revision) (DSM-IV-TR) disorders: attention-deficit/hyperactivity disorder (ADHD); disruptive behavioral disorders, including oppositional defiant disorder (ODD) and conduct disorder; autism spectrum disorders (ASDs); and mood and anxiety disorders including depression, tic disorders, and substance use disorders. In addition, suicide and mentally unhealthy days are also addressed within this report (Perou et al., 2013).

Findings from the *Mental Health Surveillance among Children—United States, 2005–2011 Report* indicate that attention-deficit/hyperactivity disorder (ADHD) is the most prevalent parent-reported diagnosis among children aged 3 to 17 years (6.8%), followed by behavioral or conduct problems (3.5%), anxiety (3.0%), depression (2.1%), autism spectrum disorders (1.1%), and Tourette syndrome (0.2% among children between the ages of 6 to 17 years) (Perou et al., 2013). An estimated 4.7% of adolescents aged 12–17 report an illicit drug use disorder in the past year, 4.2% report an alcohol abuse disorder in the past year, and 2.8% report cigarette dependence in the past year. The overall suicide rate for persons between the ages of 10 and 19 is 4.5 per 100,000 persons. Lastly, approximately 8% of adolescents between the ages of 12 and 17 report more than 14 mentally unhealthy days in the past month (Perou et al., 2013) (see Table 6.2). However, research regarding Latina/o youth indicates that they demonstrate high rates of anxiety, depressive symptoms, suicide ideation and attempts, and experimentation with illicit drugs. Experts suggest that differences in parental self-reports and clinical bias also contribute to challenges in identifying psychological disorders and mental health disparities among Latina/o children (Cross, Bazron, Dennis, & Isaacs, 1989; Morgan, Staff, Hillemeier, Farkas, & Maczuga, 2013; Pumariega, Rogers, & Roth, 2005). For example, Latina/o children from kindergarten to eighth grade are less likely to receive an ADHD diagnosis (56%) and less likely to receive multimodality treatment for ADHD (Pumariega et al., 2005).

ADHD, ODD, and Conduct Disorder

ADHD, ODD, and conduct disorder are a set of behavioral disorders that frequently co-occur. Data from the 2007 NSCH indicate that ADHD is the most prevalent parent-reported diagnosis among children aged 3 to 17 years (6.8%), with prevalence rates that are higher among males (9.6%) than among females (3.8%) and among the insured (7.1%) than among the uninsured (3.5%). There are also age differences, children aged 12–17 (8.8%) and 6–11 (7.5%), demonstrate higher prevalence rates than their peers between the ages of 3 and 5 (1.1%). Multiracial (10.2%) children also report higher prevalence of ADHD than their African American/Black

Table 6.2 Estimated Prevalence and Number of Children with Mental Disorders, Including Latina/o Children—NHIS, NSCH, NSDUH, and NHANES, United States, 2007–2011

Condition	Surveillance System and Years	Age Range (Years)	Sample Size (Number of persons surveyed)	Weighted Prevalence (%)	Weighted Number of Children	Prevalence among Latina/o Children
Attention-deficit/ hyperactivity disorder	NHIS 2007–2008	3–17	14,970	7.6 (ever)	4,718,000	4.1
	NHIS 2009–2010	3–17	18,411	8.5 (ever)	5,232,000	4.6
	NHIS 2011	3–17	10,554	8.4 (ever)	5,246,000	5.6
	NSCH 2007	3–17	78,042	8.9 (ever)	5,482,000	5.4
	NSCH 2007	3–17	78,042	6.8 (current)	4,188,000	4.0
Behavioral or conduct problems	NSCH 2007	3–17	78,042	4.6 (ever)	2,833,000	3.9
	NSCH 2007	3–17	78,042	3.5 (ever)	2,156,000	3.2
Autism spectrum disorders	NHIS 2007–2008	3–17	14,970	0.8 (ever autism)	485,000	0.5
	NHIS 2009–2010	3–17	18,411	1.1 (ever autism)	667,000	0.7
	NSCH 2007	3–17	78,042	1.8 (ever ASD)	1,109,000	1.3
	NSCH 2007	3–17	78,042	1.1 (current ASD)	678,000	1.0
Depression	NHIS 2007	4–17	7,103	3.0 (past year)	1,706,000	2.4
	NSCH 2007	3–17	78,042	3.9 (ever)	2,402,000	3.9
	NSCH 2007	3–17	78,042	2.1 (current)	1,293,000	1.8

	Survey	Age	Sample	Measure	Estimate	Percent
	NSDUH 2010–2011	12–17	45,500	12.8 (lifetime)	3,106,000	13.0
	NSDUH 2010–2011	12–17	45,500	8.1 (MDE past year)	1,961,000	7.9
	NHANES 2007–2010	12–17	1,782	6.7 (PHQ-9, past two weeks)	1,708,000	5.7
Anxiety	NHIS 2007	4–17	7,103	2.6 (phobia, past year)	1,515,000	2.5
	NSCH 2007	3–17	78,042	4.7 (ever)	2,895,000	4.6
	NSCH 2007	3–17	78,042	3.0 (current)	1,848,000	2.6
Alcohol use disorder	NSDUH 2010–2011	12–17	45,500	4.2 (past year)	1,028,000	4.5
Illicit drug use disorder	NSDUH 2010–2011	12–17	45,500	4.7 (past year)	1,155,000	20.9
Cigarette dependence	NSDUH 2010–2011	6–17	64,034	2.8 (past month)	691,000	1.8
Tourette syndrome	NSCH 2007	12–17	3,312	0.3 (ever)	148,000	0.2
	NSCH 2007		64,034	0.2 (current)	99,000	—
≥14 mentally unhealthy days	NHANES 2005–2010	12–17	3,312	8.3 (past 30 days)	1,995,000	4.9

Note: MDE=major depressive episode; NHANES=National Health and Nutrition Examination Survey; NHIS=National Health Interview Survey; NSCH=National Survey of Children's Health; NSDUH=National Survey on Drug Use and Health; PHQ-9=nine-item Patient Health Questionnaire.
Source: Centers for Disease Control and Prevention (2013). Mental health surveillance among children—United States, 2005–2011. *Morbidity and Mortality Weekly Report (MMWR) Supplement, 62*, 1–35.

(7.7%), White/European American (7.6%), Latina/o (4.0%), and Other (3.0%) peers (Perou et al., 2013).

Data from the 2007 NSCH also indicate that 3.5% of children aged 3–17 years have a current parent-reported diagnosis of behavioral or conduct problems, with higher prevalence rates among males (4.6%) than among females (2.2%). However, there are no differences in insurance coverage (3.5% insured vs. 3.3% uninsured). There are also age differences, as children aged 12–17 (4.2%) and 6–11 (3.8%) demonstrate greater prevalence of a diagnosis of behavioral or conduct problems than their peers between the ages of 3 and 5 (1.3%). African American/Black (6.0%) and Multiracial (4.0) children also report higher prevalence rates than Latina/o (3.2%), White/European American (3.0%), and Other (1.6%) children (Perou et al., 2013).

Despite these findings suggesting a lower prevalence of ADHD among Latina/o youth, smaller studies suggest that compared to their White/European American counterparts, Latina/o children from kindergarten to eighth grade are less likely to receive an ADHD diagnosis (56%) and also less likely to take prescription medication (Morgan et al., 2013). Unfortunately, they are also less likely to receive multimodality treatment for ADHD (Pumariega et al., 2005). However, it is also hypothesized cultural factors, play a role. For example, Arcia, Castillo, and Fernández (2004) reported that Cuban, Dominican, and Puerto Rican mothers whose children exhibit disruptive behaviors, including symptoms of ADHD, ODD, and conduct disorder often use terms such as *nervios* (nerves) and anxiety to describe their children's disruptive behaviors and temperament traits.

Anxiety Disorders

Parental self-reports from the 2007 NSCH indicate that 3.0% of children aged 3–17 years have a diagnosis of anxiety, with higher prevalence rates among males (3.4%) than among females (2.6%) and among those who are insured (3.1%) than among the uninsured (1.7%). Higher prevalence rates are observed among children aged 12–17 (4.1%) and 6–11 (2.9%), as compared with those aged 3–5 (1.0%). Multiracial (4.7%) and White/European American (3.4%) children demonstrate greater prevalence of an anxiety disorder as compared with their Latina/o (2.6%), African American/Black (2.2%), and Other (2.0%) peers (Perou et al., 2013).

However, despite the low prevalence of anxiety among Latina/o youth, caution is warranted, as other research suggests that Latina/o adolescents experience high rates of anxiety. For example, in a study examining differences in internalizing and externalizing behaviors among Latina/o (i.e., Cuban, Mexican, and Puerto Rican), African American, and White/

European American middle school students from Connecticut (McLaughlin, Hilt, & Nolen-Hoeksema, 2016), indicated that Latina/os, particularly Latinas, report higher levels of anxiety symptoms than their counterparts and high levels of separation anxiety and worry, regardless of gender. In addition, Latinas report the highest levels of global anxiety symptoms and physical symptoms of anxiety. Latina/o adolescents also report higher levels of polyvictimization and trauma-related mental health symptoms (i.e., symptoms of post-traumatic stress and depression) than their White/ European American peers (Andrews et al., 2015), perhaps due to neighborhood disadvantage (Rubens, Gudiño, Fite, & Grande, 2016), exposure to unique migration stressors (Potochnick & Perreria, 2010), discrimination (Smokowski & Bacallao, 2007; Smokowski et al., 2007), and social problems (Smokowski et al., 2007). In addition, Latina/o children may express negative affective and anxious states (Varela & Hensely-Maloney, 2009), through idioms of distress, such as *nervios* (nerves) and *ataques de nervios* (ataque of nerves; Arcia et al., 2004; Guarnaccia et al., 2005b; López et al., 2009; López, Ramirez, Guarnaccia, Canino, & Bird, 2011).

Depression

Unfortunately, Latina/o adolescents have among the highest rates of depressive symptoms and suicide ideation and attempts, and this persistent disparity was documented in the 1960s (Romero et al., 2014a). Parental self-reports from the 2007 NSCH indicate that 2.1% of children aged 3–17 years have a current diagnosis of depression but there are no differences based on gender (2.1% of males and 2.0% of females) or insurance status (2.1% of insured and 1.8% of uninsured). However, there are age differences; children aged 12–17 (3.5%) report higher prevalence of depression as compared with children aged 6–11 (1.4%) and 3–5 (0.5%). Multiracial (3.5%) children demonstrate greater prevalence of depression, followed by African American/Black (2.2%), White/European American (2.1%), Latina/o (1.8%), and Other (1.4%) (Perou et al., 2013).

Data from the 2010–2011 NSDUH suggests greater prevalence of lifetime major depressive disorder among adolescents. For example, 18% of adolescents aged 12–17 report a lifetime major depressive disorder, as do females (18.2% vs. 7.7%). However, prevalence rates do not differ based on insurance coverage (14.5% uninsured vs. 12.7% insured). Multiracial (16.2%) adolescents report greater prevalence of lifetime major depressive disorder than their White/European American (13.2%), Latina/o (13.0%), Other (11.7%), and African American/Black (11.1%) peers (Perou et al., 2013).

While these studies do not indicate a high prevalence of depression among Latina/o children, there is a large body of research that supports the prevalence of depression among Latina/o youth, particularly Latinas (see Romero et al., 2013). For example, Romero et al. (2014a) suggest that the high rates of depression among Latinas have been an *enduring epidemic* for the past 30 years. Equally problematic is the lack of research that examines within-group differences among Latina adolescents. Bámaca-Colbert, Plunkett, and Espinosa-Hernández (2011) indicate that overall family dynamics (i.e., conflict and family functioning and parent–adolescent relationship qualities (i.e., support, inconsistent discipline) may contribute to the risk of depression among Latina adolescents. Also, romantic and peer relationship qualities (i.e., duration, intensity, support) can also minimize or enhance depressive symptoms. Moreover, cultural factors, such as acculturative stress and discrimination can also exacerbate their risk of depression (p. 53).

Autism Spectrum Disorders

Data from the 2007 NSCH indicate that 1.1% of children aged 3–17 years have a parent-reported diagnosis of current autism or autism spectrum disorder (ASD), with higher prevalence rates among males (1.7%) than among females (0.4%). There are similar prevalence rates among children aged 6–11 (1.4%), 12–17 (1.0%), and 3–5 (0.9%). White/European American (1.3%) and Latina/o (1.0%) children report a similar prevalence of current autism or autism spectrum disorder as well as among Multiracial (0.7), Other (0.7%), and African American/Black (0.6%) children (Perou et al., 2013). However, Magaña, Lopez, and Machalicek (2017) note that the prevalence of ASD among Latina/o children increased by 110% between 2002 and 2008, compared to a 70% increase for White/European American children. They note that Latina/o children are diagnosed later and are less likely to receive specialty autism services than their White/European American counterparts and that Latina/o families seek additional information regarding autism and assisting their children and require additional social and financial support.

Tic Disorders

In comparison to other psychological disorders among children, large studies regarding Tourette syndrome are limited. Parental self-reports from the 2007 NSCH provide current estimates of Tourette syndrome. Data indicate that 0.2% of children aged 6–17 years have a current parent-reported diagnosis of Tourette syndrome, with higher prevalence rates among males than among females (0.4% vs. 0.2%) and higher prevalence rates among children aged 12–17 than among children aged 6–11 (0.4% vs. 0.2%). White/European American children (0.4%) demonstrate higher prevalence than Latina/o (0.2%) or African American (0.2%) peers. Among children with a diagnosis of Tourette syndrome, 79% also demonstrate a diagnosis of at least one other mental disorder (ADHD, behavioral problems, depression, anxiety, or ASD) (Perou et al., 2013).

Substance Use Disorders and Substance Use

Although not all Latina/o adolescents use drugs and alcohol, the current substance use patterns among Latina/o adolescents are alarming. According to the 2010–2011 NSDUH, an estimated 4.7% of adolescents aged 12–17 report an illicit drug use disorder in the past year. Males (4.8%) and females (4.6%) report similar prevalence but uninsured adolescents (5.1%) report greater prevalence than insured (4.7%) adolescents. Multiracial (6.4%) and Latina/o (5.7%) adolescents report greater illicit drug use disorder than their White/European American (4.6%), African American/Black (4.1%), and Other (2.8%) peers (Perou et al., 2013). The 2010–2011 NSDUH also indicates that an estimated 4.2% of adolescents aged 12–17 report past-year alcohol abuse disorder, with higher prevalence rates among females (4.7%) than among males (3.7%) and among uninsured (5.9%) than among insured (4.0) adolescents. Multiracial adolescents (6.4%) report greater prevalence of illicit drug use disorder than Latina/o (5.7%), White/European American (4.6%), Other (2.7%), and African American/Black (2.4%) adolescents (Perou et al., 2013). Lastly, the 2010–2011 NSDUH estimates that 2.8% of adolescents aged 12–17 report having cigarette dependence in the past year. Prevalence rates are higher among males (3.0%) than among females (2.5%) and among uninsured (3.7%) than among insured (2.7%) adolescents. Multiracial (4.1%) and White/European American (3.6%) adolescents report higher prevalence of cigarette dependence than Latina/o (1.8%), African American/Black (1.6%), and Other (1.2%) adolescents (Perou et al., 2013).

The 2015 Youth Risk Behavior Surveillance System (YRBSS; Kann et al., 2016) is a nationally representative sample of high school students from public and private schools ($N=15,624$). Of the total sample, 63.2% report prior alcohol consumption, and females report higher rates (65.3%) than males (61.4%). Latina/os (65.9%) and White/European Americans (65.3%) report greater alcohol consumption than African Americans (54.4%), as well as higher marijuana use (45.6%) than African Americans (45.5%) and White/European Americans (35.2%) (Kann et al., 2016). The YRBSS also aids in our understanding of substance use among Latina/o adolescents, and it indicates that they are disproportionally involved in *early* substance use (see Table 6.3). For example, as compared with their White/European American and African American peers, Latina/os demonstrate earlier use of cigarettes, electronic vapor products, and alcohol and experiment with illicit

Table 6.3 Youth Risk Behavior Surveillance (YRBSS)—United States, 2015

	White/European American			Black/African American			Latina/o		
	Female	Male	Total	Female	Male	Total	Female	Male	Total
Cigarette/Tobacco/Electronic Vapor									
Ever tried cigarette smoking	30.4	33.2	**31.8**	29.5	30.6	**30.1**	32.7	37.8	**35.2**
Smoked a whole cigarette before age 13	5.3	6.6	**6.0**	3.8	10.1	**7.0**	4.9	9.2	**7.1**
Current cigarette use	12.2	12.7	**12.4**	3.7	9.1	**6.5**	7.1	11.3	**9.2**
Ever tried electronic vapor products	42.3	44.0	**43.2**	37.7	46.5	**42.4**	51.2	52.6	**51.9**
Current electronic vapor use	24.2	26.3	**25.2**	14.5	21.2	**18.0**	25.0	27.4	**26.3**
Alcohol									
Ever drank alcohol	66.7	64.0	**65.3**	57.9	51.0	**54.4**	68.6	63.4	**65.9**
Drank alcohol before age 13	11.7	17.3	**14.5**	16.9	18.7	**18.0**	19.0	23.6	**21.3**
Current alcohol use	35.3	35.2	**35.2**	25.9	22.1	**23.8**	35.6	33.4	**34.4**
Largest no. of drinks in a row was ≥10	2.4	6.6	**4.5**	1.0	3.2	**2.1**	3.6	6.5	**5.1**

Marijuana

Ever used marijuana	34.3	36.2	35.2	40.5	49.7	45.5	45.3	46.0	45.6
Current marijuana use	18.7	21.2	19.9	22.1	31.3	27.1	23.5	25.5	24.5

Other Drugs

Ever used hallucinogens	4.7	8.1	6.4	1.9	6.7	4.7	6.1	7.4	6.8
Ever used cocaine	3.3	5.0	4.1	1.8	5.3	3.8	6.6	9.4	8.0
Ever used ecstasy	4.0	4.7	4.3	2.5	5.9	4.3	4.1	7.8	6.1
Ever used inhalants	5.9	6.9	6.4	5.9	7.1	6.8	8.3	7.1	7.8
Ever used heroine	0.8	1.7	1.3	1.5	3.8	2.7	1.9	3.2	2.6
Ever used methamphetamines	1.7	2.5	2.1	1.4	3.9	2.8	4.0	4.7	4.4
Ever took steroids without a doctor's prescription	1.8	3.6	2.7	3.6	4.8	4.5	3.9	4.1	4.1
Ever took prescription drugs without a doctor's prescription	15.9	17.1	16.5	10.7	18.1	14.8	16.5	18.4	17.5

Source: Kann, H., McManus, T., Harris, W. A., Shanklin, S. L., Flint, K. H., Hawkins, J., Stephanie. . . . & Zaza, S. (2016). Youth Risk Behavior Surveillance—United States, 2015. *MMWR: Morbidity & Mortality Weekly Report, 65,* 1–174.

drugs at higher rates than their peers. In addition to marijuana, they have the highest prevalence of smoking a cigarette (7.1%) and alcohol consumption (21.3%) before age 13. They also demonstrate greater experimentation with illicit substances than their White/European American and Black/African American peers, including hallucinogens (6.8%), cocaine (8.0%), ecstasy (6.1%), inhalants (7.8%), and methamphetamines (4.4%) (Kann et al., 2016).

Unfortunately, there are few studies that examine the independent effects of gender, ethnicity, and acculturation on drinking behavior among Latina/o adolescents. However, using data from National Longitudinal Study of Adolescent Health to Adult Health (Add Health), Wahl and Eitle (2010) examined alcohol use and binge drinking among a diverse sample of adolescents, including White/European Americans ($N=6,792$), Mexican Americans ($N=910$), Cuban Americans ($N=290$), and Puerto Ricans ($N=336$). Their findings indicate significant gender differences in alcohol use among first generation Mexican American and Puerto Ricans and second generation Cuban American male adolescents. Binge drinking differs significantly by gender among first-generation Mexican American and Cuban American adolescents and third-generation Puerto Rican male adolescents. In each case, males are more likely to use alcohol and binge drink than their female counterparts.

These findings underscore the need include Latina/o adolescents from diverse heritage groups within large studies and risk and protective factors, given that they are at greater risk for problems that are associated with substance use, such as academic failure, incarceration, and poor mental health (Okamoto, Ritt-Olson, Soto, Baezconde-Garbanati, & Unger, 2009). Protective factors include engagement in prosocial activities such as academics and organized after-school activities; the ability to contribute meaningfully to one's family, school, and community; recognition of contributions by teachers and family; strong bonds with family members and school; and a strong ethnic identity. Conversely, risk factors include peer pressure, stress, developmental influences, and negative role models, as well as discrimination, acculturation, family influences, access to illicit substances, misperceptions about risks of drug use, reduced social disapproval of drug use, and ethnic identity (Castro et al., 2009; Catalano, Haggerty, Hawkins, & Elgin, 2011; Molina et al., 2016; Okamoto et al., 2009; Romero & Roberts, 2003; Schinke, Hopkins, & Wahlstrom, 2016; Vaughan, Gassman, Jun, & Seitz de Martinez, 2015). For instance, perceived discrimination is particularly stressful for Latina/o adolescents, and it is hypothesized that their substance use is a means to cope with discrimination and therefore consequently associated with both lifetime and recent use of cigarettes, alcohol, marijuana, and inhalants among Latina/o adolescents (Okamoto et al., 2009).

Number of Mentally Unhealthy Days

Depression is a prominent risk indicator for suicide, and as previously discussed, Latina/os demonstrate alarming rates of depression (Romero et al., 2014a). The 2005–2010 NHANES indicates that approximately 8% of adolescents between the ages of 12 and 17 report more than 14 mentally unhealthy days in the past month. More than 14 mentally unhealthy days are reported by more females (10%) than males (6.7%). White/European American (9.6%) adolescents also more often report more than 14 mentally unhealthy days than their African American (6.6%) and Mexican American (4.9%) peers (Perou et al., 2013). However, the YRBSS suggests that 29.9% of adolescents feel sad or hopeless for two or more weeks and no longer engage in their usual activities, and females (39.8%) report greater sadness and hopelessness than males (20.3%). Latina/os (35.3%) report greater sadness and hopelessness than their White/European American (28.6%) or African American (25.2%) peers (Kann et al., 2016). The implications of their depressive symptoms are discussed in the next section because of the epidemic of Latina suicide.

Suicide

Suicide among Latina/o adolescents is an epidemic and a national health and mental health concern. According to the 2010 NVSS, the overall suicide rate for young persons between the ages of 10 and 19 is 4.5 per 100,000 persons. Gender differences exist, as males demonstrate higher rates of suicide deaths (6.9%, $N=1,503$) than females (2.0%, $N=423$). Also, adolescents between the ages of 15 and 19 (7.5%) demonstrate greater rates of suicide deaths, as compared with adolescents between the ages of 10 and 14 (1.3%). White/European Americans (5.3%) and Others (5.3%) also demonstrate greater rates of suicide deaths as compared with Latina/os (3.3%) and African American/Blacks (1.6%). Methods of suicide include hanging/suffocation (2.2%), firearms (1.8%), poisoning (0.3%), and other (0.3%) (Perou et al., 2013).

The 2015 YRBSS indicates alarming suicide rates (Kann et al., 2016). Findings indicate that 17.7% of adolescents report suicidal ideation during the past year, and gender differences exist, as females (23.4%) demonstrate greater suicidal ideation than males (12.2%). Latina/os (18.8%) and White/European Americans (17.2%) report greater suicidal ideation than African American/Blacks (14.5%). Latinas demonstrate significantly higher suicidal ideation (25.6%) than Latinos (12.4%). In terms of suicide plans, 14.6% of adolescents made suicide plans during the past year, with higher rates among Latina/o (15.7%) than their White/European American (13.9%)

and African American/Black (13.7%) peers. Unfortunately, Latinas (20.7%) report significantly higher rates of suicide plans than Latinos (10.9%).

The same study suggests that 8.6% of high school students attempted suicide during the past year, with higher rates among Latina/os (11.3%) and African American (8.9%) adolescents as compared with their White/European American (6.8%) peers. Suicide attempts are twice as high among Latinas (15.1%) as compared with Latinos (7.6%) (Kann et al., 2016). Studies such as the YRBSS are also helpful in identifying differences in suicidal ideation among Latina/o adolescents, but given the diversity among this population, the need to examine differences in heritage groups is also paramount.

Zayas and colleagues (2005) developed a conceptual model to guide research and intervention programs on Latina suicide. Their model postulates that interactions between family functioning, adolescent development, and cultural traditions may lead to emotional vulnerability and psychosocial functioning. In addition, the distinctive mother–daughter relationship also plays a central role in the adolescent's behavior. Thus, a suicide attempt is influenced by a combination of these factors and mediated by a Latina's subjective experience of adolescent–family crisis. Similarly, Romero et al. (2014a) propose that the multiracial feminist framework (Arellano & Ayala-Alcantar, 2004; Baca-Zinn & Dill, 1996) offers a gendered perspective that focuses on the resilience, equality, and empowerment of Latinas. They note that despite the epidemic of Latina depressive symptoms and suicide attempts, it is important to recognize that Latinas often emerge as resilient. Furthermore, young Latinas are "active agents in negotiating their identities, families, peers, and schools" and their close family connections and communication, positive ethnic identity, religiosity/spirituality, biculturalism/bilingualism, and engaged coping styles are sources of cultural strength and resilience (pp. 48–49). While recognizing the realities of their inequalities as women of color, Romero et al. (2014a) note that they refuse to portray Latina adolescents as victims of their culture, class, or families and therefore focus on their strengths so that prevention efforts, treatment, policies, and schools also focus on these important areas.

IDIOMS OF DISTRESS

In addition to understanding the factors that shape mental health disorders among Latina/os, it is equally important to examine prominent idioms of distress, as they may present with symptoms that diverge from mainstream nosology. Idioms of distress reflect a broad range of expressions in which cultural groups experience, express, and cope with their feelings of distress (Aguilar-Gaxiola, Kramer, Resendez, & Magaña, 2008). Despite regional and linguistic variations among Latina/os, idioms of distress are culturally sanctioned constructions of physical, psychosocial, or psychospiritual distress (Guarnaccia et al., 2003; Salgado de Snyder et al., 2000). Furthermore, idioms of distress among Latina/os are culturally accepted illnesses that signal distress through a variety of somatic and physical symptoms. They also evolve from a context characterized by social oppression and enable disenfranchised Latina/os to express their anger and powerlessness (Salgado de Snyder et al., 2000).

Scholars recommend assessing for idioms of distress among Latina/o clients, as well as the exploring trauma, dissociative features, and suicide risk (Lewis-Fernandez et al., 2010). Although the DSM-5 focuses largely on *susto* (fright), *nervios* (nerves), and *ataque de nervios* (attack of nerves), other idioms are also recognized. (See Chapter 2 for a discussion of other idioms.) Comas-Díaz (2012b) suggests that other idioms are also recognized within Latin America, such as *patatús* (dizzy spell), *salazón* (physical state of dehydration), *corriente de aire* (health risk due to a stream of air), *cuerpo cortado* (malaise, flu symptoms), *muscarañas* (daydreaming, lack of focus), *telele* (an *ataque* due to unfinished work), and *fiaca* (laziness).

In terms of psychological stressors, scholars also often focus on *susto* (fright), *nervios* (nerves), and *ataque de nervios* (attack of nerves). These syndromes are clinically important because of their associations with a variety of mental health disorders, including depression, anxiety, and panic disorder (Durà-Vilà & Hodes, 2012; Guarnaccia et al., 2003; Salgado de Snyder et al., 2000; Weller et al., 2008). It is important to recognize that there are multiple models of distress that influence clinical presentations and help-seeking behavior. Thus, mental health providers must familiarize themselves with these idioms of distress to avoid misdiagnosis of their Latina/o clients. However, it is also prudent to avoid taking these translations at face value, as their English translations do not have the same connotation.

Ataques de Nervios

Ataques de nervios, often referred to as *ataques*, were first attributed to distress among Puerto Ricans, but research indicates that other Latina/os also experience *ataques* (Guarnaccia et al., 2010; Lewis-Fernández et al., 2009, 2010). *Ataques* involves a loss of control in several important domains of experience, including emotional expressions, bodily sensations, action dimensions, and changes in consciousness. The loss of control is precipitated by stressful events, such as interpersonal conflict or the death of a loved one (Guarnaccia, Rivera, Franco, & Neighbors, 1996). While presentation of *ataques* vary, common symptoms include the following: shouting uncontrollably, attacks of crying, trembling, difficulty breathing, dizziness, a feeling of the mind going "blank" and numbness or tingling sensations, and becoming verbally and physically abusive. Dissociative symptoms, suicidal ideation, and seizures can also occur (Lewis-Fernández et al., 2010). Epidemiological studies report an estimated prevalence of 14% among Puerto Ricans who reside on the Island (Guarnaccia, Canino, Rubio-Stipec, & Bravo, 1993). Among Island children, lifetime prevalence ranges from 9% among children in community settings and 26% in clinical settings (Guarnaccia et al., 2005b). Prevalence rates of diverse Latina/os range from 9% among Mexicans and Cubans (Guarnaccia et al., 2010) to 44% among Dominican, Mexican, and Central and South American outpatients (Lewis-Fernández et al., 2010).

Ataques are interpreted as an outlet for expressing anger, upset, frustration, or sadness at the stressful event, but their expression is also a culturally sanctioned mechanism to escape from the stressful event and a way to elicit assistance and sympathy from others (De la Cancela, Guarnaccia, & Carrillo, 1986; Durà-Vilà & Hodes, 2012). Studies of *ataques* among Puerto Ricans indicate that age and gender are associated with an *ataque* endorsement (Guarnaccia et al., 1993, 2005), as well as a divorced marital status (Guarnaccia et al., 1996, 2005b, 2010). In addition, *ataques* are associated with diverse anxiety, depressive, and somatoform disorders (Guarnaccia et al., 1993, 2005b), as well as higher rates of use of general medical and specialty mental health services (Guarnaccia et al., 2010). Studies of community samples indicate that lifetime endorsement of *ataques* is associated with greater suicidal ideation, disability due to mental health problems, trauma, and the use of outpatient psychiatric services (Lewis-Fernández et al., 2009). In their examination of psychiatric outpatients, including Dominican, Mexican, and Central and South Americans, Lewis-Fernández et al. (2010) also reported a comorbid relationship between *ataques* and dissociative symptoms and disorders

However, to fully understand *ataques*, it is important to examine the social, political, and economic circumstances of Latina/os (Guarnaccia et al., 2010), as social vulnerability also creates a sense of hopelessness and lack of control due to the effects of migration and the pressure to assimilate (De la Cancela et al., 1986). *Ataques* is also associated with somatic complaints among Latina/o children and worse outcomes among mainland children (López, Ramirez, Guarnaccia, Canino, & Bird, 2011; López et al., 2009). For example, among Puerto Rican children residing in the Bronx and San Juan, Puerto Rico, *ataques* is associated with asthma, headaches, stomachaches, and a history of seizures or epilepsy (López et al., 2011). Site comparisons also indicate that children from San Juan demonstrate a higher-risk profile because of their increased likelihood of a diagnosed injury than children from the Bronx (24% vs. 5%). However, children from the Bronx are at risk for greater somatic complaints as compared with those without *ataques* at this site, perhaps because of greater exposure to risk factors such as violence and stress (López et al., 2011).

Nervios

Nervios (nerves) is often described by Latina/os to refer to chronic dysphoric mood states that accompany somatic complaints (Durà-Vilà & Hodes, 2012) and *nervios* is described as a less extreme form of *ataque de nervios* (Weller et al., 2008). Common symptoms include nervousness, sleep disturbances, tearfulness, difficulties concentrating, irritability, and somatic symptoms such as headaches, chest pains, stomach disturbances, tingling sensations, dizziness, and high/low blood pressure. *Nervios* are often triggered by stressful events, such as anger, grief, and illness (Durà-Vilà & Hodes, 2012; Weller et al., 2008). There are variations in rates of *nervios* by geographic region, including prevalence that ranges from 17.1% to 63% among Latina/os from the United States, Mexico, and Central America (Baer et al., 2003; O'Connor, Stoecklin-Marois, & Schenker, 2015; Weller et al., 2008).

Cultural and social contexts are also important in understanding the experience of *nervios* among Latina/os, as they are socially sanctioned expressions and reactions to adverse circumstances such as family discord (Durà-Vilà & Hodes, 2012) and a coping strategy to temporarily free oneself from dealing with multiple roles and responsibilities (Durà-Vilà & Hodes, 2012; Salgado de Snyder et al., 2000). *Nervios* also occurs among individuals with subordinate social roles, such as women or the poor (Weller et al., 2008). For example, among Mexican and Central American male farmworkers in California, O'Connor et al. (2015) report that income, drug use, poor self-rated physical health, high perceived stress, depressive symptoms, and poor housing conditions are strongly associated with *nervios*. Lamentably, poor housing conditions, such as home disrepair, increase the risk of *nervios*. The presence of home disrepair, water leaks, mold, and cockroaches are individually associated with *nervios* among Mexican and Central American male farmworkers.

There are also different types of *nervios*. For example, Guarnaccia et al. (2003) developed a popular Puerto Rican nosology of *nervios* to prevent misdiagnosis among Puerto Ricans and other Latina/os who present with *nervios* and *ataques*. In addition, the development of a popular nosology allows for the focus of the interpersonal, social, political, economic, and spiritual sources of distress (Guarnaccia et al., 2003, p. 330). This classification includes being a nervous person since childhood (*ser nervioso desde chiquito*), suffering from nerves (*padecer de los nervios*), and being sick from nerves (*estar enfermo de los nervios*).

Susto

Susto (fright) is described as an experience of fright, with regional variations in symptoms and treatment among Latina/os (Weller et al., 2002). Common symptoms include restlessness during sleep, shaking/trembling, agitation, general malaise, listlessness, loss of appetite, weight loss, crying, bad dreams, and somatic complaints including muscle aches and pains (Durà-Vilà & Hodes, 2012; Weller et al., 2008). *Susto* is often attributed to frightening experiences that cause a loss of vital substance or force that results in disconnection from the body (Glazer, Baer, Weller, Garcia de Alba, & Liebowitz, 2004). Prevalence rates of susto also vary, as rural Guatemalans report a 37% lifetime prevalence of *susto*, Mexican residents from Guadalajara report a prevalence of 58%, and Mexican Americans from Texas report a prevalence of 59% (Weller et al., 2008). However, 70.1% of Mexican migrant farmworkers report a lifetime prevalence of *nervios* and 22.3 report a current episode (Donlan & Lee, 2010).

The failure to fulfill important social roles and expectations may also contribute to the expression of *susto*. For example, female Mexican migrant farmworkers report greater depression severity scores and greater current and lifetime prevalence of *susto*. As a group, Mexican migrant farmworkers with lifetime prevalence of *susto* also report greater suicidal ideation or thoughts of suicide (Donlan & Lee, 2010). Although *susto* is no longer conceptualized as soul loss but as the loss of a vital force, certain Latina/os may equate soul loss with death (Glazer et al., 2004; Weller et al., 2002) or diabetes (Weller et al., 2002), and these perceptions may reflect the chronic and debilitating nature of *susto*. For example, in their landmark study of *susto* among *mestizo* and indigenous adults in Mexico, Rubel, O'Nell, and Collado-Ardón (1984) found that personal or social stress is a necessary condition for *susto* and not a frightening experience because of the link with greater stress and physical disease, as well as increased mortality. Similarly, Baer et al. (2003) found that *susto* is associated with an increased risk of comorbidity and increased mortality.

It is interesting to note that the small number of studies that examine co-occurrence of idioms of distress among Latinos support the existence of the co-occurrence of *susto*, *mal de ojo*, *empacho*, and *ataques de nervios* among Latina/o primary care patients in Texas (Bayles & Katerndahl, 2009), *coraje*, *nervios*, and *susto* among Mexican migrant farmworkers (Donlan & Lee, 2010), and *nervios* and *susto* among adults from Guadalajara, Mexico

(Weller et al., 2002, 2010). These studies suggest that these idioms of distress are distinct but that they are also chronic conditions. For example, Donlan and Lee (2010) indicate that among *coraje, nervios,* and *susto,* the relationship between current and lifetime prevalence is statistically significant, with strong effect sizes that range between .48 and .69, and *nervios* is more likely to recur. Since these idioms of distress are associated with stressors in the social environment and chronic stress, they reflect the realities of vulnerabilities associated with their economic, social, and political circumstances. Thus, these vulnerabilities have both health and mental health implications for Latina/os and highlight the need to recognize the need for early identification and adequate intervention of idioms of distress to effectively prevent psychological disorders and physical illness (Salgado de Snyder et al., 2000).

CONCLUSION

Our review highlights the protective and risk factors that impact the mental health of Latina/os. Epidemiological studies from the NLAAS are particularly helpful in identifying differences in lifetime mental health disorders among Latina/o heritage groups and differences based on demographic variables. However, these studies are neither recent nor based on DSM-5 criteria. Thus, large-scale epidemiological studies based on DSM-5 criteria are warranted, including studies that focus on LGBTQIA Latina/o adults and youth. While findings from the Mental Health Surveillance among Children Report are helpful, they are limited in their parental self-reports and small samples of Latina/os. Alike Latina/o adults, large-scale epidemiological studies on Latina/o children and adolescents are also warranted to also examine within-group differences and the role of demographic and cultural variables. An understanding of idioms of distress is also imperative, as it is important to note that the manifestation of somatic symptoms among Latina/os is not always indicative of psychopathology. Instead, they are indicative of a "cry for help" and precursors to serious medical and mental health outcomes, particularly among Latina/os with limited resources and multiple demands (Salgado de Snyder et al., 2000).

Chapter 7

Mental Health Barriers among Latina/os

It is inherently better to prevent an illness from occurring in the first place than to need to treat it once it develops. Just as other areas of medicine have promoted healthy lifestyles and thereby have reduced the incidence of conditions such as heart disease and some cancers, so now is the time for mental health providers, researchers, and policy makers to focus more on promoting mental health and preventing mental and behavioral disorders. Following this course will yield incalculable benefits, not only in terms of societal costs, but also in the significant decrease of human suffering.
—David Satcher, Surgeon General U.S. Department of Health & Human Services, 2001

Unfortunately, Latina/os experience formidable barriers to access effective mental health services. The Surgeon General's supplemental report *Mental Health: A Report of the Surgeon General* (U.S. Department of Health & Human Services [USDHHS], 2001) concluded that ethnic minorities bear a significant burden from their unmet mental health needs and consequently experience greater loss to their overall health and productivity (p. 3). In particular, disparities are manifested among Latina/os in their need for mental health services, limited availability of bilingual mental health providers, limited accessibility to culturally responsive mental health services, low utilization of mental health services, inappropriate diagnoses and outcomes, and inadequate representation within clinical trials. Despite the subsequent attention to these disparities, mental health disparities among Latina/os and other ethnic minorities have not significantly diminished. Latina/os continue to demonstrate low utilization rates and encounter significant mental health barriers (Bledsoe, 2008; Caldwell, Couture, & Nowotny, 2008; Echeverry, 1997; Kouyoumdjian, Zamboanga, & Hansen, 2003; USDHHS, 2001c; Vega & Lopez, 2001).

Latina/os also demonstrate an unmet need, as they are more likely to use mental health services in crisis situations and report lower satisfaction when they pursue mental health services (Aguilar-Gaxiola et al., 2012; Caldwell et al., 2008). They also experience premature termination and substandard mental health care (Aguilar-Gaxiola et al., 2012; Alegría et al., 2002; Caldwell et al., 2008; Kouyoumdjian et al., 2003; USDHHS, 2001c). However, it is particularly challenging to identify differences in mental health disparities among Latina/o heritage groups, as few studies have examined within-group differences. Most studies combine these various groups into a pan-ethnic category (Bledsoe, 2008), despite critical demographic and sociocultural differences and potentially different patterns of mental health seeking across these groups (Alegría et al. 2007a,b,c; Cho, Kim, & Velez-Ortiz, 2014a). Thus, this chapter discusses mental health utilization among Latina/os and the various individual, cultural, organizational, and societal factors that contribute to their mental health barriers. In addition, we provide recommendations to address these mental health barriers.

Mental health disparities and demographic differences also exist among Latina/o youth and their White/European American peers. For example, Kataoka, Zhang, and Wells (2002) report that within the past year, 79% of children between the ages of 6 to 17 did not utilize any mental health service, and the unmet needs of Latina/o children are even higher (88%) than those of their White/European American counterparts (see Figure 7.1). An examination of at-risk Latina/o youth (Hough et al., 2002) also indicates that although more than half (55.6%) of Latina/o adolescents use specialty outpatient services, their rates are lower than those of their White/European American peers (73.2%). In addition, they enter specialty mental health services at a later age and make significantly fewer specialty mental health service visits. Latina/o adolescents are also significantly less likely to use specialty mental health services than their White/European peers independent of diagnosis, gender, age, and service sector (Hough et al., 2002).

MENTAL HEALTH UTILIZATION RATES OF LATINA/OS

A significant body of research illustrates that Latina/os generally underutilize mental health services (Aguilar-Gaxiola et al., 2012; Cook, McGuire, & Miranda, 2007; USDHHS, 2001c; Vega, Rodriguez, & Gruskin, 2009) than

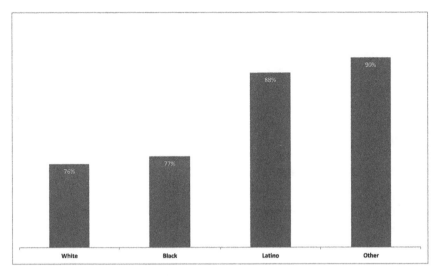

Figure 7.1 Unmet Children's Mental Health Needs, by Race/Ethnicity.

Source: Kataoka, S. H., Zhang, L., & Wells, K. B. (2002). Unmet need for mental health care among US children: Variation by ethnicity and insurance status. *American Journal of Psychiatry, 159*, 1548–1555.

White/European Americans. For instance, Latina/os experience more mental health disparities as compared with their White/European American counterparts (Aguilar-Gaxiola et al., 2012; Alegría et al., 2002, 2008a; Cook et al., 2007; USDHHS, 2001; Vega et al., 2009). Poor Latina/os have lower access to formal mental health services than poor White/European Americans. Language fluency, cultural differences such as self-reliance, access to Medicaid specialty services in Latina/o neighborhoods, differences in recognition of mental health problems, and lower quality of mental health care contribute to inequalities in formal mental health services among Latina/os (Aguilar-Gaxiola et al., 2012; Alegría et al., 2008).

There are racial/ethnic differences in crisis visits and psychiatric hospitalizations. Latina/os demonstrate disproportionately lower rates of psychiatric hospitalizations as compared with other ethnic/racial groups (Camacho et al., 2012; USDHHS, 2001). Latina/os with mental disorders are less likely than White/European Americans to utilize mental health services, but are more likely to delay treatment (Alegría et al., 2008b). Once they enter treatment, the services they receive are inadequate as compared with those for White/European Americans (Alegría et al., 2008b; Cook et al., 2007), resulting in premature termination (USDHHS, 2001c). For example, data from the National Institute of Mental Health Collaborative Psychiatric Epidemiology Surveys (CPES) (Alegría et al., 2008b) indicate significant underdetection of depression among less acculturated individuals. Among Latina/os with a depressive disorder in the past year, 63.7% did not enter treatment, as compared with 40.2% of White/European Americas. In addition, when they enter treatment they are significantly less likely to receive adequate care. These findings highlight that even after adjusting for socioeconomic variables, such as poverty, insurance coverage, and education, Latina/o ethnicity independently affects access to depression treatment.

There are also differences in utilization rates among Latina/o heritage groups. For example, data from the National Latina/o and Asian American Study (NLAAS) indicate that overall mental health service use and specialty service use are significantly higher among Puerto Ricans than among Mexicans, Cubans, and Other Latina/os (Alegría et al., 2007a). One in five Puerto Ricans report past-year mental health service use and specialty service, in contrast to 1 in every 10 Mexicans. Cultural factors such as nativity, language, age at migration, years of residence in the United States, and generational status are associated with use of mental health services. However, stratified analysis according to past-year psychiatric diagnoses indicates that associations hold only among those without psychological disorders. Mexicans are less likely than Other Latina/os to report satisfaction with their mental health services, and immigrants with 5 or fewer years of U.S. residence report less satisfaction than Latina/os with more than 20 years of U.S. residence (Alegría et al., 2007a).

Data from the 2002–2003 Medical Expenditure Panel Survey (MEPS) indicate diverse utilization patterns among Latina/os in their use of mental health care, including specialty and nonspecialty mental health services (Berdahl & Stone, 2009). Lower English language proficiency is associated with lower use of specialist use and any type of mental health care. Cubans are twice as likely as White/European Americans to visit a nonspecialist mental health care provider after controlling for language and years in the United States. Puerto Ricans are more likely to use mental health services than other Latinos. Among Latina/o heritage groups, Mexicans have the lowest odds of using any type of mental health care. While English language proficiency and time in the United States partially explain lower use relative to White/European Americans, they do not fully explain these disparities. González et al. (2010) also observed differences among Latina/o heritage groups in their examination of past-year depression pharmacotherapy and psychotherapy. Mexican Americans are less likely to receive pharmacological therapy, psychotherapy, and combined therapies than Puerto Ricans and White/European Americans. In addition, Mexican Americans are less likely to report guideline-concordant pharmacological therapy and psychotherapy.

Data from the Mexican American Prevalence and Services Study (MAPPS; Vega et al., 1998) indicate that only 64.7% of U.S.-born Mexican Americans received any services for their recent psychiatric disorders. The underutilization by Mexican immigrants is even more pronounced, as 80% with a diagnosable disorder remain untreated. In their examination of unauthorized and documented immigrant Latina/os, Pérez and Fortuna (2005) report that although unauthorized Latina/os have a significantly greater number of concurrent psychosocial stressors, they use fewer mental health visits (4.4) than their documented (7.9) or U.S.-born (13.3) counterparts. However, they keep their appointments at similar rates as documented and U.S.-born Latina/os (74%, 77%, & 69% respectively).

Differences in mental health utilization among Latina/os are also due to language preferences. For instance, Folsom et al. (2007) examined the effect of language preference on mental health service utilization among Latina/os and White/European Americans who initiated treatment for schizophrenia, bipolar disorder, or major depression in San Diego County's Adult and Older Adult Mental Health Services system between 2001 and 2004. Spanish-speaking Latina/os differ from English-speaking Latina/os on most demographic, clinical, and service use measures, while few differences exist between English-speaking Latina/os and White/European Americans. In particular, Spanish-speaking Latina/os are less likely to enter mental health services through emergency care or incarceration but are more likely to enter mental health services through outpatient treatment than English-speaking Latina/os and White/European Americans. However, these groups do not differ in their duration of their treatment or inpatient care (Folsom et al., 2007).

RELIANCE UPON PRIMARY CARE SETTINGS

Both immigrant and U.S.-born Mexican Americans disproportionately use the general medical sector for their mental health problems (Vega et al., 1998). While White/European Americans utilize outpatient mental health services, Latina/os may prefer to use emergency department and primary care settings because they are more accessible and less stigmatizing (Caldwell et al., 2008). Their emergency department visits may also indicate that they are in crisis and the chronic nature of their condition. However, high patient loads, inconsistent training levels, and financial disincentives place general practitioners at a disadvantage in diagnosing and treating mental health disorders among Latina/os and other ethnic minorities. When Latina/os seek treatment through emergency departments, they face a greater risk of misdiagnosis and of receiving inferior services (Caldwell et al., 2008). Their risk for misdiagnosis is also amplified by differences in self-reports of distress.

For example, differences in their expression of depression may lead to misdiagnosis within medical settings. Furthermore, because of their limited psychiatric training, physicians face the burden of recognizing and accurately diagnosing mental health disorders among their Latina/o patients (Vega et al., 2001).

Nonadherence to psychotropic medication use among Latina/os is also troublesome. For example, in a review of psychotropic medication (e.g., antipsychotics, mood stabilizers, and antidepressants) nonadherence, Lanouette, Folsom, Sciolla, and Jeste (2009) found significant ethnic/racial differences in nonadherence. Latina/os (41%) and African Americans (43%) have lower nonadherence as compared with White/European Americans (31%). In the four studies that examine solely Latina/os, their mean nonadherence rate is even higher, at 44%. Risk factors for nonadherence include being a monolingual Spanish speaker, low socioeconomic status, the lack of health insurance, and barriers to accessing high-quality care. However, protective factors are also observed, including family support, older age, being more proactive in one's care, and eight or more visits with a therapist in the past year (Lanouette et al., 2009). Unfortunately, Latina/o immigrants perceive that psychotropic medications are addictive, and these beliefs may contribute to their poor adherence or misrepresentation to their physicians (Watson et al., 2013). Latina/o immigrants report that their nonadherence is also exacerbated by their interactions with physicians who do not adequately explain the purpose of their medications and their proper use.

BARRIERS TO MENTAL HEALTH AMONG LATINA/OS

Contextualizing barriers among Latina/os can aid in identifying common factors that influence their mental health service utilization. However, because of the vast differences among Latina/os, including the influences that place individuals and families at risk for psychological difficulties, one cannot assume that these factors affect all Latina/os, but they are useful to consider within culturally competent assessments and interventions (Bledsoe, 2008). Nonetheless, these barriers can be contextualized through the use of an ecological perspective to understand the influence of individual, cultural, organizational, and societal factors (Bledsoe, 2008). Interestingly, there is significant overlap between the medical and mental health barriers of Latina/os (see Chapter 3), as these barriers interact and impact their physical health and mental health. These contextual barriers include individual, cultural, and organizational barriers (see Table 7.1).

Table 7.1 Barriers to Mental Health Services

Individual Barriers
Poverty
Lack of health insurance
Age
Gender
Education
Limited English proficiency
Low health literacy

Cultural Barriers
Reliance upon family members
Religious beliefs
Preference for non–mental health resources
Stigma
Self-reliance

Organizational Barriers
Limited transportation
Geographic location of mental health facilities
Cost and economic burden of mental health treatment
Distrust of the mental health system
Discrimination
Shortage of Spanish-speaking mental health providers

Individual Barriers

Individual mental health barriers among Latina/os include poverty, lack of health insurance, age, gender, education, limited English proficiency, and low health literacy.

Poverty: Poverty is a major barrier to access to mental health services, particularly as 23.5% of Latina/os live below the poverty line (see Chapter 1) and comprise the highest percentage of uninsured persons within the United States (23.7%), surpassing that of the total uninsured population (Stepler & Brown, 2016). Only 19% of uninsured Latina/os seek mental health services compared with 38 to 51% of insured Latina/os (Alegría et al., 2007a). In addition, a higher percentage of foreign-born Latinos are uninsured (41.7%) than U.S.-born Latina/os (14.0%) (Stepler & Brown, 2016). Unfortunately, unauthorized Latina/o immigrants have limited access to health and social services. Latina/os are more likely to work in low-wage occupations that provide limited socioeconomic mobility and insurance benefits. If health coverage is available from employers, it is not easily affordable (American Cancer Society, 2015) or adequate (Valdez, Dvorscek, Budge, & Esmond, 2011). The purchase of health insurance also poses economic hardships, as health insurance is viewed in terms of costs and benefits rather than risks and benefits (Martinez & Carter-Pokras, 2006).

Lack of health insurance: As with poverty, the lack of insurance is a major mental health barrier. Unfortunately, the lack of insurance creates a decreased likelihood of having a primary care provider, preventive services, referrals, early detection, and adequate treatment (Betancourt, Carrillo, Green, & Maina, 2004). Vega and Lopez (2001) suggest that private insurance is also important for the increased use of mental health specialty providers, as the availability of public insurance does not increase the use of mental health services among Latina/os. In addition, they suggest that the likelihood of visiting a mental health specialist is two times greater among individuals with private insurance compared to those with public insurance.

Age: There is differential availability of mental health services among various age groups, with insufficient services for young and elderly Latina/os, who often present with multiple needs and problems (Bledsoe, 2008; Dupree, Herrera, Tyson, Yang, & King-Kallimanis, 2010; Echeverry, 1997). For instance, Latina/o children experience a higher rate of unmet needs and mental health utilization than their White/European American counterparts (Lopez, Bergren, & Painter, 2008). Similarly, while the elderly comprise a smaller proportion of Latina/os, elderly Latina/os also present with significant unmet needs for mental health services (Barrio et al., 2008), as well as challenges that may compete with their mental health concerns, such as poverty and physical health problems (Bledsoe, 2008; Echeverry, 1997; Dupree et al., 2010).

Gender: Gender is also a barrier, as Latinos are less likely to seek mental health treatment because of cultural notions that it is emasculating for them to seek mental health treatment (Bledsoe, 2008; Echeverry, 1997; Rastogi, Massey-Hastings, & Wieling, 2012) or beliefs that their mental health concerns are best handled within the family rather than within mental health settings (Cabassa, 2007; Cho et al., 2014). Thus, it is not surprising that Latinos may attempt to hide or camouflage their psychological symptoms (Caldwell et al., 2008). They are also more likely to express negative attitudes toward mental health treatments (Cabassa, 2007) and less likely than Latinas to use mental health services from either mental health or medical sectors (Peifer, Hu, & Vega, 2000). For example, Peifer et al. (2000) found that Mexican women are 3.1 times more likely than Mexican men to use mental health services.

Educational level: Educational level is also associated with mental health barriers. For example, among Latina/os of Mexican origin, those with 11 years of education or fewer are less likely to use mental health services than their peers with more than 11 years of education (Peifer et al., 2000). Berdahl and Stone (2009) also found that high school and college graduates are more likely to utilize mental health care. In addition, professional graduates are more than two and a half times as likely to use any type of mental health service compared to high school dropouts. The education effect is also larger for specialty mental health care. It is hypothesized that educational level is associated with knowledge of available resources, income, degree of acculturation, and English proficiency (Bledsoe, 2008; Echeverry, 1997). An understanding of mental health treatment is associated with higher levels of educational attainment, and this understanding is also associated with the utilization of mental health services (Echeverry, 1997).

Limited English proficiency: Linguistic barriers also pose problems with mental health treatment and create challenges for Latina/os to access mental health care. Linguistic barriers also create difficulties for Latina/os with limited English proficiency (LEP) to communicate with mental health staff and providers (Mercado-Crespo et al., 2010; Sentell, Shumway, & Snowden, 2007). Most mental health services are provided in English, because of the limited number of Spanish-speaking mental health providers (Bledsoe, 2008; Echeverry, 1997; Kouyoumdjian et al., 2003; USDHHS, 2001c; Vega & Lopez, 2001). While in treatment, Latina/os with LEP face the risk of misdiagnosis and inappropriate treatment, as well as dissatisfaction and premature termination (Kouyoumdjian et al., 2003).

Latina/os with LEP rely on English-speaking family members to act as interpreters and this reliance for interpretation and translation compromises their confidentiality, particularly when discussing sensitive topics such as abuse (Mercado-Crespo et al., 2010). Thus, among Spanish-speaking Latina/os, language is one of the most important factors that influence the clinical encounter and quality of care. Given that mental health treatment largely relies upon direct verbal communication, language barriers are particularly problematic (Kim et al., 2011). While mental health facilities may provide interpreters, Latina/os with LEP prefer to work with a Spanish-speaking mental health provider to avoid language barriers (Rastogi et al., 2012).

Other research supports how LEP creates barriers for Latina/os. For example, NLAAS data indicate that LEP is a barrier to mental health service use among Latina/o immigrants with psychological disorders (Kim et al., 2011). Less than 20% of the total immigrant population utilize any type of mental health services, and those with limited English proficiency are less likely to use mental health services compared to their counterparts with English proficiency. Mental health services require extensive verbal expression of one's thoughts and feelings, which not only reflect language barriers, but cultural barriers as well. Thus, for monolingual Spanish-speaking Latina/os, immigrants, English proficiency plays a critical role in their ability to access mental health treatment and quality of care (Kim et al., 2011).

Low health literacy: The low health literacy of Latina/o immigrants acts as a mental health barrier. For example, they may lack knowledge regarding psychological disorders and possess a limited understanding of the symptoms of psychological disorders (Caldwell et al., 2008; Mercado-Crespo et al., 2010; Rastogi et al., 2012; Watson et al., 2013). Latina/os are also unfamiliar with the process of locating a mental health professional and the therapeutic process, and this lack of information acts as a barrier to seeking treatment (Watson et al., 2013). They may also experience intimidation by the complex nature of the U.S. mental health system (Mercado-Crespo et al., 2010). Others may perceive mental health services as being solely for the wealthy or privileged, as in their countries of origin. Even among Latina/os who are aware of the provision of mental health services, they may experience intimidation by the uncertainty of entering into an unknown environment.

Cultural Barriers to Mental Health among Latina/os

Cultural barriers such as reliance on family members, religious beliefs, preferences for non–mental health resources, stigma, and self-reliance also create significant cultural mental health barriers for Latina/os (Bledsoe, 2008; Echeverry, 1997; Falicov, 1999; Kouyoumdjian et al., 2003; Mercado-Crespo et al., 2010). Unfortunately, these barriers deter Latina/os from seeking mental health services.

Reliance upon family members: As a collective group, family relationships are often important to Latina/os, and family members provide strong support during periods of emotional and psychological difficulties (Bledsoe, 2008; Echeverry, 1997; Falicov, 1999, 2014; Kouyoumdjian et al., 2003). Thus, Latina/os may prefer to consult with their family and friends for emotional support, rather than mental health providers (Bledsoe, 2008; Cabassa, 2007; Dupree et al., 2010; Kouyoumdjian et al., 2003). However, while family members and social networks may offer support, some scholars argue that extended family support systems may also serve as a barrier to seeking mental health resources because psychological problems are dealt within the privacy of the family (Guarnaccia, Martinez, & Acosta, 2005). Latina/os with mental health disorders may not pursue mental health services because of their reluctance to share family secrets and because of the belief that doing so is a betrayal of trust (Caldwell et al., 2008). They may also fear that their families will experience stigma and shame because of their mental illness. Thus, family members may attempt to dissuade individuals from seeking help by minimizing their pathology (Rastogi et al., 2012).

Religious beliefs and preferences for non–mental health resources: Religious beliefs that dictate that only God can solve a problem or illness may deter Latina/os from seeking mental health services, even after other options prove unsuccessful. Similarly, Latina/os of certain faiths may believe that prayer is the most appropriate mechanism to resolve a problem and may also consult with religious leaders or clergy (Bledsoe, 2008; Echeverry, 1997; Peifer et al., 2000; Rastogi et al., 2012; Vargas et al., 2015). Latina/os in need of psychological care may prefer other types of resources rather than seeking mental health providers. These resources may include alternative healers or other sources of help, such as natural remedies (Bledsoe, 2008; Echeverry, 1997) or medications from their countries of origin that are often prescribed by a pharmacist or social networks (Watson et al., 2013); this is particularly so among poor, low acculturated or rural Latina/os. These preferences are also related to cultural beliefs regarding mental illness and treatment, as Latina/os may view their physical and psychological concerns as inseparable (Bledsoe, 2008; Echeverry, 1997; Falicov, 2013).

Stigma: A significant mental health barrier among Latina/os is stigma, as they are often concerned about the stigma associated with mental illness (Mercado-Crespo et al., 2010; Sentell, Shumway, & Snowden, 2007; Vargas et al., 2015). Unfortunately, Latina/os often perceive that working with a mental health provider is an admission of weakness or instability, as only the insane require mental health services (Bledsoe, 2008; Echeverry, 1997; Kouyoumdjian et al., 2003; Rastogi et al., 2012; Vargas et al., 2015). These perspectives are also associated with the stigma associated with mental illness. Research suggests that Latina/os often seek a physician or a nontraditional healer for their psychological difficulties (see Chapter 8) to avoid the stigma of seeing a mental health provider (Kouyoumdjian et al., 2003; Rastogi et al., 2012). Furthermore, older Latina/os are reluctant to enter therapy because they fear being labeled as mentally ill (Barrio et al., 2008).

Many of the stigmas and taboos associated with mental illness are due to low mental health literacy (Caplan & Cordero, 2015; Watson et al., 2013), such as myths and misinformation regarding the etiology of psychological disorders, as well as its consequences (Mercado-Crespo et al., 2010; Watson et al., 2013). Latina/os may perceive that mental illness is due to a person's weakness or lack of character (Aguilar-Gaxiola et al., 2012; Caplan & Cordero, 2015; Mercado-Crespo et al., 2010; Vargas et al., 2015). Other explanations may include spiritual or religious attributions, such as punishment from God, witchcraft, demonic possession, or the loss of one's soul (Caplan & Cordero, 2015). For instance, the label of *locura* (madness) is also associated with negative connotations. A person who is labeled *loco* is perceived as severely mentally ill, potentially violent, and incurable (Guarnaccia, Martinez, & Acosta, 2002). Thus, mental help seeking is associated with being *loco/loca* (Rastogi et al., 2012; Vargas et al., 2015). Similarly, the stigma of seeking psychiatric help also extends into beliefs that one is "not all right in the head *(no estar bien de la cabeza)*" (Vargas et al., 2015). However, the label of *nervios* (nerves) is less stigmatizing within one's family or community (see Chapter 6).

Stigma is also correlated with a decreased quality of care (Vega, Rodriguez, & Ang, 2010). Stigmatizing beliefs about depression can serve as a barrier to the recognition of symptoms, seeking treatment, and treatment adherence among Latina/os. Studies regarding the use of antidepressants indicate that the stigma of antidepressant use implies social deficiencies, such as weakness or an inability to cope, and the presence of severe problems or a severe mental disorder (Cabassa, 2007; Interian, Martinez, Guarnaccia, Vega, & Escobar, 2007; Vargas et al., 2015). In addition, using antidepressants is viewed as equivalent to the use of illicit drugs (Interian et al., 2007); antidepressants are perceived to be addictive (Cabassa & Hansen, 2007; Cabassa, Zayas, & Hansen, 2006; Watson et al., 2013) or that they cause organ damage (Vargas et al., 2015). Among low-income and Spanish-speaking Latina/os in primary care for depression (Vega et al., 2010), patients who report higher levels of perceived stigma are less likely to disclose their depression diagnosis to their family and friends and also less likely to take their antidepressants. They are also less likely to manage their depression and more likely to miss their appointments. Others may fear stereotyping and resist their diagnosis and treatment and thus deflect disclosure of depression and their use of antidepressants (Interian et al., 2007).

Differences in acculturation and age may also contribute to perceptions regarding the mentally ill and stigma. For example, Rojas-Vilches, Negy, and Reig-Ferrer (2011) examined attitudes toward seeking therapy between Puerto Rican and Cuban young adults and their parents. Parents report that social stigma is attached to mental illness and mental health treatment, and parents who perceive that mental illness is untreatable are less willing to seek professional help. Conversely, young adults do not endorse these beliefs and demonstrate greater willingness to seek therapy. Although within-group differences are not observed between Puerto Ricans and Cubans, differences in acculturation remain. For both young adults and their parents, increased acculturation is associated with less pejorative attitudes toward mental illness and therapy (Rojas-Vilches et al., 2011).

Self-reliance: Self-reliant attitudes (preference to solve emotional problems on one's own) also act as a barrier to seeking care and are also associated with lower use of mental health treatment. Latina/os who prefer to solve problems on their own are less likely to seek formal mental health care (Berdahl & Stone, 2009). For example, in a community sample of Puerto Ricans who reside in low-income areas in Puerto Rico, Ortega and Alegría (2002) found that participants who identify as self-reliant are 40% less likely to seek mental health treatment; they perceive that mental health services are ineffective in curing their mental health problems. They are also uncomfortable if their family members learn that they are in treatment. A self-reliant attitude is also observed among diverse (i.e., Dominican Republic, Mexico, Ecuador, and other Latin American countries) foreign-born Latina/os from New York (Vargas et al., 2015), who indicate that one should *poner de su parte* (put forth effort). These perceptions highlight the importance of being strong to cope with life problems and coping with the assistance of family members and not the mental health care system.

Organizational Barriers to Mental Health among Latino/as

Organizational factors such as limited transportation, geographic location of mental health facilities, cost and economic burden, distrust of mental health facilities, and limited numbers of Spanish-speaking mental health providers also create mental health barriers for Latina/os (Barrio et al., 2008; Caldwell et al., 2008; Echeverry, 1997). Unfortunately, the U.S. mental health care system is inherently complex, underfunded, and bureaucratic.

Limited transportation and geographic location of mental health facilities: Access to mental health services is impeded by challenges with transportation. New immigrants who are unfamiliar with their geographical area or who are unfamiliar with public transportation are unlikely to seek help (Caldwell et al., 2008). Transportation is also a challenge for Latinas who do not drive or lack child care and must often travel with their children. The lack of transportation and limited mobility make it difficult to travel to mental health facilities, particularly facilities that require significant travel (Caldwell et al., 2008) and facilities that are far from a bus or subway stop may also create hardships. Limited hours of operation and the timing of visits also create difficulties, particularly for Latina/os who work during traditional office hours (Martinez & Carter-Pokras, 2006) or those who work far longer than an eight-hour workday, such as farmworkers (Aguilar-Gaxiola et al., 2012).

Cost and economic burden: Mental health treatment may amplify the economic burden of Latina/os, particularly those who are unable to leave their place of employment for their mental health needs because they lack leave benefits (Valdez et al., 2011) or flexible work schedules. Similarly, Latina/os employed in low-wage positions do not have the ability to take time off from work to attend a therapy session, as doing so may entail financial hardships. For example, migrant workers are reluctant to take time off for their health care, as the disruption in their workday decreases their income and threatens their livelihood (Aguilar-Gaxiola et al., 2012). Thus, cost is also a significant barrier to access to mental health services and may result in treatment delays, as a large number of Latina/os lack sufficient health insurance coverage or financial resources to afford mental health care (Bledsoe, 2008; Cabassa & Hansen, 2007; Cabassa et al., 2006; Echeverry, 1997; Kouyoumdjian et al., 2003; USDHHS, 2001c; Vega & Lopez, 2001).

Insurance copayments or deductibles are often unaffordable (Bledsoe, 2008; Cabassa & Hansen, 2007; Cabassa et al., 2006; Echeverry, 1997), and even among Latina/os with insurance, their copay may also create a financial hardship. Because service providers do not offer child care, the lack of child care poses difficulties and contributes to missed appointments or premature termination (Caldwell et al., 2008). In addition, other challenges, such as family responsibilities, may take precedence over a therapy session. Thus, the amount of time, effort, money, and potential frustration associated with an appointment may outweigh the perceived benefit of seeking mental health services (Caldwell et al., 2008).

Distrust of the mental health system: Regrettably, Latina/os are often distrustful of the mental health system (Falicov, 1999; Vega & Lopez, 2001) because of the legacy of racism within medical and mental health institutions and the poor quality of mental health services for Latina/o immigrants. In addition, anti-immigrant sentiments and policies also distance Latina/os from mental health care (Bledsoe, 2008; Vega & Lopez, 2001). For instance, unauthorized Latina/os may avoid seeking services because they fear that mental health providers will report their legal status to immigration authorities, resulting in deportation (Bledsoe, 2008; Cabassa, 2007; Echeverry, 1997; Watson et al., 2013). For instance, Latina/o community members from the Midwest (Rastogi et al., 2012) express fear that a visit to a mental health provider will create legal problems due to misperceptions that the government can access their clinical records or that their visit will lead to an investigation by the Department of Child and Family Services. Among Latina/o immigrants, distrust is attributed to the poor quality of mental health services, often because of long wait periods, difficulties accessing mental health services, limited hours of operation, fear of deportation, and lack of Spanish-speaking bilingual and bicultural services (Aguilar-Gaxiola et al., 2012; Cabassa & Hansen, 2007; Mercado-Crespo, 2010).

Discrimination: Latina/os are also concerned about discrimination within mental health settings (Aguilar-Gaxiola, 2012; Bledsoe, 2008; USDHHS,

2001), due to both racial and cultural bias (Guarnaccia et al., 2005). Unfortunately, experiences of discrimination within clinical settings (Guarnaccia, Martinez, & Acosta, 2002) and ineffective mainstream mental health approaches contribute to client dissatisfaction and premature termination among Latina/os (Kouyoumdjian et al., 2003). For example, when they pursue mental health services, Latina/os often encounter Eurocentric services that are insensitive and incongruent with their cultural and spiritual experiences (Comas-Díaz, 2006). The lack of culturally sensitive mental health providers, assessments, and treatment approaches also play a vital role in their skepticism regarding the efficacy of mainstream mental health approaches and further contribute to the mental health disparities of Latina/os (Comas-Díaz, 2006; Kouyoumdjian et al., 2003; Rastogi et al., 2012).

Limited Spanish-speaking mental health providers: The shortage of mental health facilities and specialized providers, particularly within rural areas is also problematic (Aguilar-Gaxiola et al., 2012). Furthermore, the limited availability of bilingual and bicultural services is also a significant mental health barrier, particularly among monolingual Spanish-speaking Latina/os or individuals who prefer to work with a Spanish-speaking provider (Bledsoe, 2008; Cabassa & Hansen, 2007; Cabassa et al., 2006; Echeverry, 1997; Kouyoumdjian et al., 2003; Mercado-Crespo et al., 2011; Rastogi et al., 2012; USDHHS, 2001c; Vega & Lopez, 2001). Even highly acculturated, middle-class Latinos may prefer to work with a bilingual/bicultural mental health provider who is familiar with their cultural background and unique worldviews (Bledsoe, 2008; Echeverry, 1997), such as *simpatia*. For example, it is often difficult for Latina/os to build a strong therapeutic alliance with mental health providers who are perceived as detached, as they traditionally value mental health providers who are warm, personal, and encouraging (Rastogi et al., 2012). The detached behavior of providers leads to dissatisfaction and premature termination of treatment. Furthermore, the shortage of bilingual and bicultural mental health providers often translates into language barriers and results in miscommunication (Aguilar-Gaxiola et al., 2012). Unfortunately, the limited number of bilingual and bicultural mental health providers contributes to the unmet mental health needs of Latina/os, particularly monolingual immigrants (Aguilar-Gaxiola et al., 2012; Barrio et al., 2008; Falicov, 2014; Rastogi et al., 2012).

WAYS TO ADDRESS MENTAL HEALTH BARRIERS AMONG LATINA/OS

Latina/o experts provide directives to address the mental health disparities of Latina/os. These directives include the consideration of cultural strengths among Latina/os, the integration of Latina/o cultural values, community outreach, the elimination of organizational barriers, community-oriented approaches, and cultural adaptations and culturally appropriate diagnostic tools and assessments (Aguilar-Gaxiola et al., 2012; Arredondo et al., 2014; Falicov, 2013; Santiago-Rivera et al., 2002; Sue & Sue, 2016).

Integration of Latina/o Cultural Strengths and Values within Clinical Work

An ethical imperative of clinical work with Latina/os is the need for multicultural counseling competencies (Arredondo et al., 2014; Santiago-Rivera et al., 2002; Sue, Arredondo, & McDavis, 1992; Sue & Sue, 2016), including awareness of one's own values and biases, self-awareness of client's worldview, and culturally appropriate intervention strategies. Thus, Santiago-Rivera et al. (2002) suggest that Latina/o-specific competencies include the following:

- Understanding the concepts and terms of *personalismo, familismo, respeto, dignidad,* and *orgullo,* and their meaning for relationship building with clients of Latina/o heritage.
- Recognition of the role of spirituality and formalized religion for individual Latina/o clients.
- The ability to determine the counseling approach that is best suited for the individual client based on the presenting issue(s), and expected outcomes from counseling, previous experience in counseling, levels of acculturation, migration issues, gender role socialization, socioeconomic status, educational attainment, language proficiency (e.g., level of English language–speaking ability), and ethnic/racial identity status.
- The ability to describe one's own level of ethnic/racial identity as it may facilitate or impede the counseling alliance with individuals of varying Latina/o heritage and phenotype.
- The ability to identify and modify approaches to be culturally effective (p. 17).

Mental health interventions with Latina/os must reflect cultural sensitivity through clinical approaches and program activities that build upon the cultural strengths of Latina/os. These strengths include cultural values such as *confianza, familismo, personalismo, respeto,* and others (Adames & Chavez-Dueñas, 2017; Añez et al., 2005; Arredondo et al., 2014; Buki, Salazar, & Pitton, 2009; Falicov, 2013; Santiago-Rivera et al., 2002; Tovar, 2017) (see Chapter 1). While adherence to these cultural values differs among Latina/os due to acculturation, ethnic identity, and other factors (Adames & Chavez-Dueñas, 2017; Añez et al., 2005), cumulatively, these values emphasize courtesy, kindness, formal friendliness, respect, and recognition

Table 7.2 Cultural Values That Influence Mental Health Treatment

Familismo (Familism): A value that places a strong emphasis on familial ideals and involves broad networks of support that extend beyond the nuclear family to include aunts, uncles, grandparents, godparents, and other close family friends.

Respeto (Respect): A value that reveals the hierarchical structures that may exist in Latina/o communities, and contributes to differential behaviors toward others based on a number of factors, such as age, gender, social or economic status, and authority.

Dignidad (Dignity): A value that recognizes that individuals are inherently worthy and worthy of respect.

Confianza (Trust): A value in which individuals are invested in establishing relationships that are based on reciprocal trust.

Personalismo/Simpatia (Being Personal): A value that places considerable emphasis on the personal, smooth, interactions of individuals while avoiding conflict or confrontation.

Vergüenza (Shame): The value of being cognizant of not engaging in behaviors that may humiliate or dishonor one's self, family, or social group.

Amabilidad (Amiable): A value in which a person is pleasant, helpful, and cordial. It differs from *personalismo*, as it highlights when the individual goes "the extra mile" to help others while focusing on their needs and well-being.

Lealtad (Loyal): A value that is an essential element in the development of trust in human relationships. It connotes that the other person has demonstrated a strong emotional connection, commitment, and loyalty to an individual, family, and/or social group.

Obedencia (Obedience): An important cultural value for Latina/o parents who seek to teach their children to follow the guidance of elders, teachers, and other adults in order to develop a behavioral pattern that is consistent with cultural and social norms and expectations.

Responsabilidad (Responsibility): A value that describes the socialization of individuals in which a significant emphasis is placed on developing a strong sense of accountability for one's actions, making a commitment to following through with one's word and/or promises, and being reliable to others.

Ser trabajador (Strong Work Ethic): A traditional cultural value that emphasizes the importance of being productive, hardworking, and diligent in the completion of tasks.

Honestidad (Honesty): A value in which individuals strive to be sincere with their words, feelings, and actions.

Humilidad (Humility): A characteristic in which an individual does not focus on his or her own triumph and virtues but does recognize his or her own shortcomings.

Source: Adames & Chavez-Dueñas (2017). *Cultural foundations and interventions in Latino/a mental health: History, theory, and within-group differences.* New York: Routledge.

of the family's importance (see Table 7.2). When these values are not recognized within the clinical encounter, this neglect creates barriers to treatment and adversely impacts the therapeutic alliance. Mental health providers are perceived as uncaring, arrogant, and indifferent, resulting in decreased satisfaction, noncompliance, premature termination, and potential conflict. For instance, *confianza* (trust and intimacy) plays an important role within clinical work with Latina/os, as it is often based on the application of *personalismo* and *respeto* (Añez et al., 2005; Arredondo et al., 2014; Falicov, 2013; Santiago-Rivera et al., 2002). *Confianza* with Latina/os is created through the gradual development of a meaningful relationship that is characterized by warmth, patience, and kindness (Falicov, 2013). Santiago-Rivera et al. (2002) identify these behaviors as *interpersonal etiquette* and discuss how these value orientations are often prominent among Latina/o interpersonal relationships and influence the clinical encounter. In addition, they provide recommendations for the application of interpersonal etiquette to facilitate rapport (see Table 7.3).

Table 7.3 The Application of Latina/o Interpersonal Etiquette to Facilitate Rapport

---

- Begin counseling in a formal style, and then proceed into more informal verbal and nonverbal interactions.
- Address adults with formal titles: Mr. and Mrs.
- Allow proximity in seating arrangements and personal communication.
- Follow a hierarchical approach to greetings, starting with males or elders and adults before children.
- Recognize differences in last names and possible differences in a client's recorded name.
- It is important to note than in Spanish-speaking countries, individuals keep both parents' surnames, but in the United States, typically only the father's surname is used.
- Maintain a flexible time frame without rushing the visit or conducting time-pressured sessions.
- Start with *platica* (personable small talk), a necessary prerequisite before engaging in serious conversations.
- Educate Latina/o clients about the counseling process and structure.
- To ensure rapport, present sensitive issues with an apology or recognition that the question or message is potentially offensive or strong (e.g., "Please excuse me but I need to ask you certain questions that may be difficult to answer, but it is important for the treatment").

Source: Santiago-Rivera, Arredondo & Gallardo-Cooper (2002). *Counseling Latinos and la familia: A practical guide* (Vol. 17). Thousand Oaks, CA: Sage.

A mental health provider who fails to establish a personal connection through *platica* or appropriate self-disclosure runs the risk of being perceived as *frio* (cold) (Añez et al., 2005). In addition, during the first clinical encounter mental health providers should use formal titles, such as *Señora* or *Doña* (Mrs.), as well as *Señor* or *Don* (Mr.), rather than first names. Also the formal use of *usted* (formal you) rather than *tu* (informal you) with immigrant or older Latina/os (Añez et al., 2005; Falicov, 2013) is important, since *respeto* is an intricate aspect of interpersonal relationships among Latina/os. A general recommendation is to address Latina/os formally unless told to do otherwise during the initial contact, since *falta de respeto* (act of disrespect) is considered offensive and may jeopardize the therapeutic alliance and noncompliance (Añez et al., 2005).

Flexibility and accommodation are also paramount to building a solid therapeutic alliance with Latina/os (Falicov, 2013). For instance, it is not uncommon for Latina/os to ask for advice. Although mental health providers are often uncomfortable providing advice, Falicov (2013) indicates that generalized, nonspecific advice or a reassuring word can aid in alliance building and build trust. Flexibility is also warranted in one's interactions with Latina/os. Given the low health literacy among Latina/os with limited English proficiency, mental health providers must avoid using clinical jargon, provide educational materials, and create a welcoming mental health environment (Valdez et al., 2011). The elimination of these barriers can be accomplished by employing a diverse workforce of mental health professions and staff who demonstrate *respeto*, *dignidad*, and *personalismo*. (See Adames & Chavez-Dueñas [2017] for a review of how these values manifest within therapy.) Because Latina/os are subjected to discrimination and harassment, they may experience *vergüenza* (fear of being judged), as well as feel vulnerable or physically exposed (Adames & Chavez-Dueñas, 2017). Thus, treating clients with *dignidad* (dignity) and demonstrating that they are inherently worthy (Santiago-Rivera et al., 2002) is a fundamental element of therapy. Asking about specific and detailed information related to a client's life also models important Latina/o cultural values and creates a caring environment needed to maintain Latina/o clients in therapy (Falicov, 2013).

Moreover, despite time constraints, clinicians must take the time to ensure that their Latina/o clients understand the process of therapy, as they may perceive that counseling is similar to a medical visit and solely entails a one-time visit (Santiago-Rivera et al., 2002). In addition, cultural sensitivity entails open discussions regarding other concerns, such as mental health barriers. This entails a discussion regarding the client's mental health beliefs, cultural values, stigma, and other related areas. Discussions regarding confidentiality are also important to ensure that clients understand the type of information that is recorded and who has access to such information (Adames, & Chavez-Dueñas, 2017; Arredondo et al., 2014; Falicov, 2013; Gallardo, 2012), particularly as unauthorized Latina/os may fear that their personal information will be released to the immigration authorities. Similarly, discussions regarding the parameters of confidentiality, mandates of abuse reporting, informed consent, and the role of the counselor are paramount, to ensure high standards of ethical mental health practice (Santiago-Rivera et al., 2002).

Community Outreach

Given the low mental health literacy of Latina/os, it is essential to dispel myths regarding mental illness and provide helpful information regarding how to secure mental health services. In addition, since unauthorized Latina/os may avoid seeking services because they fear deportation, outreach efforts should also dispel this myth. Materials should include colorful graphics and materials with messages for individuals with low literacy and limited knowledge regarding mental health. These materials are perceived as highly credible when they are culturally relevant and emphasize the family (Buki et al., 2009). They are also efficacious when they include visually appealing pictures and illustrations and convey linguistically simple messages. Literacy issues are also confounded when mental health instruction and materials are designed for relatively educated individuals with high English literacy. Furthermore, Spanish-language materials that are direct translations from English are often inappropriate, as they lack linguistic and cultural relevance. Other Spanish translations tend to be written at a high reading level and are inappropriate for low-level readers (Elder, Ayala, Parra-Medina, & Talavera, 2009). Thus, these materials must contain nontechnical and user-friendly language that is written at a fifth-grade level to allow for greater comprehension.

Pictorial messages and testimonials, such as telenovelas are also appealing to Latina/os (Arellano-Morales et al., 2016; Buki et al., 2009). The telenovela (Spanish soap opera) is a popular form of entertainment among Spanish-speaking Latina/os. Mental health facilities should develop a telenovela to provide information regarding mental illness and address myths to Spanish-speaking Latina/os. In addition, a public service announcement (PSA) featuring a mental health hotline should accompany the telenovela. Similarly, mental health providers should utilize *fotonovelas* to educate Latina/os regarding mental illness and treatment (Hernandez & Organista, 2013). *Fotonovelas* are a traditional print medium that are popular in Latin America and contain sequential photographs accompanied by dialogue bubbles to depict a story and contain a moral message. They can also serve as useful outreach tools for distribution at health fairs, schools, or other locations that Latina/os frequent, such as churches or grocery stores for Spanish-speaking Latina/os (Mercado-Crespo et al., 2010).

Latina/os utilize the same technologies as their White/European American counterparts but they appear to use them differently, and place greater importance on linguistic and cultural factors (Victorson et al., 2014). Thus, electronic mental health outreach and interventions with Latina/os must include tailored messages and interventions that incorporate their unique cultural norms and values (Arellano-Morales et al., 2016; Victorson et al., 2014). Traditional forums such as public service announcements for radio and television, live interviews, and the placement of ads and articles within bilingual and Spanish community newspapers will certainly aid in the mental health promotion of Latina/os (Mercado-Crespo et al., 2010). However, given the increased the use of smartphone and mobile devices among Latina/os cell phone–mediated interventions hold promise for hard-to-reach populations and warrant further consideration (Victorson et al., 2014). Social media also holds great promise for mental health promotion among Latinos. Multiple social media platforms such as Facebook, YouTube, Twitter, and other popular social networking sites can aid in mental health efforts and increase their understanding of mental health.

The Elimination of Organizational Barriers

Mental health organizations must work toward eliminating their organizational barriers, such as cost. Thus, free or low cost services are warranted, particularly as mental health services can create financial hardships for Latina/os. Limited hours of operation also create hardships and challenges for Latina/os, particularly those with inflexible work schedules. Thus, flexible hours are warranted to accommodate Latina/os who work during traditional office hours, as well as those with limited child care options. Transportation is also challenging for Latina/os with limited mobility, and mental health organizations should consider providing transportation services or free vouchers for transportation. However, offering home visits or mental health services within the local community, such as faith-based organizations, schools, or community centers, easily eliminates issues of transportation, childcare, and lack of access (Falicov, 2013).

Due to the financial and organizational barriers that prevent Latina/os from accessing mental health services, it is vital to increase health care coverage among Latina/o immigrants, through the integration of mental health services into primary health care facilities. Similarly, the increased health coverage and mental health utilization of unauthorized Latina/os is imperative to their well-being. Pérez and Fortuna (2005) suggest that since they are ineligible for many needed services, agencies, clinics, and hospitals that work with unauthorized Latina/os must identify appropriate and viable treatment options, such as free brief treatment. Organizations must also identify additional funding sources and collaborate with other agencies that provide treatment to unauthorized Latina/os. Furthermore, supplementing mental health care with case management services can also aid in decreasing mental health disparities among Latina/os (Cabassa & Hansen, 2007; Cabassa et al., 2006; USDHHS, 2001). For instance, combined case-management and depression care may be effective for low-income and/or low-acculturated Latina/os, who may require assistance navigating the health care system and encounter multiple social and economic demands that prevent them from accessing and engaging in treatment (Cabassa & Hansen, 2007; Cabassa et al., 2006).

Mental health facilities must also employ bilingual and bicultural Latina/o mental health providers and staff to meet the mental health needs of Latina/os (Falicov, 2013). While the exact number of Spanish-speaking mental health providers is unknown, a report from the American Psychological Association (Lin, Nigrinis, Christidis, & Stamm, 2015) indicates that among the 83,142 active psychologists in 2013, only 4,140 were Latina/os, including 689 Latinos and 3,451 Latinas. Colleges and universities should focus on recruiting greater numbers of bilingual Latina/os into the mental health profession. In addition, increased governmental funding is needed to provide scholarships and grants for education and training for these Latina/o mental health professionals.

Indeed, there is a significant need to develop a cadre of bilingual mental health professionals and infrastructures to ensure their success (Delgado-Romero, Espino, Werther, & González, 2011; Mercado-Crespo et al., 2010). Delgado-Romero et al. (2011) indicate that most bilingual and bicultural trainees are trained in generalist mental health programs that seldom employ Latina/o faculty. However, there are a small number of bilingual training programs, such as the Psychological Services for Spanish Speaking Populations (PSSP) program at Our Lady of the Lake University in San Antonio, Texas. As an APA-accredited program, PSSP trains bilingual mental health providers to become equally competent in English and Spanish through its curriculum and a cultural-immersion summer component in Mexico (Romero-Delgado et al., 2011). In California, a small number of colleges offer training experiences with Latina/os, such as the Marriage & Family Therapy (MFT) program at Pacific Oaks College in Pasadena, CA. Their MFT program offers a Latina/Latino Family Studies Specialization. Similarly, Pepperdine University, in Malibu, CA, offers a Master of Arts in Clinical Psychology with an emphasis in Marriage and Family Therapy with

Latinas/os. This program is administered through Aliento, The Center for Latina/o Communities, at the Irvine Graduate Campus.

However, given the dearth of bilingual Latina/o mental health providers, mental health and primary care facilities must ensure that their translators provide accurate and clinically relevant translations (Falicov, 2013). In addition, mental health facilities must provide their staff with regular cultural competency training and continue to focus on eliminating other barriers within their infrastructure that contribute to mental health care disparities (Aguilar-Gaxiola et al., 2012; Buki & Piedra, 2011; Caldwell, 2008; Daniel, 2010; Sue, 2001; Valdez et al., 2011). However, in addition to employing bilingual mental health providers and translators, mental health organizations must embrace organizational philosophies and policies that continuously strive for cultural and linguistic competence, a welcoming environment, social justice perspectives, and efficacious and Latina/o-centered mental health practices for Latina/o clients (see Chapter 10).

Community-Based Approaches

Community-based approaches hold promise in reducing mental health barriers and stigma and can also reach a large number of Latina/os through culturally responsive interventions (Falicov, 2013). *Promotoras de salud* (lay health educators), also known as *promotoras*, are a key strategy for the health promotion of Latina/os within community-based approaches (Arellano-Morales et al., 2016) and aid in increasing access and preventive health services (see Chapter 3). However, *promotoras* are also helpful in reducing the mental health barriers of Latina/os. They function as bridges between the community and the mental health care system. For instance, they offer personalized support, such as *personalismo*, and engender *confianza* as community members (Mercado-Crespo et al., 2010; Rhodes, Foley, Zometa, & Bloom, 2007). They are often natural helpers who are trained to engage in numerous roles such as role models, advocates, and health providers. For instance, *promotoras* and support groups are needed for older Spanish-speaking Latina/os who experience social isolation because of their limited English proficiency and poverty. Barrio et al. (2008) suggest that the creation of senior centers and community groups in convenient locations where Latina/o elders reside are important to provide comprehensive services to address their limited transportation, reliance on family members, and social isolation. In addition, the use of *promotoras* can help address the fragmentation of physical, social, and mental health services.

Community-based participatory research (CBPR) is a method to address the mental health disparities of Latina/os. In collaboration with community members, researchers can integrate cultural and social factors that are associated with increased mental health equity. For example, the Latino Strategic Planning Workgroup and the Concilio engaged in CBPR to identify strategies to reduce the mental health disparities of Latina/os in California through the identification of community-defined, strengths-based approaches (Aguilar-Gaxiola et al., 2012). Their extensive work identified the following core community-identified strategies to improve community services and treatment: (1) peer support and mentoring programs that focus on education and support services; (2) family psychoeducational curricula to increase involvement of the family and extended family and promote health and wellness; (3) promote wellness and illness management, and favor community-based strategies that integrate mental health services and other health and social services; (4) employ community capacity-building strategies that promote the connection of community-based strengths and health improvements in Latino behavioral health outcomes; (5) create a meaningful educational campaign to reduce stigma and exclusion at various levels; and (6) include best practices in integrated services that are culturally and linguistically competent to strengthen treatment effectiveness (Aguilar-Gaxiola et al., 2012).

Undoubtedly, because Latina/os prefer to utilize primary care settings for their mental health, there is a significant need for integrated mental health care (Cabassa & Hansen, 2007; Cabassa et al., 2006; Caldwell et al., 2008; Holden et al., 2014). This integration offers the opportunity to decrease their mental health disparities, particularly as they are more likely to report mental health problems in primary care settings than in mental health settings. Also, because primary care settings offer the opportunity for comprehensive medical and mental health care on site, there are significant benefits for Latina/os, such as increased compliance and follow-up because of the increased collaboration among professionals and increased access, as well as decreased stigma of mental illness (Benuto & O'Donohue, 2016; Holden et al., 2014; Willerton et al., 2008). For instance, providing therapy, such as medical family therapy, within primary care settings can decrease fear and stigma among Latina/os, since therapy is provided as a natural part of comprehensive health care (Willerton et al., 2008). Also, family therapists and other mental health professionals are better equipped to work with Latina/o clients within a medical context and can sensitively address contextual and systemic factors that impact their well-being. However, because many Latina/os seek mental health treatment from primary health care providers rather than from mental health providers, health providers should receive additional training in Latina/o mental health, to understand the importance of building rapport. For instance, insufficient time spent with older Latina/os violates their expectations of their relationship with their provider (Barrio et al., 2008). Training should help providers recognize the various presentations of distress among Latina/os, such as idioms of distress or depression. In addition, they should address the issue of mental health stigma and promote empowerment (Vega et al., 2010).

School-based mental health services are also important to Latina/o children and adolescents, particularly as they can also reduce stigma and schools have natural access to families that are reluctant to seek mental health services in traditional settings (Beehler, Birman, & Campbell, 2012; Kataoka et al., 2003). For example, the implementation of Cultural Adjustment and Trauma Services (CATS), is a comprehensive school-based mental health service program of the International Institute of New Jersey and targets immigrant Latina/o children and other immigrant youth with significant trauma exposure and/or cultural adjustment needs. CATS provides evidence-based clinical services within schools, including cognitive–behavior therapy (CBT) and trauma focused-CBT, family services, psychoeducation, supportive therapy, as well as outreach services and outreach and tangible support services, including job placement and food pantries. Outcomes suggest that CATS aids in improved functioning and reduced PTSD symptoms among immigrant youth and impacts multiple levels of their ecology (Beehler et al., 2012).

Culturally Appropriate Diagnostic Tools and Treatment

The limited availability of valid and culturally appropriate diagnostic tools for use with both English- and Spanish-speaking Latina/os poses challenges in the assessment and treatment process (American Psychological Association [APA], 2012; Benuto, 2016; Geisinger, 2015; Paniagua, 2014), particularly among mental health providers who tend to rely upon established testing and established assessment strategies and measures (see Geisinger, 2015). For example, clinical bias emerges when Eurocentric models of illness are utilized and result in misdiagnosis and limited attention to their resilience (APA, 2012). Furthermore, scholars recommend the importance of considering social, cultural, and linguistic contexts of Latina/os and immigrant clients and the coexistence of pathology and resilience within all phases of assessment, diagnosis, and treatment (APA, 2012). A solution to these limitations is the incorporation of a multidimensional framework in which culture, context, and social domains are addressed within the assessment process and treatment (Santiago-Rivera et al., 2002) through the use of a culture-centered clinical interview. Santiago-Rivera et al. (2002) developed the Culture-Centered Clinical Interview (CCCI), which is easily applied to individual, couples, or family therapy. Its semi-structured format also provides flexibility and allows for a Latina/o-centered treatment plan.

In addition, contextual approaches are also important, as they consider how internal and external factors impact a client's presenting problems. For example, the revised Cultural Formulation Interview (American Psychiatric Association, 2013) is featured within the *Diagnostic and Statistical Manual of Mental Disorders*, 5th ed. (DSM-5) and provides a standardized approach to cultural assessment. The Cultural Formulation Interview (CFI) includes three semi-structured interviews, including a core 16-item questionnaire; the CFI-Information Version; and 12 supplementary models that expand on these basic assessments. Lewis-Fernández and colleagues (2016) also provide clinicians with guidance and 12 supplementary modules and videos on subjects such as immigrants and refugees, coping and help seeking, through the development of the *Handbook on the Cultural Formulation Interview*.

The CFI enables providers to account for the influence of culture within their clinical work with Latina/os, an increased understanding of their presenting concerns through increased culturally sensitive and comprehensive assessment, and improved treatment planning and outcomes. In particular, the CFI allows for the systematic assessment of the following: (1) client's cultural identity; (2) client's conceptualizations of distress; (3) psychosocial stressors and cultural features of vulnerability and resilience; (4) cultural features of the relationship between the client and clinician; and (5) overall cultural assessment (APA, 2013). The use of the CFI is particularly useful for clinicians, since particular attention is given to cultural features that help orient clinical interventions and also renders useful information regarding culturally based values, norms, and behaviors, including alternative health practices, physiological interpretations, or religious beliefs (Lewis-Fernández & Díaz, 2002).

It is critical to use strength-based approaches that focus on the resilience of Latina/os rather than deficit-based perspectives (Adames & Chavez-Dueñas, 2017; Arredondo et al., 2014; Falicov, 2013; Santiago-Rivera et al., 2002). There is a clear need for treatments that are Latina/o-centered and innovative. In addition, cultural adaptations that include significant modifications and integrate Latina/o culture to increase their relevance, as well as the increased engagement of Latina/os are clearly needed (Cardemil & Sarmiento, 2009). These modifications may result in decreased dropout rates, increased access and utilization of services, and reduced mental health disparities among Latina/os (Falicov, 2009a). For example, cultural adaptations are effective for the treatment of depression with Latina/os (Cardemil

& Sarmiento, 2009) and other psychological disorders and age cohorts (see Chapter 8).

CONCLUSION

It is quite disturbing that Latina/os experience formidable barriers to effective mental health care and that despite subsequent attention to these disparities, mental health disparities among Latina/os have not diminished significantly. There is also a complex interplay between structural, economic, and cultural factors that pose barriers to their mental health utilization. As suggested by the former Surgeon General, it is time for mental health providers, researchers, and policymakers to increase their focus on promoting mental health and preventing mental health disorders. These barriers are eliminated with increased insurance coverage, integrated behavioral care, community-based approaches, community outreach, cultural sensitivity, and bilingual and bicultural staff. Contemporary strategies that utilize individual, community, and system approaches to encourage innovative and creative ways of thinking and providing care are also needed. In addition, advocacy efforts, research endeavors, and federal funding are paramount to sustain these efforts, as the prevention and treatment of mental health disorders is a moral issue.

Chapter 8

Culture-Specific Interventions and Community Efforts

When you subscribe to an empowerment multicultural model, you recognize your clients' contextual reality, accept their experience as valuable knowledge, affirm their cultural strengths, and acknowledge their perspectives on healing.
—Lillian Comas-Díaz, 2012c

Lamentably, mental health disparities among Latina/os are complex and multidimensional (see Chapter 6). They necessitate the use of strength-based approaches that focus on their resilience (Arredondo et al., 2014) rather than the deficit-based perspectives that often applied to Latina/os (Adames & Chavez-Dueñas, 2017; Falicov, 2014). Experts also call for the conceptualization of presenting problems from a developmental and life-cycle approach, such as a stage in the lifespan for Latina/os (e.g., bicultural or bilingual development), or a specific life event, such as divorce (Arredondo et al., 2014). This approach is nonthreatening and can reduce mental health stigma, and address relevant psychocultural stressors (Arredondo et al., 2014). Furthermore, acknowledging and integrating Latina/o cultural values and/or cultural family preferences into treatment can increase the service utilization, engagement and collaboration, and retention of Latina/o clients and result in positive outcomes (Aguila-Gaxiola et al., 2012; Cardemil & Sarmiento, 2009; Falicov, 2009a; Garza & Watts, 2010; Rosales Meza & Arellano-Morales, 2014). Comas-Díaz (2012c) also highlights the importance of treatment approaches that foster the examination of oppression to promote liberation through empowering, pluralistic and holistic approaches. For Latina/os, empowerment will increase their self-efficacy, mastery, agency, and control, as these approaches will foster self-healing, the development of critical consciousness, and the ability to overcome internalized oppression. Cumulatively, these perspectives are Latina/o-centered counseling approaches (Arredondo et al., 2014). Similarly, Arredondo et al. indicate that the following factors contribute to a Latina/o-centered counseling approach: (a) the utilization of dynamic multidimensional perspectives, (b) the integration of culture and therapeutic structures, (c) the application of strengths-based models, (d) the consideration of situational and contextual interpretations, (e) the inclusion of spirituality and healing practices, and (f) the implementation of social justice directives (p. 174).

Grounded within empowerment and social justice perspectives, this chapter provides a general overview of the psychological strengths of Latina/os, the importance of a strong therapeutic alliance, and intervention frameworks/guidelines for clinical work with Latina/os. We also review the debate regarding EBPs and treatments and cultural adaptations for Latina/os, such as cognitive behavioral therapy (CBT). Lastly, culture-specific treatments and community mental health efforts with Latina/os, such as the use of *promotoras*, gender-specific groups, and interventions with Latina/o youth are also reviewed

PSYCHOLOGICAL STRENGTHS OF LATINA/OS

As noted in Chapter 1, Latina/os are descendants of advanced and resilient civilizations, and their values, traditional practices, and new strategies enable them to survive and thrive despite their numerous challenges (Adames & Chavez-Dueñas, 2017). Without minimizing these serious challenges and risks (Falicov, 2014), experts highlight the importance of utilizing strengths-based approaches and fostering resilience (Adames & Chavez-Dueñas, 2017; Arredondo et al., 2014; Falicov, 2013; Gallardo, 2012; Santiago-Rivera et al., 2002). For example, Falicov (2013) notes that many Latina/os possess the following strengths: (1) the capacity to thrive and possess resources; (2) situation triumphs; (3) loving capacities; and (4) courage to face prejudice and economic injustice (p. 28). She further notes that their strengths include strong family and community bonds, strong systems of help, healthy maintenance of cultural rituals, capacity for hard work, and pride in good parenting.

Adames and Chavez-Dueñas (2017) also identify seven psychological strengths of Latina/os that can aid in developing strengths-based approaches (see Table 8.1). In particular, these psychological strengths

Table 8.1 Seven Psychological Strengths of Latina/os

Strengths	Descriptions
Determination	The endless drive and courage to do whatever is necessary to meet one's goals, despite barriers. For instance, Latina/os will not rest until they achieve their goals, whether immigrating to the United States, purchasing a home, or earning an academic degree.
Esperanza	Faith that even during the most difficult situations one can endure these challenges. This strength is captured by the *dicho* (saying), *La esperanza es lo ultimo que muere* (Hope is the last thing that dies).
Adaptability	The ability to adapt and thrive in a variety of environments. Latina/o immigrants in the United States demonstrate an incredible capacity to adapt and thrive despite vast cultural and linguistic differences.
Strong Work Ethic	Valuing the importance of hard work, producing quality, and taking pride in one's work endeavors regardless of social status or occupation. Overall, this value is guided by producing excellence for the betterment of self, family, and community.
Connectedness to Others	Valuing the need and enjoyment of being emotionally, physically, and spiritually connected to others throughout the lifespan in order to witness and share in life's challenging and joyous times.
Collective Emotional Expression	The ability, need, and desire to share strong emotions with others. All emotions ranging from sorrow and longing, to joy and gleefulness are freely expressed by Latina/os through music, dance, spoken word, spiritual rituals, art, literature, and sporting events.
Resistance	The willpower and courage to stand firmly for one's beliefs, ideals, and practices. This strength is also demonstrated in the determination of Latina/os to defy the odds and limits that are created by oppressive systems.

From: Adames & Chavez-Dueñas (2017). *Cultural formulations and interventions in Latino/a mental health: History, theory and within group differences.* New York: Routledge.

include determination, *esperanza* (hope), adaptability, a strong work ethic, connectedness to others, collective emotional expression, and resistance (pp. 28–29). For example, they note that resistance and adaptability enable Latina/os to adapt and thrive within various environments. In addition, they possess the willpower and courage to stand firmly for their beliefs and the ability to overcome oppressive systems. Barrio et al. (2011) suggest that these cultural strengths are often underutilized in mental health settings. Arredondo and colleagues (2014) note that limited awareness or dismissal of these cultural strengths can cause a mental health provider to "fall into the psychopathology trap" and contribute to counseling attrition and perceptions of therapeutic oppression (p. 180).

Also recognizing the need to focus on strengths, Arredondo et al. (2014) created a family resilience model for strengths-based family therapy with Latina/os that is embedded within beliefs systems and family organizational patterns, as well as an ecological conceptualization of family problems. They posit that a strengths-based orientation requires an understanding of risk factors and an appreciation of personal and cultural protective factors. These protective elements are interrelated with personal and cultural assets, such as *familismo*, collectivism, social support, flexibility, and spirituality, among others. Through a Latina/o-centered ecological orientation, their model focuses on six components that reflect strengths among Latina/o families, including making meaning from adversity, a positive outlook, transcendence and spirituality, flexibility, connectedness, and social and economic resources (see Table 8.2). For example, Arredondo et al. (2014) highlight the importance of a positive outlook, and indicate that mental health providers should communicate hope and optimism and also reinforce perseverance, persistence, and action despite stressors and cultural adaptations.

THE IMPORTANCE OF ESTABLISHING A STRONG THERAPEUTIC ALLIANCE

Mental health interventions with Latina/os must reflect cultural sensitivity through clinical approaches and program activities that build on the cultural strengths of Latina/os. While recognizing that adherence to Latina/o cultural values certainly differs among Latina/os because of their significant diversity across numerous domains, cumulatively, these values emphasize courtesy, kindness, formal friendliness, respect, and recognition of the family's importance. When these values are absent from the clinical encounter, significant barriers are often created. Flexibility and accommodation are also paramount to building a solid therapeutic alliance with Latina/os (Arredondo et al., 2014; Falicov, 2013; Santiago-Rivera et al., 2002). Thus, a core element of culturally responsive clinical work is the demonstration of interpersonal etiquette (Santiago-Rivera et al., 2002), as discussed in Chapter 7.

Arredondo et al. (2014) also highlight the importance of establishing a strong therapeutic alliance with Latina/os, as clinicians are "agents of change" within the therapeutic encounter, regardless of their theoretical

Table 8.2 Strengths-Based Family Therapy with Latina/os

Resiliency Process	Component	Relevant Areas to Target in Therapy With Latina/os
Belief Systems	Making meaning from adversity	1. Approach the crisis as a family affair in which all members share in the experience, rely on their interrelatedness, and how they can contribute to the resolution ("shared challenge"). Focus on *familismo* to address immigration history, the adaptation process, prejudice, language barriers, parent–child conflict, and family conflict.
		2. Normalize adversity and contextualize problems: define the family's life stage crisis, reframe generational conflicts as cultural events, affirm emotional reactions and different styles of emotional expression, justify reactions, do not focus on pathology.
		3. Reframe the crisis or problem as a manageable event, *Si se puede* [Yes, we can do it!!]. Explore explanatory attributions: *fatalismo* (fatalism), spiritual attributions, psychocultural explanations for problems (e.g., *nervios* [nerves] due to immigration trauma), *dichos* with positive messages.
	Positive Outlook	1. Communicate hope and optimism.
		2. Identify and affirm strengths, including personal, family, and cultural strengths; spirituality; and adaptive beliefs. Identify strengths of the native and host cultures.
		3. Reinforce perseverance, persistence, and action despite stressors and cultural adaptations.
		4. Identify what can and cannot be changed; reframe what cannot be changed and focus on manageable elements; address issues of loss (loss of status, family separations, country-of-origin family and traditions), as well as focus on the here and now to solve present problems, using *fatalismo* as a way of coping with what cannot be changed.

(*continued*)

Table 8.2 Strengths-Based Family Therapy with Latina/os (*continued*)

Resiliency Process	Component	Relevant Areas to Target in Therapy With Latina/os
	Transcendence and spirituality	1. Seek purpose and existential understanding. 2. Explore sources of *fortaleza interna* (inner strength). 3. Explore healing practices, spirituality, faith, folk healing, rituals, prayers, alternative spiritual beliefs, and practices (*curanderismo* [healing practices], *espiritismo* [spiritualism], *Santería*), and church membership. 4. Provide inspiration; envision new possibilities, promote social action, model coping strategies, empower with a social justice orientation and social justice solutions, and provide models. 5. Identify transformations; lessons learned from adversity, gains, *No hay mal que por bien no venga* (There is always an upside to a downside).
Organizational patterns	Flexibility	1. Assist with adaptations, reorganization, and changes in family structure and dynamics: gender roles, expectations, working families, shared responsibilities. 2. Maintain stability and continuity through crisis: seek connections with country of origin and extended family, support preferred healing practices and rituals, seek out healers and elders in community who provide continuity of coping mechanism. 3. Provide authoritative leadership; be an active therapist, give advice, model communication and coping strategies, advocate for clients, educate, seek out resources in the community. 4. Consider alternative medicine methods (la *botánica* [botanical, folk healing store where natural healing medication can be purchased], folk healing practices). 5. Provide ecological therapeutic interventions.

(*continued*)

Table 8.2 Strengths-Based Family Therapy with Latina/os (*continued*)

Resiliency Process	Component	Relevant Areas to Target in Therapy With Latina/os
	Connectedness	1. Identify the members of the family network.
		2. Strengthen family solidarity and support (*familismo*).
		3. Reinforce values of *respeto*, boundaries, tolerance with differences, and hierarchical organization.
		4. Encourage reconciliation and reconnections with family members, social networks, and extended family members.
	Social and economic resources	1. Include extended family and *compadrazco* (kinship) in the therapeutic process for support and generalization of positive effects.
		2. Seek out supportive networks in the community, for example, churches, agencies, and institutions that are linguistically and culturally sensitive.
		3. Explore assistance with logistics to ensure compliance with treatment (transportation, flexible appointment schedules, child care, in-home services).
		4. Engage in client advocacy.
		5. Incorporate ecological interventions and community mentors (e.g., *promotoras*).

From: Arredondo, Gallardo-Cooper, Delgado-Romero, & Zapata (2014). *Culturally responsive counseling with Latinas/os*. Alexandria, VA: American Counseling Association.

orientation. They provide several recommendations to facilitate the therapeutic relationship:

- Focus on shared similarities with clients instead of emphasizing differences in order to increase your connection with them.
- Develop cultural empathy.
- Unveil your internalized personal and cultural biases.
- Disclose and ask about differences and similarities.
- Address and explore psychocultural stressors.

- Seek to communicate in the same language as your client to facilitate the quality of care, discussions regarding treatment barriers, and the therapeutic relationship.
- Be congruent with the client or family's level of formality or informality. Some families may present as more formal during the initial meeting.
- Directly check and verify with Latina/o clients that you are responding to their needs.
- Be responsive to communication style and language to facilitate engagement (Arredondo et al., 2014, pp. 160–161).

INTERVENTION FRAMEWORKS AND GUIDELINES FOR EFFICACIOUS COUNSELING WITH LATINA/OS

There are a number of frameworks and guidelines for clinical practice with Latina/os. While it is beyond the scope of this chapter to address all of these recommendations, we review several guidelines and models that are multidimensional, systemic, and holistic, rather than simply recommending techniques for the generic Latina/o client. As noted by Gallardo (2012), culturally responsive skill in therapy is not simply the implementation of techniques, but rather the process by which one engages in the therapeutic encounter (p. 105).

One of the first frameworks to integrate the cultural values and beliefs of Latina/os within clinical practice is the Multidimensional Ecosystemic Comparative Approach (MECA; Falicov, 1998). MECA incorporates the major constructs of cultural diversity and social justice. Cultural diversity is explored primarily within the domains of family organization and family life cycle. Within this domain, assessment and processes address relational stresses and other factors that impact family organization, as well as child-rearing practices, cultural ideals, and rituals. In addition, a social justice position focuses on life conditions, power differentials, and contextual discrimination that limits opportunities and impacts health and mental health. Within this domain, assessment and processes address migration and acculturation and ecological contexts, such as poverty and contextual protections. A critical component of MECA is a reflective and culturally humble stance, including the examination of personal and theoretical niches of mental health providers and supervisors and their impact on clinical practice and supervision. A number of training and narrative tools are used also in conjunction with MECA applications, such as culture-centered genograms and ecomaps (Falicov, 1998, 2013).

Another model that is designed to help mental health providers identify core issues that facilitate the therapeutic process, is the Latina/o Skills Identification Stage Model (L-SISM; Gallardo, 2012). The Skills Identification

Stage Model (SISM) was originally developed for clinical use with African Americans, but Gallardo (2009) adopted the model for use with Latina/o clients, resulting in the L-SISM. A key element of this model is the recognition of the multiple intersections that shape worldviews, multiple identities, and values of each Latina/o and the multidimensional and systemic perspective. The L-SISM is applicable to different therapeutic modalities and focuses on six domains that aid in developing culturally responsive interventions with Latina/o clients, and incorporates cultural domains, such as spirituality, class, gender, and sexual orientation.

The first domain, *Connecting with Clients*, focuses on *personalismo*, making small talk, using *dichos*, music, and poetry as ways to connect with clients and educate them about the therapeutic process. In addition, within this domain, mental health providers assess the client's cultural strengths and existing resources. The second domain, *Assessment*, focuses on the assessment of generational status, ethnic identity, level of acculturation, language usage, trauma, and environmental factors. This domain also entails an understanding of a client's distress from a Latina/o-centered frame of reference. The third domain, *Facilitating Awareness*, focuses on client strengths and existing resources to facilitate awareness regarding sociopolitical forces and to reframe perceptions regarding their problems. In addition, this domain focuses on traditional ways that clients cope with their presenting problems (i.e., community-specific narratives, assigned readings, etc.). The fourth domain, *Setting Goals*, focuses on the development of treatment goals, with particular attention to how a mental health provider's beliefs about Latina/os impact the therapeutic process. This domain also includes an understanding of how a client's level of education, socioeconomic status, community groups, and the expanded role of the family in helping clients achieve their treatment goals. The fifth domain, *Instigating Change*, addresses the importance of culturally adapting existing interventions and connections between the mental health provider and Latina/o communities. In addition, this domain entails social advocacy for Latina/o clients. Lastly, the sixth domain, *Feedback and Accountability*, highlights the need to understand and evaluate treatment outcomes within a Latina/o specific context and asking for client feedback (Gallardo, 2012).

To highlight the role of race, skin color, and physiognomy, in conjunction with culture, Adames and Chavez-Dueñas (2017), recently created the Culturally Responsive AND Racially Conscious Ecosystemic (CREAR-CE) Treatment Approach. The word *crear* is a Spanish verb that means to form, create, or build anew. The CREAR-CE Treatment Approach includes three main phases that include various domains within each phase. For example, Phase I, *Building A Culturally Racially Responsive and Racially Conscious Self*, emphasizes the importance of developing knowledge and awareness of the clinician as a cultural and racial being. Thus, this phase includes three areas, including complexity of self-knowledge and awareness (i.e., courses, journals, films/documentaries), emotional processing (i.e., engaging in difficult dialogues), and behavioral engagement (i.e., getting out of one's comfort zone and having meaningful interactions with persons who are similar and dissimilar). Phase II, *Learning Social-Cultural and Historical Foundations of Latinos/as*, includes a sophisticated understanding of a client's sociohistorical context, level of acculturation, stage/status of both racial and ethnic identity development, and traditional cultural values and worldview to provide culturally responsive and racially conscious treatment. These components include knowledge of within-group differences, historical roots, immigration patterns, skin color and physiognomy, racial and ethnic identity, acculturation, and gender. Lastly, Phase III, *Delivering Culturally Responsive and Racially Conscious Treatment*, focuses on areas that help clients connect with their personal and collective healing powers. In particular, these domains include connecting with clients, assessing racial/ethnic identity and acculturation, contextualizing the problem, developing prosocial coping skills, addressing skin color and the role of racism, and healing through liberation.

DEBATE REGARDING EVIDENCE-BASED PROGRAMS AND TREATMENTS

The integration of empirical science and clinical practice has dominated the field of mental health (Adames & Chavez-Dueñas, 2017), such as EBPs. The concept of EBPs and treatments refers to the promotion of high-quality services through robust scientific testing, whereby researchers systematically evaluate the efficacy of particular treatments in producing desired outcomes (Foxen, 2016). Such evidence is often produced through randomized clinical trials and quasi-experimental studies (Foxen, 2016). EBPs can include treatments that are considered efficacious, with different standards of research determining levels of efficacy (Bernal, Jimenez-Chafey, & Domenech Rodríguez, 2009; Castro, Barrera, & Holleran Steiker, 2010). EBPs are alluring to policymakers, funders, and many mental health practitioners since interventions are manualized, promote clear-cut standards and measurable outcomes, and promise high-quality services, accountability, and cost savings (Foxen, 2016).

However, a common criticism of EBPs is that they often fail to include Latina/os and other ethnic minorities and their efficacy with ethnic minorities are limited. Studies that document the efficacy of behavioral treatments are often based on White/European Americans and have limited generalizability to other populations. In addition, the conditions and context under which efficacy studies are conducted often differ significantly from those in many community-based settings in terms of language, resources, training staff, and other practical constraints (Foxen, 2016). Thus, there is a significant gap between the availability and relevance of EBPs for ethnic minorities (Wallis, Amaro, & Cortés, 2012). To bridge this gap, researchers and clinicians have tailored specific EBPs for specific populations and contexts, and while these efforts are slowly evolving, several Latina/o scholars suggest that cultural adaptations are needed, as they are efficacious with Latina/os (Bernal et al., 2009; Castro et al., 2010).

CULTURAL ADAPTATIONS OF EVIDENCE-BASED PRACTICES WITH LATINA/OS

Cultural adaptation refers to "the systematic modification of an evidence-based treatment (EBT) or intervention protocol to consider language, culture, and context in such a way that is compatible with the client's cultural patterns, meaning, and values" (Bernal et al., 2009, p. 362). As with EBPs, there are also debates regarding cultural adaptations as well, including the cost, lack of empirical evidence that mainstream programs do not work for ethnic minorities, and similarities in risk factors among majority and minorities groups (Foxen, 2016). Nonetheless, others argue that adaptations are required when a program or intervention is mismatched with a new target community (Castro, Barrera, & Martinez, 2004; Wallis et al., 2012).

When interventions designed for White/European Americans are used with Latina/os, these interventions are problematic, since they lack community buy-in and result in low participation. The intervention may also conflict with Latina/o cultural values, beliefs, and norms and potentially result in high dropout rates and low efficacy (Wallis et al., 2012). Cultural adaptations are considered a middle ground between two extreme positions, including a universal top-down approach that views an intervention's content as applicable to all groups and does not require alterations. Conversely, a culture-specific approach is a bottom-up approach that emphasizes culturally grounded content that includes the values, beliefs, and practices of a specific group (Barrera et al., 2012, p. 197).

In their edited book, Domenech Rodríguez and Bernal (2012) offer exemplars of cultural adaptations of conventional EBPs for a variety of psychological problems for various racial/ethnic groups, including Latina/os. In addition, there are several models to guide cultural adaptations that were independently developed but nonetheless demonstrate consensus (Barrera & Castro, 2006; Domenech Rodríguez, Baumann, & Schwartz, 2011; Domenech Rodríguez & Weiling, 2004; Kumpfer, Pinyuchon, Melo, & Whiteside, 2008). For example, Barrera, Castro, Strycker, and Toobert (2013) propose that cultural adaptations can be organized into five stages:

information gathering, preliminary design, preliminary testing, refinement, and final trial. In addition, ecological validity helps to increase the congruence between a client's experience and elements of the treatment. If the criteria of ecological validity are met, then one can assume that the treatment is aligned with the client's culture, language, and worldview (Domenech Rodríguez et al., 2011; Domenech Rodríguez & Bernal, 2012).

For example, in their pilot study Ramos and Alegría (2014) evaluated the acceptability, feasibility, and efficacy of a brief depression intervention for Latina/os, entitled the *Engagement and Counseling for Latinos* (ECLA) intervention. They offer a detailed description of how they follow Barrera et al.'s (2013) five-stage approach (i.e., information gathering, preliminary adaptation, preliminary testing, adaptation, and refinement). Their process of cultural adaptation includes accommodations for health literacy of a brief telephone cognitive behavioral depression intervention for Central and South American and Caribbean immigrants in low-resource settings. They also detail how feedback from key stakeholders, such as clinicians and participants, enable them to modify program materials including the addition of visual aids, *dichos*, *personalismo*, and other culturally relevant values and proverbs.

One of the most widely used frameworks for culturally centered interventions with Latina/os, is the ecological validity model (Bernal, Bonilla, & Bellido, 1995; Bernal & Sáez-Santiago, 2006). This model outlines eight broad areas for consideration in culturally adapting an intervention: language, persons, metaphors, content, concepts, goals, methods, and context (Bernal et al., 1995; Bernal & Sáez-Santiago, 2006). In particular, these cultural dimensions in the adaptation process also include the following: (a) language, the language used in an intervention is culturally appropriate and syntonic; (b) persons, culturally centered interventions consider the role of ethnic and racial similarities and differences in the client–therapist dyad; (c) metaphors, the use of symbols and concepts such as refrains or *dichos*; (d) content/deep structure, including cultural knowledge, cultural values, beliefs, norms, worldviews, lifestyles, customs, and traditions; (e) concepts, treatment is compatible with culture and conceptualized in a way that is compatible with client's beliefs systems; (f) goals, treatment goals are matched with client's cultural values and traditions to reduce behavioral resistance; (g) methods/delivery, include decisions regarding type of intervention, program location, materials, and presentation strategies; and (h) personal context/environment, includes a client's immediate environment and sociocultural–historical contexts, including acculturation, enculturation, acculturative stress, migration, availability of social supports, and a client's culture of origin, and a community's infrastructure (Domenech Rodríguez & Bernal, 2012).

CULTURE-SPECIFIC TREATMENTS FOR USE WITH LATINA/OS

Additional forms of integrating culture into therapy involve therapies known as either culture-specific therapies or culturally centered therapies (Cardemil & Sarmiento, 2009; Falicov, 2009a). These therapies are based on the assumption that cultures have their own healing approaches and that traditional forms of psychotherapy are inappropriate, as they impose and are rooted within White middle-class values (Cardemil & Sarmiento, 2009; Falicov, 2009a). These types of therapies are also "theoretically incongruent to provide a traditional form of psychotherapy for culturally specific expressions of distress" (Cardemil & Sarmiento, 2009, p. 337). Strengths of culturally centered therapies consist of their focus on wellness and their ability to validate and address psychosocial and sociocultural stressors within the lives of Latina/os. Additionally, Cardemil and Sarmiento (2009) identify the congruence between conceptualization of the problem and treatment approach as an important strength. These therapies offer much promise because they are grounded within Latina/o culture and thus, may provide culture-specific healing that may not be achieved through other types of treatments. Still, it is important to recognize that the specificity may limit the generalizability of these treatments.

Examples of culture-specific therapies include *cuento* therapy (Costantino, Malgady, & Rogler, 1986), a groundbreaking therapy based on Puerto Rican folklore. These researchers developed a storytelling technique with a moral message rooted in folktales for Puerto Rican children. In their landmark study, they compared three methods, including (a) *cuento* therapy; (b) play therapy; and (c) no therapy, among 210 children with maladaptive behaviors and their mothers. Results indicate that compared to the other groups, the *cuento* approach is superior in reducing children's trait anxiety, even one year later.

Although the use of metaphors is long-standing (Santiago-Rivera, Arredondo, & Gallardo-Cooper, 2002), Maria Zuñiga (1992) was among the first practitioners to address the efficacy of *dichos* with Latinos. She notes that as sayings or idioms in Spanish, *dichos* reveal the psychology of a people and their worldviews. She uses *dichos* in clinical settings as therapeutic tools to reduce client resistance, reframe problems, increase client motivation, make points, and address client's feelings. *Dichos* are also utilized with hospitalized Spanish-speaking psychiatric patients (Aviera, 1996). The use of *dichos* contributes to positive attitudes toward therapy and increased functioning. In particular, *dichos* enable clients to engage in discussions regarding a wide range of issues, facilitate increased rapport, motivation, and insight, and also assist in exploring cultural values and identity (Aviera, 1996).

José Szapocznik and his associates developed culturally sensitive family therapies for Cuban families, including a combination of structural and strategic family therapy models. Their pioneering work includes *Brief Strategic Family Therapy, Family Effectiveness Training,* and *Bicultural Effectiveness Training* to increase family functioning among Cuban families to resolve intergenerational and acculturation conflicts (Szapocznik & Kurtines, 1993; Szapocznik et al., 1984, 1986, 1997). For example, as a family treatment model Brief Strategic Family Therapy (BSFT; Szapocznik, Hervis, & Schwartz, 2003) was developed and tested for four decades with Cuban families at the University of Miami's Center for Family Studies, with Cuban adolescents with behavior problems, such as substance abuse, delinquency, association with antisocial peers, and unsafe sexual behaviors (Horigian, Anderson, & Szapocznik, 2016). BSFT is an integrative model that combines structural and strategic family therapy techniques to address systemic/relational (primarily family) interactions that are associated with adolescent problem behaviors. BSFT is a present problem–focused, directive, and practical approach, and as a short-term program, it is implemented in 12 to 16 sessions that are typically delivered once a week for 1½ hours over a four-month period (Horigian et al., 2016).

Other culturally sensitive therapies include increased literacy of psychosis. Lopez and colleagues (2009) developed a 35-minute psychoeducational program to increase literacy about psychosis among Spanish-speaking Latina/os. The program uses popular cultural icons derived from music, art, and videos, as well as a mnemonic device, *La CLAve* (The Clue). *La CLAve* increases (a) knowledge of psychosis, (b) efficacy beliefs that one can identify psychosis in others, (c) attributions to mental illness, and (d) seeking professional help. Symptoms are described in nontechnical language to facilitate recall of the symptoms of psychosis and to enhance their belief that they can identify psychosis in others. Pre- and post-testing data indicate that *La CLAve* is well received by community residents ($N=57$) and family caregivers ($N=38$), with increased knowledge of psychotic symptoms for both groups. In addition, the three-week follow-up indicates a degree of stability among participants' knowledge of psychosis.

Also focusing on schizophrenia, Barrio and Yamada (2010) developed a *Culturally Based Family Intervention with Mexican American Families* (CFIMA) based on their three-year iterative intervention development process that is guided by a cultural exchange framework and findings from an ethnographic study. CFIMA is piloted as multifamily group 16-session intervention with 59 Mexican American families. The intervention process focuses on the transaction exchange of knowledge, attitudes, and practices that occur between Latina/o families and service providers. In particular, the three stages of cultural exchange include cultural assessments, cultural accommodations, and cultural integration of strengths and resources. Preliminary evidence indicates that CFIMA effectively increases illness knowledge and reduces family burden. Because of their enhanced knowledge, participants experience a sense of empowerment to become more assertive about seeking mental health treatment and express a renewed sense of pride in their Mexican heritage to become active in the treatment process. Interestingly, their increased knowledge enables them to teach other family members, friends, neighbors, and co-workers about mental illness and the importance of culture (Barrio, Hernández, & Barragán, 2011)

Unfortunately, there are few culture-specific programs for elderly Latina/os. Costantino, Malgady, and Primavera (2009) investigate a new two-factor construct, termed *cultural congruence*, which is related to cultural competence in the delivery of mental health services to ethnic minority clients. Their participants include older immigrants—largely Puerto Rican and Dominican clients ($N=272$)—who receive mental health services either through integrated primary care or referral to specialized mental health care. Findings indicate that cultural congruence predicts treatment outcomes (reduction of symptoms) independent of treatment and moderates depression, suicidality, anxiety, and physical health criteria. Cultural congruence increases with the enhanced specialty referral model rather than the integrated primary care model.

Similarly, *Un Nuevo Amanecer* (A New Dawn) is an evidence-based depression treatment program for Latina/o older adults and elders (age 60 years and older) with depression (Chavez-Korell et al., 2012). As an EBP, *Un Nuevo Amanecer* was originally designed for older adults from a Midwestern primary care setting. Although relatively little adaptation of the clinical protocol is required, which facilitates fidelity to the evidence-based model, major cultural adaptations are required. Cultural adaptations include (a) adapting treatment to a community center setting to improve Latina/o elders' access, retention, and outcomes; (b) language adaptation of all materials and services into Spanish; (c) the consideration of illiteracy and low literacy adaptations of treatment materials; (d) decreasing the ratio of clients; and (e) culturally sensitive and appropriate treatment activities. The preliminary data provide support that *Un Nuevo Amanecer* clients report significantly reduced depressive symptoms (Chavez-Korell et al., 2012).

The Use of Cognitive Behavioral Therapy with Latina/os

Several authors (Cardemil, Kim, Pinedo, & Miller, 2005; Comas-Díaz, 1981; Interian, Allen, Gara, & Escobar, 2008; Interian & Diaz-Martinez, 2007; Organista & Muñoz, 1996) advocate for the use of culturally responsive CBT for Latino/as with anxiety and depression. They propose that CBT is particularly suitable for Latino/as because of its directive, problem-solving approach that fits well with traditional expectations of immediate symptom relief and guidance. In addition, its didactic style helps to quickly orient clients to treatment and aides in demystifying therapy and alleviating stigma (Organista & Muñoz, 1996). Indeed, both individual and group CBT effectively reduce anxiety and depression in Latino/as (Cardemil et al., 2005; Comas-Díaz, 1981; Interian et al., 2008; Miranda et al., 2003). However, in their review of culturally adapted CBT interventions with Latina/os, Benuto and O'Donohue (2015) suggest that these interventions demonstrate basic methodological limitations and fail to employ the gold standard practices associated with randomized clinical trials. They also lack consensus regarding what adaptations or modifications are necessary and instead rely on generalizations for culturally sensitive interventions with Latina/os.

While CBT is a useful treatment, researchers emphasize tailoring content, goals, and methods to Latina/o culture, as this impacts the cognitive and behavioral process, facilitates cognitive restructuring, and contributes to improved access and outcomes (Organista, 2000; Organista & Muñoz, 1996). Cultural adaptations to CBT include the use of *dichos* to help clients understand the importance of active and behavioral coping strategies (Interian & Diaz-Martinez, 2007; Organista, 2000) and the incorporation of Latina/o spiritual beliefs that address the importance of shifting into a more active direction (Organista, 2000; Organista & Muñoz, 1996). Additionally, the *dicho "poner de su parte"* (Doing your/their part) is used when framing the purpose of implementing behavioral techniques within therapy. The use of this proverb with Latina/o clients allows them to recognize that this aspect of therapy provides an opportunity to *poner de su parte* to improve their mental health and functioning (Interian & Diaz-Martinez, 2007).

Culturally competent CBT is framed within a model originally proposed by Rogler, Malgady, Costantino, and Blumenthal (1987). Their model includes culturally competent interventions with Latina/os to ensure ease of access, strategies that are compatible with Latina/o culture, and the adaptation of traditional treatment approaches. Recommendations for culturally adapting CBT include consideration of each client's unique ethnocultural background and treatment expectations, as well as culturally relevant interpersonal styles, values, and metaphors/language that are captured with *dichos*. For example, being able to *desahogarse* and *poner de su parte* appear to represent the language that many clients use to describe valued methods of coping, which therapists, in turn, can integrate into the CBT process. Finally, Interian and Díaz-Martínez (2007) propose case conceptualization as a method for adapting to the problem complexity that a number of Latina/o clients are likely to experience. For instance, when conducting CBT with Latina/os, the issue of high problem complexity is particularly relevant, as they are likely to experience multiple stressors due to migration, greater challenges associated with socioeconomic difficulties, and perhaps difficult circumstances that prompt their immigration to the United States.

CBT is also efficacious with Latina/o youth and the treatment of depression. For instance, Rosselló, Bernal, and Rivera-Medina (2008) compared individual therapy to group formats of cognitive behavioral therapy and interpersonal psychotherapy for the treatment of depression in Puerto Rican adolescents. Their participants include 112 adolescents from San Juan, Puerto Rico, who are randomly assigned to four conditions (Cognitive Behavioral Treatment-Individual [CBT-I], Cognitive Behavioral Treatment-Group [CBT-G], Interpersonal Treatment-Individual [IPT-I], and Interpersonal Treatment-Group [IPT-G]). The individual treatment conditions consist of 12 one-hour therapy sessions held once a week for 12 weeks. The group treatment also consists of 12 sessions that are two hours in length and held over a 12-week period. CBT and IPT are provided in both group and individual formats. CBT and IPT are culturally and developmentally adapted to Puerto Rican adolescents and adapted to group formats. Detailed manuals are prepared for the four therapy conditions to ensure treatment integrity. Findings suggest that CBT and IPT are robust treatments in both group and individual formats. However, CBT produces significantly greater decreases in depressive symptoms and improved self-concept than IPT. Rosselló et al. (2008) suggest that CBT appears to offer faster symptom relief, because it is structured and concrete and its directive approach is consonant with the cultural value of *respeto*.

Group CBT is also beneficial for reducing substance abuse among Latina/o adolescents. In a randomized clinical trial, Burrow-Sánchez, Minami, and Hops (2015) compared the efficacy of an empirically supported standard version of a group-based cognitive behavioral treatment (S-CBT) to a culturally accommodated version (A-CBT) with adolescents of Mexican descent. Their participants ($N=70$) were primarily male and largely recruited from the juvenile justice system. The *Cultural Accommodation Model* (CAM-SAT) guided the culturally accommodated treatment for substance abuse treatment. Participants were randomly assigned to one of two group-based treatment conditions (S-CBT$=36$; A-CBT$=34$). Although both groups demonstrate significantly decreased substance use, the results do not support a time–treatment condition interaction. However, outcomes are moderated by ethnic identity and *familismo*. Latina/o adolescents with greater affiliation to their ethnic identity and parental *familismo* appear to receive greater benefits from a culturally accommodated substance abuse treatment than peers with less affiliation.

Group CBT is also beneficial for the reduction of depression and anxiety among Latina/os, such as migrant farmworkers. For example, Hovey, Hurtado, and Seligman (2014) evaluated a culturally responsive cognitive behavioral support group for Mexican migrant farmworkers in Colorado. They assessed for changes in migrant farmworker stress, anxiety, depressive symptoms, hopelessness, and self-esteem at the end of treatment and at six-month follow-up. Six women with elevated depression and migrant farmworker stress underwent a six-session intervention conducted in Spanish by a licensed clinical psychologist and a *promotora*. Weekly sessions are held in the evenings at a local church for 1½ hours and transportation is provided.

Rather than being called "group treatment," the group is framed as an opportunity for the participants to discuss their difficulties as farmworkers. Each session focuses on issues that are identified by the participants as being relevant, and the group leaders utilize culturally valued interactions in their interventions. These considerations help strengthen comfort, trust, and alliances; decrease possible stigma and premature termination and dropout; and enhance the effectiveness of the CBT techniques. The emphasis on problem solving, assertiveness, and skill building appears to contribute to participants' increase in coping competence by helping them regain a sense of control and thus alleviate their learned helplessness. Furthermore, findings indicate increased self-esteem and reduced stress, anxiety, and depressive symptoms. Findings also provide support for the use of culturally responsive support groups as an effective short-term intervention for Mexican migrant farmworkers. The use of a *promotora* appears particularly helpful to decrease stigma and promote trust, and she also serves as a role model for the participants since several can relate to her (Hovey et al., 2014).

Mental Health Interventions with *Promotoras*

The use of *promotoras* is a culturally and linguistically relevant approach to address the health and mental health disparities of Latina/os. There is a significant amount of literature suggesting that *promotoras* help improve the health, knowledge, and behaviors of Latina/os (see Chapter 3). Their success is often attributed to their roles as community advocates, role models, health advisors, and providers of social support (Elder et al., 2009). While *promotoras* largely provide health promotion and interventions with Latina/os, the use of *promotoras* for mental health efforts have increased within the past decade (Arellano-Morales, Elder, Sosa, Vaquero, & Alcantára, 2016), such as autism spectrum disorder (Magaña et al., 2017), depression literacy

(Hernandez & Organista, 2013; Unger et al., 2013), depression care (Ell et al., 2017), stress (Tran et al., 2014), coping (Perez et al., 2016), and mental health and diabetes (Reinschmidt & Chong, 2005). Indeed, *promotoras* can aid in decreasing the mental health disparities of Latina/os by specifically addressing the identified needs of the community (Castro, Balcazar, & Cota, 2008), particularly since they work without borders, such churches, homes, schools, community centers, and other locations within the community.

For example, in a randomized study, Hernandez and Organista (2013) extend the work of Unger et al. (2013), and evaluate the effectiveness of a *fotonovela* entitled *Secret Feelings*, to increase knowledge of depression and treatment among a sample of predominantly Mexican women from the San Francisco area ($N=142$) who are at risk for depression and low health literacy. The *fotonovela* is a traditional print medium found in Latin America that contains sequential photographs accompanied by dialogue bubbles to depict a simple, dramatic story (or soap opera) enveloped in a dramatic plot that contains a moral message. The experimental group is exposed to the *fotonovela* that includes a story of a depressed middle-aged mother who models how to seek treatment and discuss her mental health concerns with her family. Control group participants are exposed to a discussion of family communication and intergenerational relationships. Pretreatment and post-treatment data indicate significant gains for the experimental group in their depression-related knowledge, self-efficacy to identify the need for treatment, and reduced stigma toward antidepressants (Hernandez & Organista, 2013).

Hernandez and Organista (2013) attribute the program's success to the use of a multiservice delivery site that allows for collaboration with *promotoras*, childcare, assistance to participants who experience difficulties completing preintervention and postintervention measures, and a group format that allows participants to read aloud their *fotonovela*. These improvements are important for Latinas with low health literacy that are at risk for depression as well as Latinos, as *fotonovelas* are potentially effective mental health tools that provide health information for a stigmatized condition such as depression and may potentially motivate Latina/os to seek help (Hernandez & Organista, 2013; Unger et al., 2013).

Latina immigrants who reside in new immigrant settlement areas, such as the Southeast, often experience significant stressors and mental health disparities that are magnified by scant culturally appropriate services and limited social support. Tran et al. (2014) evaluated the impact of ALMA (*Amigas Latinas Motivando el Alma*/Latina Friends Motivating the Soul), a pilot *promotora* intervention that is offered in three North Carolina counties to improve mental health among Latinas by offering training in coping skills. The intervention, developed within a community-based participatory framework, trains *promotoras* to conduct outreach to Latinas within their social networks (*compañeras*).

Nearly two thirds of the *compañeras* are from Mexico and others are largely from South American countries ($N=58$). Preintervention and postintervention findings indicate lower levels of perceived stress and acculturation stress. The most prevalent acculturation stressors among *compañeras* are related to being away from family and friends, concerns about drugs and alcohol in their communities, and limited English proficiency. The ALMA curriculum specifically builds social networks among Latinas, which helps alleviate their loneliness and lack of support. Improvement in depressive symptoms, attitudes regarding depression treatment, and positive coping responses are also observed. Tran et al. (2014) suggest that interventions such as ALMA that focus on building self-care strategies are crucial to reducing preclinical symptoms and address health care disparities that result from unavailable or underused mental health services among immigrant Latinas.

Promotoras also aid in preventive substance abuse efforts. For example, Ayón, Peña, and Naddy (2014) developed a culturally grounded intervention that is implemented by *promotoras* to prevent substance use among Latina/o adolescents in their neighborhoods. The *Promotora* program is initiated to address the high rates of substance use among Latina/o adolescents in Arizona. Using a community-based approach informed by the Popular Education Model, *promotoras* collaborate with other parents to increase their awareness of underage drinking and to enhance their role as parents in the prevention of their children's substance use. *Promotoras* provide a one-hour educational workshop to immigrant Latina/o parents at community centers, housing developments, and school-based programs. Workshop elements include the reenactment of lived experiences, problem posing with discussions, poster presentations with pictures, and statistics. The community workshops are designed to raise parents' awareness about their role in preventing substance abuse among youths.

During the program's first year, 85 community members participated in the intervention but only 71 participants completed pre- and post-test surveys (83% response rate). Findings suggest positive results, indicating significant improvement in participants' awareness of the rates, risks, and consequences of alcohol use. Participants are better prepared to identify indicators of substance use among adolescents following the workshop. The workshop also prompts parents to think about their role in preventing alcohol abuse among youths. Participants report that good communication, parental support, and monitoring are necessary steps to prevent their children's alcohol use. Participants also report that the strengths of the workshops include the quality of information, delivery of the presentation, and that the facilitators are mothers (Ayón et al., 2014).

Promotoras also assist Spanish-speaking Latina/os with smoking cessation. For example, the intervention *Proyecto Sol*, is based on social cognitive constructs and delivered in a smoker's home by *promotoras* (Woodruff, Talavera, & Elder, 2002). Latina/o smokers ($N=313$) are randomly assigned to a three-month intervention condition or a comparison group. Comparison group participants are referred to a California Smoker's Helpline in Spanish. In addition to the use of *promotoras*, the curriculum is modified to address several cultural and linguistic barriers among Latina/os. For example, the curriculum is delivered in Spanish and at a low literacy level for Mexicans, and South and Central Americans who reside along the California border. Latina/o cultural values are also considered, including *familismo, simpatía, personalismo,* and *respeto*.

The content of *Proyecto Sol* is based on social cognitive principles including positive reinforcement, stimulus control, modeling, social support, problem solving, and practical skills and techniques for quitting, principles that are congruent with several findings associated with smoking among Latina/os. The three-month intervention includes four home visits and three telephone calls from the assigned *promotora*, and the use of a video and workbook. Although the curriculum is specific and structured, *promotoras* and participants are allowed flexibility in their timing and content, a potentially important component of culturally appropriate approaches. Findings indicate that *Proyecto Sol* is an efficacious and culturally appropriate intervention for Latina/o smokers. Intervention group participants report significantly higher postintervention smoking abstinence rates than comparison participants referred to a Spanish-language helpline. Approximately one week after the intervention, validated (by measuring carbon monoxide levels) past-week abstinence rates are more than twice as high in the intervention group (20.5%) as in the comparison group (8.7%) (Woodruff et al., 2002).

Gender-Specific Therapeutic Groups

Group work is beneficial because it enables Latina/os to overcome the stigma of mental health treatment and provides a venue that offers social support and a sense of community. For Mexican women, *comadres* play an important role, as close bonds help them to cope with daily struggles due to their significant trust and alliances (Santiago-Rivera et al., 2002). Rayle, Sand, Brucato, and Ortega (2006) developed a *comadre* approach with monolingual Spanish-speaking immigrant Mexican women to create an environment of sisterhood, trust, support, and education in their well-based pilot group. Group meetings take place at a local agency every Monday night for 10 consecutive weeks and are facilitated by two middle-aged bilingual Latinas. Bilingual child development specialists also provide childcare. The closed group meets for two hours every week and includes 10 Mexican immigrant women whose ages ranged between 25 and 53 (M=36.70; SD=7.60).

Although the pilot group is initially designed as a structured group, the participants indicate their interest in a support network versus structured lessons. The group has also become more process-focused rather than structured and psychoeducational, although holistic wellness remains a constant theme. As a wellness-based group, the facilitators focus on seven specific areas such as physical health, occupation/career wellness, emotional self-wellness, social support/relationships, acculturation experiences, spiritual wellness, and physical safety and utilize activities that illustrate important concepts in a concrete and visual manner. Voluntary, postintervention interviews indicate that a *comadre* group is beneficial and allows participants to meet other Latina immigrants who are experiencing similar challenges and establish meaningful relationships that are built on trust and honesty. The group appears to heighten their awareness of the importance of having coping resources and techniques for personal wellness, resulting in increased self-confidence and decreased isolation (Rayle et al., 2006).

Unfortunately, there are limited empirical studies that focus on the mental health treatment of Latino men. However, in partnership with *promotoras* and staff from a community-based organization that serves the needs of Latino day laborers, Moore et al. (2016) recently developed a culturally adapted and integrated behavioral intervention. Their three-session intervention combines motivational enhancement therapy (MET) and strengths-based case management (SBCM) to reduce heavy drinking among Mexican and Central American day laborers. Based on a nonconfrontational approach, MET focuses on fostering engagement and retention in treatment and helps address mental health disparities among immigrant Latinos. Strengths-based case management is also helpful and includes a process for setting and negotiating goals and uses informal resources (e.g., family, church) and formal resources (e.g., links to services) to address social needs and make positive changes.

Moore et al.'s (2016) pilot two-group randomized trial (N=29) evaluated the initial efficacy of MET/SBCM as compared with brief feedback. *Promotoras* provide MET/SBCM in Spanish at a community-based organization that operates job centers. Most intervention-group participants (12 of 14) attended all counseling sessions and are satisfied with their treatment, and most participants (25 of 29) remained in the study at 18 weeks.

Alcohol-related measures improved in both groups over time but no statistically significant differences are observed at any time point. However, the comparative effect size of MET/SBCM on weekly drinking is large at 6 weeks and moderate at 12 weeks. Post hoc analyses indicate significantly reduced drinking over time for intervention-group participants but not for control-group participants. Moore et al. (2016) attribute these positive outcomes to their community partnership, financial incentives, *promotoras* who are trusted by the participants, an intervention that addresses the cultural and social context of participants, and a convenient time and location.

Cultural factors are also important for IPV programs for Latinos, particularly in terms of content and delivery. In their qualitative study, Parra-Cardona and colleagues (2013) examine *Raíces Nuevas* (New Roots), a culturally informed version of the Spanish version of the Duluth curriculum, *Creating a Process of Change for Men Who Batter* (Paymar, Pence, & Aravena Azócar, 2002). The Duluth curriculum, embodies a feminist cognitive behavioral approach, and consists of detailed 26 weekly, two-hour sessions to promote change among men who batter. Qualitative findings confirm that the Spanish version of the Duluth curriculum is beneficial for Mexican men who participate in *Raíces Nuevas* because of the critical role of culture within the content of the intervention and method of delivery. Participants indicate the importance of a format to discuss relevant Latina/o cultural values, as well as the challenges due to racial discrimination and exclusion. Contrary to assumptions that feminist-informed batterer interventions lead to dissatisfaction among Latino men who batter, findings from this program indicate that they benefit significantly from *Raíces Nuevas*, as men are challenged to implement changes in their lives, rather than simply "talking about" these changes (Parra-Cardona et al., 2013).

Interventions with Latina/o Youth

Given the high rates of suicidal behavior among Latina adolescents, Life Is Precious was developed by Comunilife, a community-based organization in New York City and cofounded by Dr. Rosa Gil (Humensky et al., 2013). As an innovative program, Life Is Precious is designed to address risk factors among Latinas by providing comprehensive services in one location, including mental health treatment, school support, family support, and other life skills. Life Is Precious operates under the philosophy of *mi casa es su casa* (my house is your house), a place where Latinas and their families can feel at home and understood. The program serves Latina (i.e., Puerto Rican, Colombian, Dominican, Honduran, and Mexican) adolescents between the ages of 12 and 18 and operates at two sites (the Bronx and Brooklyn). Approximately 8 to 10 Latinas attend on any given day, and small groups allow staff members to provide individual attention and small-group workshops.

Life Is Precious provides various services, including the facilitation of mental health treatment, assistance with academic performance and family relationships, opportunities to participate in art and music therapy, and healthy living initiatives. Life Is Precious also collaborates with community organizations, such as a local art museum, and local colleges and universities. Interventions also target parents/caregivers to increase their understanding of U.S. teenage culture and to help them cope with their daughters' needs. Informal assessment suggests improvements in suicidal behavior, school performance, and family functioning. No attempted suicides are reported and grade improvement and college attendance are also reported. There is also improved communication among participants and family members, improved coping skills, and a high degree of satisfaction with program services. Informal assessments also suggest that Life Is Precious is generally viewed as successful by program staff, community partners, and policy practitioners.

A promising program model that addresses prevention of a number of risk-related sexual behaviors within a cultural context is *Joven Noble* (Tello, Cervantes, Cordova, & Santos, 2010). *Joven Noble* is a comprehensive youth leadership program for Latino boys and young men between the ages of 10 and 24; it includes rites of passage and character development. The 10-week program offers a curriculum that is based on the philosophy that youth need other men and women, their family, and community to care for, assist, heal, guide, and successfully prepare them for adulthood. In particular, the curriculum provides information and guidance related to a multitude of life-skill issues, including reproductive health, substance abuse, gangs, relationship violence, school, community rights and responsibilities, and leadership development.

The curriculum is deeply rooted in the customs of Latina/o culture and reinforces positive aspects of family, culture, and community. *El Joven Noble* is divided into four core teachings of development: *Conocimiento*: Acknowledgment and Positive Cultural Identity Development; *Entendimiento*: Understanding of Their Sacred Purpose; *Integracion*: Integrating Bilingual/Bicultural Values; and *Movemiento*: Safety, Security and Interconnected Trust. These four core teachings directly target four parallel risk areas that contribute to self-destructive behavior. Thus, physical, emotional, mental, and spiritual aspects of each core area serve as a basis for direction. Each stage uses a mixture of activities and teaching experiences associated with their self, family, and community. Pre- and post-test assessments of 683 adolescent Latinos indicate increased sexual abstinence and improvement across a range of risk and protective factors. The 10-week session of *El Joven Noble* appears to effectively shape the attitudes and beliefs of Latino youth. However, it is less effective in changing their perceptions regarding their cultural identity or sense of cultural esteem (Tello et al., 2010).

In a modular approach, Cervantes, Goldbach, and Santos (2011) created *Familia Adelante,* a multi-risk prevention intervention for high-risk Latina/o youth and their families that provides a psychoeducational curriculum to enhance family and peer communication, prevent/reduce substance abuse, increase knowledge about human immunodeficiency virus (HIV) infection and perceptions of harm regarding high-risk behavior, and improve school bonding and behavior. *Familia Adelante* also attempts to enhance psycho-social coping and life skills among Latina/o youth and their parents and decrease substance use and emotional problems by focusing on ways to cope with acculturative stress.

All group sessions are held at a convenient school location and conducted during after-school hours. Bilingual and bicultural staff facilitate simultaneous youth and parent group sessions that typically consist of 8 to 10 individual participants. A facilitator manual outlines each session topic and corresponding goals, learning objectives, and activities. Effect sizes of greater than 0.30 are observed across a number of risk-related factor, and many of the program effects are durable and shown through follow-up testing. Findings indicate significantly enhanced communication and perception of substance use harm and significantly reduced social norms regarding sexual behavior, HIV anxiety, and past use of marijuana and other illegal drugs. Parents consistently report improvements in their children's behavior across multiple domains over the course of the intervention and during posttest. Their children also report significant improvement in their communication with their parents and increased family attachment.

In a randomized controlled study to evaluate the efficacy of a culturally adapted version of the Early Pathways program, Fung and Fox (2014) implemented an in-home, parent–child therapy program with 137 at-risk Latina/o children (i.e., Mexican, Puerto Rican, Other, and Multiracial). Participants are under the age of six, from low-income families, and are referred for severe behavior and emotional problems. Early Pathways directly engages parent–child dyads, emphasizes parent-directed training, child-led play, psycho-education, and cognitive behavioral strategies. Services are provided in participant's homes in the Midwest. Cultural modifications include establishing community partnerships with pediatricians, nurses, and social workers to identify the needs and barriers of Latina/o families, translation of materials, bilingual services, acculturation assessments, and cultural competence training. Initial modifications are analyzed and adjusted throughout the program.

Significant differences between the immediate and delayed treatment groups on all post-test measures are observed, including high caregiver satisfaction with the intervention. More specifically, outcomes include reduced child behavior problems, increased child prosocial behaviors, improved caregiver limit setting, enhanced caregiver nurturing, improved parent–child relationships, and decreased clinical diagnoses following treatment. Findings also suggest that the in-home format is an effective way to directly observe children in their natural environment and to help improve both child behavior and parent–child interactions. In addition, community partnerships to identify specific community needs and barriers and cultural adaptations allow for increased access and culturally responsive treatment to low-income Latina/o families (Fung & Fox, 2014).

Also focusing on parent–child interactions, Matos et al. (2006) examined the efficacy of adapting *parent–child interaction therapy* (PCIT) for Puerto Rican parents of children aged 4 to 6 with hyperactivity and other significant behavior problems. Four steps are followed, including the translation and preliminary adaptation of the treatment manual and application of the treatment to nine families as part of an exploratory study using repeated measures. In addition, the treatment is revised and refined, and in-depth interviews with parents ($N=15$) and clinical psychologists ($N=5$) from Puerto Rico provide feedback on treatment process and components. Throughout this process, cultural elements and modifications are recommended for integration into the treatment protocol. Parents and psychologists conclude that PCIT components do not conflict with personal, spiritual, or cultural values held by Puerto Rican families. The only exception is the use of a time-out room. Nonetheless, parents report a high level of satisfaction, a significant reduction in children's externalizing behavior problems, and reduced parenting stress and improved parenting practices. Results from this study may inform clinicians and researchers who work with Puerto Rican families regarding relevant issues to promote their participation in behavioral family interventions and to enhance their acceptability and effectiveness (Matos et al., 2006).

School-based mental health programs for Latina/o youth are also beneficial, as the delivery of mental health services through school systems can help reduce financial and structural barriers that often prevent Latina/os from receiving needed services. For example, Kataoka et al. (2003) pilot-tested a school mental health program for Latina/o immigrant students (e.g., Mexico, El Salvador, Guatemala, and others) who were exposed to community violence. The Los Angeles Unified School District (LAUSD) developed the Mental Health for Immigrants Program (MHIP), a trauma-focused and culturally sensitive program for their large immigrant student body, and developed a collaborative partnership with research clinicians from local academic institutions and educational specialists.

In their quasi-experimental study, 198 students (3rd through 8th) with trauma-related depression and/or posttraumatic stress disorder symptoms are compared to their wait-listed peers. The intervention consists of manual-based, eight-session, group cognitive behavioral therapy delivered in Spanish by bilingual, bicultural school social workers. Parents and teachers are also eligible to receive psychoeducation and support services. After adjusting for covariates, students in the intervention group ($N=152$) demonstrate decreased posttraumatic stress disorder and depressive symptoms as compared with the wait-listed group ($N=47$) at 3-month follow-up. The delivery of the Mental Health for Immigrants Program within a school setting appears to help decrease the significant unmet mental health needs of Latina/o immigrant children and minimizes stigma that is often associated with mental health services (Kataoka et al., 2003).

CONCLUSION

In this chapter we highlight how cultural strengths and resources of Latina/o families are important assets that warrant utilization within clinical practice. The integration of their psychological strengths can aid in the development of strengths-based approaches. Although various Latina/o-centered approaches to counseling are available, approaches that foster liberation and resilience are essential. We underscore the importance of building a strong therapeutic alliance in which mental health providers recognize the strengths and resources of their Latina/o clients. These Latina/o-centered approaches offer much promise because they are grounded within Latina/o culture and increase their access to mental health care when they are provided in locations and times that are convenient for Latina/o clients. They also appear to eliminate other logistical barriers, such as transportation, cost, and literacy, and language.

Chapter 9

Nontraditional Mental Health Practices

The role that indigenous healing plays in clients' lives must be recognized because healers affect the mental health and psychological functioning of clients. It is necessary to form therapeutic alliances with the client as well as the indigenous healer, and this may require that counselors begin by taking an inventory of their perceptions of indigenous healers and also participate in a form of indigenous healing.

—Yeh, Hunter, Madan-Bahel, Chiang, and Arora, 2004

Vontress (2001) argues that the culture in which individuals are socialized determines their beliefs regarding the nature of their problems and that their healing practices are also outcomes of their worldviews. Among Latina/os, these worldviews often reflect that the body, mind, and spirit are interconnected and illness is derived from disequilibrium from various sources, including natural, social, spiritual, or psychological disturbances (Avila & Parker, 1999; Sutherland, 2014) (see Chapter 7). Healing for these disturbances may include conventional medicine and mental health treatment, diverse healing methods such as massage, acupuncture, meditation, burning incense, and aroma therapy (Constantine, Myers, Kindaichi, & Moore, 2004) or indigenous healing practices such as *Espiritismo, Santería*, and *Curanderismo. Espiritismo, Santería*, and *Curanderismo* are three of the largest syncretized (e.g. blending of beliefs, symbols, and ceremonies) and healing faith traditions among Latina/os that demonstrate the worldviews and spirituality of Latina/os, including the amalgamation of animism, mysticism, and Christianity (Hoogasian & Lijtmaer, 2010).

Healing traditions emerge from the cultural context of Latina/os and evolve to meet their needs (Comas-Díaz, 2006, 2012 a,b,c). These healing traditions provide cultural stability and continuity (Comas-Díaz, 1981, 2012a; Falicov, 2009b; Hoogasian & Gloria, 2015; McNeill & Cervantes, 2008; Trotter & Chavira, 1997) and enable Latina/os to cope with their social environments (Comas-Díaz, 2012a,c; Koss-Chionino, 2013). For example, these healing traditions are representative of the struggle for agency and survival from historical wounds and loss (Sutherland, 2014). Furthermore, as healing and spiritual systems, they assume a holistic approach and function as an informal mental health system (Delgado & Humm-Delgado, 1982; Gloria & Peregoy, 1996; Sandoval, 1979) during periods of crisis (Comas-Díaz, 1981, 2012a). Although the healing and spiritual practices of Latina/os are constantly evolving and incorporating new elements and theologies (Comas-Díaz, 2006, 2014), indigenous healing methods are salient, since they reflect the cultural perspectives and worldviews of Latina/os regarding their conceptualizations of health and illness (Holliday, 2008; Martinez et al., 2014; McNeill & Cervantes, 2008; McNeill, Esquivel, Carrasco, & Mendoza, 2008; Ramirez, 1998; Valdez, 2014). This chapter provides a general discussion of the spiritual and indigenous practices of Latina/os and a general overview of *Curanderismo*, *Santería*, and *Espiritismo* and their application to Latina/o mental health. In addition, we address spirituality, social justice, and treatment implications.

It is estimated that 50–75% of Mexican Americans practice or hold values that are consistent with *Curanderismo* (Tafur, Crowe, & Torres 2009), and there are more than one million practitioners of *Santería* in the United States and Latin America (González-Whippler, 2002). In addition, there are 70 spiritist centers in the United States that assist thousands of *Espiritismo* believers (Hoogasian & Gloria, 2015). Therefore, it is important to integrate the spiritual belief systems of Latina/os into the therapeutic process because spirituality permeates the lives of Latina/os (Cervantes, 2008; Comas-Díaz, 2006; Falicov, 2009b; McNeill & Cervantes, 2008). Unfortunately, healing methods play a critical role in the healing process of Latina/os, they are often marginalized by the scientific community (Avila & Parker, 1999; Chávez, 2016) or devalued within the field of mental health (Constantine et al., 2004; McNeill & Cervantes, 2008; Parks, Zea, & Mason, 2014; Valdez, 2014; Yeh et al., 2004).

Furthermore, mental health providers often marginalize the spiritual systems of Latina/os because they are not as easily recognized as traditional Christian-based spiritual systems. Unfortunately, Western mental health providers experience heightened uneasiness when they work with clients who engage in indigenous healing systems (Hoogasian & Lijtmaer, 2010). It is important to regard indigenous-based spiritual systems as equal to Christianity or other traditional religions (Cervantes & McNeill, 2008, p. 305). Failure to respect and integrate the spiritual systems of Latina/os will create resistance and lack of treatment adherence, as well as failure to assess their impact on a client's view of mental illness (Baez & Hernandez, 2001). It is not surprising that Latina/os may deny or underreport such beliefs and practices if they fear their providers are biased (Baez & Hernandez, 2001) or because certain practices are kept secret due to fear of stigma (Parks et al., 2014). Latina/o scholars highlight how mental health providers must become sensitive to the enduring presence of spirituality and the use of indigenous practices. Thus, they should develop "respectful curiosity" toward possible uses of these resources, rather than regarding these practices as useless magic and superstition (Falicov, 1999). For example, respectful interventions reflect a willingness to explore references to alternative spiritual beliefs, expressed interest in nontraditional healing practices or consultations with nontraditional healers, dignified references to spiritual practitioners, and welcomed therapeutic input from spiritual sources (Baez & Hernandez, 2001).

THE ROLE OF INDIGENOUS HEALERS

Healers such as *espiritistas*, *curandera/os*, and *santera/os*, are regarded as trusted healers, spiritual advisors, and counselors (Comas-Díaz, 2006, 2008). They function as culturally responsive mental health providers by addressing the specific needs of their clients and the use of culture-specific methods to diagnose and treat their presenting concerns. As sanctioned healers, they are well known within their communities and share similar experiences and holistic concerns with their clients, as well as similar beliefs regarding the causes of pathology (Harris, Velásquez, White, & Renteria, 2004; Martinez et al., 2014; McNeill & Cervantes, 2008; Trotter & Chavira, 1997). They provide immediate relief during periods of crisis, involve family and community members, communicate with the supernatural, and restore harmony through the use of rituals and other curative methods (Harris et al., 2004; Hernandez-Ramdwar, 2014; McNeill & Cervantes, 2008; Valdez, 2014). Comas-Díaz (2012b, c) also notes that many elements of indigenous healers are embedded in humanism and attempt to foster cultural strengths and traditions to address internalized colonization and oppression. In addition, these elements promote personal and collective healing and liberation. For example, within Western psychotherapy, the role of the mental health provider is that of a clinician and expert, rather than a healer, teacher, or guide.

Usage, knowledge, and exposure to these healers vary among Latina/os based on their socialization, acculturation, social class, and geographic location (McNeill & Cervantes, 2008). There are also varied perspectives regarding indigenous healers. For instance, some Latina/os are ambivalent and skeptical about these healers. They may regard them as quacks, charlatans, or unscrupulous healers who exploit gullible persons or endanger their client's health through ineffective or dangerous practices (Baez & Hernandez, 2001; Trotter & Chavira, 1997). Misperceptions and stereotypes regarding indigenous healers pertain to superstitions, and individuals may also attribute these powers to the devil or black magic (Baez & Hernandez, 2002). Thus, Latina/os may perceive that the practices of indigenous healers are in direct opposition to the Church and it is best to avoid them since they are diabolic (Trotter & Chavira, 1997).

Conversely, Latina/os may hold positive views toward these healers and seek them out because of their culturally salient theories of illness and therapeutic approaches, as well as their *cultural empathy* (Lopez, 2005). Historically, traditional folk medicine and not modern medicine served as a main resource for Latina/os who resided in rural areas or those who lacked medical resources (Hoogasian & Lijtmaer, 2010; Lopez, 2005). The bureaucratic and impersonal nature of health and mental health care systems also contributed to their high dissatisfaction and preference for indigenous healers, such as *curandera/os* (Applewhite, 1995). However, scholars suggest that the help-seeking behaviors of Latina/os are not uniform, as Latina/os may utilize both indigenous healers and mental health providers (Applewhite, 1995; Baez & Hernandez, 2001; Pasquali, 1994). They also demonstrate a spectrum of belief and practice in *Santería* and *Espiritismo*, ranging from near disbelief to fervent devotion (Baez & Hernandez, 2001). While the use of indigenous healers is often attributed to poverty, less education, or region, Latina/os with higher SES may also utilize these healers, often secretly (Falicov, 2009b). Multicultural experts also identify similarities among indigenous healers and mental health providers (see Comas-Díaz, 2012c), including the existence of (1) a trained healer whose healing powers are accepted by a sufferer and his/her network, (2) a sufferer who seeks relief from the healer, and (3) systematic contact between the healer and sufferer, where the healer attempts to reduce distress by changing the sufferer's behavior.

Although the healing methods and roles of indigenous healers may differ, four curative activities are often observed. Ramirez (1998) suggests the following four specific categories of curative activities:

1. Confession, atonement, and absolution to rid the body of sin and guilt that can cause illness and maladjustment. Thus, healing occurs through prayer or ritual cleanings, such as *limpias*, where the body is sprinkled with holy water.

2. Restoration of balance, wholeness, and harmony through self-control. Illness and maladjustment are viewed as a lack of self-control, since individuals allow feelings, emotions, or desires to act unconstrained, creating unbalance or fragmentation. Curative rituals may include the elimination of negative elements from their body or confronting the evil spirit that possessed them or took their soul.

3. Involvement of family and community in treatment occurs as family members and close friends may accompany a patient to the healer's residence and commit to support the reintegration of the patient into the family, community, and culture. Doing so allows for the restoration of the family and community's wholeness and harmony.

4. Communication with the supernatural separates healers apart from others, as they are said to have the capacity to directly communicate with the spirit world or facilitate communication between the patient and supernatural world.

INDIGENOUS HEALING

The spirituality of Latina/os is the product of Native American animism, mysticism of African slaves, and European Christianity. This syncretism suggests that among Latina/os, illness is due to disconnection from self, culture, and community (Comas-Díaz, 2006). In a book by McNeill and Cervantes (2008), the authors highlight how the integration of spiritual practices are salient for efficacious clinical work with Latina/os. They also suggest that Latina/os are increasingly claiming their *mestiza/o* cultural roots, including indigenous and African American influences, practices, and spiritual consciousness that were previously hidden, oppressed, and devalued.

For Latina/os, traditions such as *Día de los Muertos* (Day of the Dead) may remain an integral part of their lives, as they provide strength, resilience, and comfort during challenging periods. For many, these traditions represent a spiritual practice in response to a history of colonization, displacement, class stratification, and other forms of oppression (Comas-Díaz, 2006; McNeill & Cervantes, 2008; Ramirez, 1998)). Regrettably, the destruction of the *mestiza/o* spiritual framework and subsequent cataclysmic events also resulted in the denial of indigenous roots and spirituality (Cervantes, 2008). The search for indigenous spirituality, such as *mestiza/o* spirituality, is a critical link to the rediscovery of indigenous/spiritual beliefs. Therefore, the "return of the soul" is an important element for the healing of Latina/os (Cervantes, 2008, p. 9). Similarly, Comas-Díaz (2006) suggests that "calling back the spirit" allows for the development of spiritual resilience and empowerment through the affirmation of ethnic roots and practices (p. 440).

These perspectives are easily traced to indigenous worldviews, such as those of the Aztecs. The Aztecs demonstrated an ethnopharmacological system that surpassed the Europeans, as well as a sophisticated public health system. As an advanced society, they also demonstrated sophisticated medical specialties, including psychiatry (Padilla, 1980, 1984). For instance, insanity was classified into two main categories, including active and passive insanity. Active insanity, known as *xolopeyotl*, was due to the abuse of narcotic and/or poisonous green plants and fungi, including jimson weed, peyote, and hallucinogenic mushrooms. Remedies for active insanity included herbal antitoxins, purgatives, and withdrawal, remedies that are currently utilized for the treatment of alcohol and substance abuse (Padilla, 1980, 1984). Passive insanity, known as *tlahuiliscayotl*, included illnesses that currently resemble mania, schizophrenia, and depression. Passive insanity was treated by *tonalpouohqui*, who were special healers. The *tonalpouohqui* were trained to diagnose and treat mental illness and utilized catharsis, dream interpretation, and psychotherapy; their personal attributes were a determining factor of successful outcomes (Padilla, 1980, 1984).

Among the Aztecs, mental illness implied possession by evil spirits or punishment for sinful behavior, and conceptions of psychopathology included social, physiological, and psychological elements (Padilla, 1980, 1984). Socially, the presence of a disturbed individual was said to disrupt a community's equilibrium and affected the entire community through the loss of crops as a result of bad weather or invasion by an enemy. Thus, it was important to cure the mentally ill and restore the community's equilibrium. The entire community was expected to participate in the health attainment of the mentally ill. Physiologically, the heart was the origin of feelings, passions, and emotions, and the Aztecs believed that the heart was responsible for an individual's affective and behavioral functioning. A person with the most severe type of emotional disturbance was regarded as a *yollopoliuhqui* and said to have lost his/her heart; these persons also received assistance from a *tonalpouohqui* (Padilla, 1980, 1984).

Curanderismo

Curanderismo is the most widely studied belief system in the social sciences (Applewhite, 1995; Harris et al., 2004) and is often identified as a healing and spiritual practice of Mexicans and Mexican Americans, although *curandera/os* exist within other areas of Latin America and the Caribbean. The term *curanderismo*, is derived from the Spanish verb, *curar*, meaning to cure. As a holistic system of healing, *curanderismo* places a strong emphasis on the social, psychological, and spiritual factors that contribute to poor health and illness (Harris et al., 2004; Trotter & Chavira, 1997). The racial and cultural mixture between indigenous peoples and Spanish colonizers during the 16th century resulted in the evolution of *curanderismo* (Chávez, 2016). Important Mesoamerican ritualistic, religious, medical, and anthropological concepts are integrated within *curanderismo*, as well as a wealth of herbal and medicinal concepts from indigenous groups (Ortiz, Davis, & McNeill, 2008), and Spanish and African healing methods (Avila & Parker, 1999). Trotter and Chavira (1997) suggest that *curanderismo* was shaped by at least six major historical influences, including Judeo-Christian religious beliefs, symbols and rituals; early Arabic medicine and health practices that were combined with Greek humoral medicine, medieval and European witchcraft, Native American herbal traditions and health practices, modern beliefs about spiritualism and psychic phenomena, and scientific medicine (p. 25).

Thus, *curanderismo* integrates folk and medical beliefs, and rituals that address spiritual, psychological, and physical issues. It involves three aspects, such as faith in natural and supernatural elements, a view that God's divine influences all areas of one's life, and the belief that individuals can metaphysically employ the powers of healing, such as *curandera/os* (Applewhite, 1995). *Curandera/os* have the metaphysical gift of healing, due to their God-given gift, known as *el don*. Ideologically, they share an understanding of health and illness as a manifestation of an interactive process among three main dimensions, including religious and/or spiritual, affective-emotional, and somatic dimensions. This multidimensionality is expressed through three concepts that include the *espiritu* (spirit), *alma* (soul), and *cuerpo* (body) (Zacharias, 2006). The *espiritu* plays a central role in health and illness and well as mental health and psychological disorders. Because the *espiritu* level is a guardian of mental and somatic health, if it is unable to fulfill its protective function, affective and somatic dysfunction occurs (Zacharias, 2006). Diagnosis of mental illness also reflects this three-dimensional structure and often includes causal assumptions about pathology.

Trotter and Chavira's (1997) ethnographic work provides careful attention to the various approaches to healing through the perspectives of *curandera/os* from the Rio Grande Valley of Texas. They note how *curandera/os* possess multiple specialty areas that overlap, since they often address physical, spiritual, mental, and emotional components to diagnose and treat illness (Tafur et al., 2009). For example, these specializations include *yerbera/os* (herbalists), *parteras* (midwives), *sobadera/os* and *hueseros* (bone and muscle specialists), *espiritualista/os* (psychic mediums), and *señoras* (card reading) (Ortiz et al., 2008; Tafur et al., 2009). *Curanderismo* includes three levels of treatment—*nivel material* (material level), *nivel espiritual* (spiritual level), and *nivel mental* (mental level). While these levels are not mutually exclusive and are similar in their treatment, they require a different gift and specialized training (Trotter & Chavira, 1997).

Ortiz et al. (2008) highlight that while modern medicine is "high tech" because of advances in science and technology, and perhaps better at curing biological contagion and physical injury, *curanderismo* is "high touch" and equally effective. The use of tactile contact within healing and therapeutic elements helps decrease social isolation. In particular, healing touch through *masaje* (massage), *barridas* (spiritual sweeping), *soba* (rubbing), and *ventosa* (cupping glass) allow for healers to "do more than cure the psychic fragmentation and social alienation that a sick person often suffers. Touch demonstrates acceptance to a person whose shame at personal weakness may endanger his identity" (p. 283). Furthermore, the use of tactile objects, the laying of hands, and words of blessings also provide comfort, fortitude, and protection.

In his examination of *curandera/os*, Zacharias (2006) found that *curandera/o* diagnose and treat the following culture-bound syndromes: *susto* (fright), *mal aire* (negative air/vibrations), *mal de ojo* (evil eye), *envidia* (envy of others), *sentimientos fuertes* (vehement feelings), *brujería* (witchcraft), and *falta de fé* (lack of faith). Their therapeutic methods also reflect multidimensional approaches, including ritual healing methods that often include spiritual and other symbolic interventions, such as sensory and corporal stimulation. In particular, the extensive use of spirituality, altered states of consciousness, and bifocal ritual interventions (shift of therapeutic focus within a ritual between sensorial experience and abstract-symbolic meaning) aid in successful outcomes (Zacharias, 2006).

Important interpersonal qualities of *curandera/os* include being empathic, genuine, caring, confident in their personal manner, and competent to render traditional services (Ortiz & Torres, 2007). Their ability to develop rapport and to use the language and beliefs of their clients contribute to their success. Furthermore, their ability to use culturally and socially appropriate therapeutic techniques is also vital. *Curanderismo* combines self-reliance with cultural relevance and family systems to provide Latina/os with stability and continuity in an era of social disruption due to urban and technological changes (Trotter & Chavira, 1997).

Curandera/os provide valuable counseling services that resemble traditional social work and psychological services, as they tend to focus on courtship, marital, financial, legal, social, and business relationships (Chávez, 2016; Trotter & Chavira, 1997). They often use their knowledge of their client's background, along with their own understanding of psychology to provide advice. In addition, they activate the natural support systems that currently exist in the community, such as their families and peer groups, to support their client's designated therapy. *Curandera/os* also capitalize on their patients' faith and belief systems, religious and spiritual aspects of the healing process, through the use of everyday products and resources that their clients can easily attain, such as herbs, fruits, eggs, and oils (Trotter & Chavira, 1997).

Chávez (2016) suggests that the use of *pláticas* (talking) as a therapeutic tool that stresses *personalismo* enables *curandera/os* to gather data about the presenting concern and establish equal, warm, and genuine relationships with their clients. Through *pláticas they* provide guidance on self-care, prescribe herbs, and provide advice. Furthermore, Chávez (2016) suggests that the practice of *curanderismo* is humanistic through the practice of *plática* and strategic or open-process-type questioning. This process emphasizes personal agency because it empowers clients to define their problem, make self-determined decisions, and take personal responsibility to improve their own lives and well-being.

Espiritismo

According to Comas-Díaz (1981, 2012c), *Espiritismo* is a religion and folk psychotherapy, while others argue that it is a spiritual belief system (Harwood, 1977). *Espiritismo* is often identified as a healing and spiritual practice among Puerto Ricans, although believers also include other Latina/os. Spiritism originated in the 1850s with the work of Allan Kardec (pseudonym for Léon Dénizarth Hippolyte Rivail), a French philosopher and educator who believed that spirits are reincarnated in order to achieve spiritual progress (Fernandez, Murphy, & Paravisini-Gebert, 2011). Puerto Rican intellectuals who studied in Europe and later returned to Puerto Rico introduced spiritism during the 19th century (Molina, 1996). They held an interest in *espiritismo* as a philosophical system that provided a social and moral developmental framework. Conversely, working-class Puerto Ricans became interested in *espiritismo* because it offered a framework for understanding, healing, and treating illness. They syncretized *espiritismo* with popular Catholicism, *curanderismo*, herbal medicine, and other indigenous and African healing practices (Molina, 1996). *Espiritismo* differs from spiritism, as it is primarily used as a folk healing and spiritual development practice among Puerto Ricans (Comas-Díaz, 2012c). In the Caribbean region, *espiritismo* also emerged as an affirmation of one's ethnic roots and as a coping mechanism against social discontent (Comas-Díaz, 2012c; Soto Espinoza, 2014). Thus, *espiritismo* enables Latina/os to cope with powerlessness and oppression.

A foundation of *espiritismo* is the view of a spirit world that constantly interacts with the material world (*mundo material*). The spirit world is inhabited by spirits who are classified by a hierarchy of moral development, and this hierarchy includes 3 levels and 10 grades of spiritual development (Harwood, 1977). The lowest level of spirits includes dark or turbulent spirits in need of light and redemption because of their excessive attachment to the material world and interest in harming human beings. Conversely, pure spirits are at the highest level because they have achieved spiritual perfection and are able to protect humans from the negative influence of ignorant spirits (Fernandez et al., 2011; Molina, 1996; Soto Espinoza, 2014). In order to progress from one level to the next, spirits must undergo trials (*pruebas*). Communication between spirits and humans is an essential aspect of *espiritismo*, as mediums or *espiritistas* serve as intermediaries between the spirit and material world through a trance. *Espiritistas* must engage in a process to develop their faculties (*desarrollo de facultades*) and various capacities to successfully communicate with the spirits, as well as receive help from them.

Espiritistas treat a wide range of concerns, including family relationships, psychosomatic concerns, sleep disturbances, hallucinations, nervous conditions, psychotic behavior, and others (Comas-Díaz, 1981; Koss-Chionio, 2013; Moreira-Almeida & Koss-Chioino, 2009). Mental or physical illness is attributed to ignorant spirits who can control a person's thoughts and actions, and lead to the experience of an "*obsesión*" (obsession). A person experiencing an *obsesión* is under the influence of an ignorant spirit and subjected to the spirit's will. In addition, ignorant spirits can create physical disturbances, such as headaches or even major illness. Comas-Díaz (1981) suggests that individuals are not regarded as sick and blamed for their symptoms but instead are viewed as suffering from a *causa*. Those who experience auditory and visual hallucinations are not pathologized but rather confer prestige, as these symptoms are regarded as *facultades espirituales*, which are a preamble for becoming an *espiritista*. The practice of *espiritismo* is fluid and can take place within an *espiritista*'s home or a spiritual center, known as a *centro espiritista*. A *centro* includes spiritually developed individuals who seek to help the spiritually ill and increase their *facultades* (Comas-Díaz, 1981). A session often begins with a reading from Allan Kardec's (1957) *The Gospel According to Spiritism* (El Evangelio Según Espiritismo) and *Collection of Selected Prayers* (Coleccion De Oraciónes Escogidas, 1975). These prayers request the presence of spirit guides, the education of ignorant spirits, and support for the health of the infirm (Comas-Díaz, 1981).

Espiritistas believe that individuals are composed of spirit and matter and that illness has a material (physical) or spiritual *causa* (cause) or both (Comas-Díaz, 1981). *Espiritistas* attempt to diagnose clients through their communication with the spirits (*buscando la causa*). If a *causa* is material, and not spiritual, *espiritistas* often refer their clients to health professionals.

However, spiritual *causas* require educating or giving light to the spirit who is responsible for the problem in order to discontinue its harm. The *espiritista* must divine which symptoms are produced by the ignorant spirit in order to create dialogue and a healing process. If the ignorant spirit follows the *espiritista*'s advice, the *causa* is relieved but it must repent for its affliction. Clients must also engage in the working of the *causa* through a number of activities and rituals (Comas-Díaz, 1981; Fernandez et al., 2011). *Espiritistas* view their client's problems as part of their spiritual development (Comas-Díaz, 2012c), and unlike traditional mental health providers, they search for spiritual causes and their treatment emphasizes spiritual development. See Table 9.1 for a comparison of salient differences between mental health providers and *espiritistas*.

Methods for diagnosis may include prayers, card reading, spirit writing, spirit communication through a cup of water, and seeing revelations concerning the afflicted person. After a diagnosis, an *espiritista* engages in working the cause (*trabajando la causa*) through possession by the *causa* spirit; this work continues until the *causa* demonstrates repentance and spiritual development (Comas-Díaz, 1981; Fernandez et al., 2011). Other rituals may include lighting candles and reading prayers, group healing sessions

Table 9.1 Differences between Mainstream Psychotherapy and *Espiritismo*

Psychotherapy	*Espiritismo*
Diagnosis	**Diagnosis**
Diagnostic intake	Searching for the spiritual cause
Client verbalizes problems	*Espiritista* channels (divines) problems
Client receives diagnostic label	Sufferer is viewed as evolving spiritually
Treatment	**Treatment**
Psychotherapy, psychopharmacology	Rituals, prayers, possession, *remedios*
Clinician may or many not communicate culturally and linguistically	*Espiritista* communicates both culturally and linguistically
Family may or may not be involved	Nuclear/extended family is involved
Clients are responsible for their behavior	Sufferers are not responsible for their behavior
Focus on adaptation and reduction of problems	Emphasis on spiritual development
Absence of spiritual component	Presence of spiritual components

Source: Comas-Díaz, L. (2012). *Multicultural care: A clinician's guide to cultural competence.* Washington, DC: American Psychological Association.

involving family members, house cleansings, herbal remedies, the use of protective fetishes to ward off evil, and personal cleansing through the use of herbal baths (Comas-Díaz, 1981). These curative processes are said to exorcise (*despojar*) or give light (*dando luz*) to the spirits in order to resolve the client's problem. In addition, treatment may include spiritual development (*desarrollo spiritual*) or the development of one's spiritual faculties (Comas-Díaz, 1981).

As a mental health system, *espiritismo* reflects the cultural values and circumstances of Latina/os (Comas-Díaz, 1981). The ability to develop rapport and use the language and beliefs of their clients contribute to the success of *espiritistas*. Furthermore, their ability to use culturally and socially appropriate therapeutic techniques is also vital. The integration of family members is also an integral component of spiritual treatment. For example, in their examination of Puerto Rican and Brazilian *espiritualistas*, Moreira-Almeida and Koss-Chioino (2009) found that they often achieved positive results, such as decreased symptoms and/or improved social adjustment, among clients diagnosed with schizophrenia or psychotic symptoms. Symptoms were not regarded as disordered or crazy but instead were attributed to spirits and their possession. *Espiritualistas* demonstrated uncritical acceptance, showed no fear, and encouraged patients to value their hallucinations and delusions. The elimination of stigma provided hope for family members, decreased shame and guilt, and increased patients' social integration. In addition, *espiritualistas* maintained close and continuous relationships with their patients and family members over the years and reactivated their relationships during the first signs of a patient's relapse or heightened agitation (Moreira-Almeida & Koss-Chioino, 2009).

Santería

Santería, also known *Lukumí, Ifá,* or *Regla de Ocha,* is a traditional healing system that is utilized by various Latina/os (McNeill et al., 2008). It functions as a religion and health care system throughout Latin America and the Caribbean (Gloria & Peregoy, 1996; Hernandez-Ramdwar, 2014; Rosario & De la Rosa, 2013). Estimates suggest that over 100 million persons practice *Santería* in the United States and Latin America (González-Whippler, 2002). As an organized religion, *Santería* emerged from Cuba as a direct result of the slave trade in the 16th century, the religious practices of the Yoruba (González-Whippler, 2002), and subsequent sociocultural shifts (Holliday, 2008). The word *Santería* derives from the Spanish word, *santo,* meaning saint (Martinez et al., 2014), and emerged as a derogatory and Eurocentric term to distinguish between stigmatized popular expressions of Catholicism from Orthodox-Catholic practices in Spanish colonized

Cuba (Rosario & De la Rosa, 2013) and their heavy worship of Catholic saints (Martinez et al., 2014).

Because the Spanish colonizers considered the religious practices of the African slaves as idolatrous and sacrilegious, the slaves hid their Yoruba-based religion by masking their beliefs under Catholicism (Holliday, 2008). The development of *Santería* enabled them to avoid persecution and maintain their religion by worshiping Catholic saints that were representations of Yoruba divinities, known as *Orishas. Santería* was also cloaked in secrecy because of the legacy of persecution and scrutiny during the diaspora due to fear, general misunderstanding, and racism (Hernandez-Ramdwar, 2014). However, Hernandez-Ramdwar (2014) suggests that *Santería* has become revitalized in contemporary Cuba because of a faltering health care system, governmental support, and interest in *Santería* among foreign travelers.

In addition to various African influences, native precolonial Latin American and Caribbean Indian beliefs and practices also contributed to theological epistemologies of *Santería* (Rosario & De la Rosa, 2013). The acceptance of *Santería* in Latin America was facilitated by the widespread influence of Kardec's spiritualist beliefs and distinct Mexican Spiritualism, the salience of venerating unorthodox folk saints, and the prevalent practices of *curanderismo* that have comparable ritual elements (Ortiz et al., 2008; Rosario & De la Rosa, 2013). *Santería* is largely an oral tradition, as knowledge is conveyed through tightly knit kinship relations that are formed between novices called *Iyawos* (godchildren) and priests and priestesses (godparents), called *Santera/os* (González-Whippler, 2002; Holliday, 2008). The metaphysical and social family that develops among *iyawos* and *santera/ os* is through an initiation process that results in reciprocity and strong social ties (Holliday, 2008). For instance, *santera/os* direct the spiritual development of their godchildren, who in return provide support through labor and/or resources.

A person's life is viewed as a spiritual phenomenon that is maintained through healing practices that are based on interdependence between physical and spiritual dimensions (Ortiz et al., 2008). *Orishas* interact with the world and humankind as emissaries of the Creator and Supreme Being, *Olodumare/Olorun/Olofi*, who is the ultimate embodiment of a spiritual-mystical energy or power, known as *aché* (Fernandez et al., 2011; Hernandez-Ramdwar, 2014; Ortiz et al., 2008). *Olodumare* designated a number of *orishas* to rule over different aspects of life and nature. At birth, individuals are assigned a spiritual guide who serves as a protector and guardian angel. Thus, at birth individuals receive a plant, an animal, and a stone that serve as spiritual allies (Fernandez et al., 2011; Pasquali, 1994). As protective guides, the *orishas* aid their followers and provide direction for an

Table 9.2 The Most Commonly Cited and Used *Orishas* in *Santería*

Orisha	Saint	Feast Day	Attribute/Power	Representation in Nature	Color(s)/Offerings/Symbols
Olofi; Olodumare; Olorun			Creator and source of all power		Invoked in selected prayers
Eleggua	Saint Anthony of Padua, Anima Sola, or Niño de Atocha	January 6 or June 13 (contested)	Owner of destiny and the crossroads; trickster; warrior deity	Corners; crossroads	Red and black; roasted corn, smoked possum; blood of young roosters; cement head with cowrie shells representing eyes and mouth
Obatalá	Jesus of Nazareth, or the Virgin—Our Lady of Mercy	September 24	Son of Olofi—father of the *orishas*; god of peace and wisdom	Fatherhood, all white substances	White; silver bell called "agogo," white pigeons and other four-legged white animals. *Iruke* (horsetail with a braided handle)
Changó	Saint Barbara	December 4	An impulsive and warrior-like god; promiscuous and womanizer	Fire; thunder and lightning	Red and white; apples, bananas, the double-edged ax; blood of rams, lambs, goats, and roosters
Ogún	Saint Peter	June 29	God of iron and warrior deity; owner of metals	Iron; steel	Green and black; offerings placed in the railroad tracks; knives, railroad spikes, horseshoes; blood of roosters, pigeons, etc.

Ochosi	Saint Norbert	June 6	God of justice and warrior deity	All game animals	Gold and blue: the crossbow, deer antlers, handcuffs, blood of pigeons, etc.
Babalú-Ayé	Saint Lazarus	December 17	God of illnesses and skin diseases	Smallpox; leg ailments	Black, purple, and yellow; crutches, cigars, pennies
Yemayá	The Virgin—Our Lady of Regla	September 7	Goddess of the Oceans; primordial mother of the *santos*	The ocean	Blue; seashells, canoes, corals; water-melons, sugar cane syrup, pork rinds; blood of ducks
Oshún	The Virgin—Our Lady of Charity	September 8	Goddess of the rivers, sensuality, love, and money	Rivers	Yellow and gold; mirrors, gold, copper; blood of hens and female goats; fans, mirrors
Oyá	The Virgin—Our Lady of La Candelaria or Saint Theresa	February 2	Goddess of the cemetery and death; impulsive and mighty	Wind, cemeteries/burial grounds	Nine colors; eggplants; offerings placed in cemeteries; horsetail
Orúnmila	Saint Francis of Assisi	October 4	Divination		Table of Ifá

Source: Adapted from Holliday (2008) and Martínez, Taylor, Calvert, Hirsch, & Webster (2014).

enhanced spiritual and material life (Ortiz et al., 2008). Among the various *orishas*, seven form a pantheon, known as the Seven African Powers, including the following: Obatalá (peace and purification), Eleguá (messenger), Orula (divination), Changó (passion and enemies), Ogún (war and employment), Yemayá (maternity and womanhood), and Ochun (love) (Ortiz et al., 2008).

Each *orisha* is known for a specific human trait, specific attributes, and an association with a force of nature. Further, they are associated with the attributes or qualities of a specific Catholic saint (see Table 9.2), particularly due to statues and lithographs of Catholic iconography. For instance, Changó, the Yoruba orisha of fire and thunder is identified with Santa Barbara, the patroness of Spanish artillery, due to her iconographic representations. She is dressed in red (Changó's symbolic color), and identified with thundering artillery cannons (Fernandez et al., 2011; Sandoval, 1979). Thus, the similarities between saints and orishas provide a basis for syncretism (Fernandez et al., 2011; Pasquali, 1994; Sandoval, 1979). Orishas also have their own colors and ornaments, such as specific necklaces (*collares*) and bracelets (*pulsos*), as well as a feast day for worship and celebration with specific foods, plants, explicit chants, drum rhythms, dance movements, and sacred narratives. For example on the feast day of Santa Barbara, followers gather for a vigil and smoke cigars because Changó enjoys the taste and smell of cigars. Because the symbolic colors of Changó and Santa Barbara are red, red candles and flowers are also displayed. The ritual later concludes with music, rum, the presentation of red applies, and the smoking of cigars (Pasquali, 1994).

A basic premise of *Santería* is the notion of spiritual balance and its association with health and illness, as physical and mental health are not divorced from the metaphysical. The cause of illness is often attributed to malevolent supernatural forces and the protection of one's health involves averting or neutralizing these negative supernatural forces (Pasquali, 1994). Maintaining a harmonious connection with ancestors or spirits of deceased family members is also important. Failure to remember the departed or behavior that dishonors their memory may result in punishment, resulting in disruptions such as chronic illness, general misfortune, accidents, etc. Similarly, each orisha is believed to cause specific afflictions, illnesses, and disruptions if followers fail to engage in proper worship of their orisha. For example, Obatala punishes with paralysis and birth deformities while Oya is associated with marital separation (Martinez et al., 2014).

A major feature of *Santería* is the magical abilities of skilled *santera/os*, particularly *babalawos* or high priests (Baez & Hernandez, 2001). While they each introduce variations in their rituals and mythology (Hernandez-Ramdwar, 2014), González-Whippler (2002) suggests that the magical feats of *santera/os* include the elimination of negative influences, the curing of illnesses, securing employment, improving one's financial condition, and attracting a lover or spouse, as well as subduing an enemy. *Santera/os* are particularly appealing since their work is directed to ameliorate problems that are unresolvable through ordinary means. Thus, individuals consult *santera/os* for a variety of reasons, including physical illness, nervous conditions, and life problems (McNeill et al., 2008).

Santera/os also assume various roles based on their client's needs, as they can act as a physician, psychologist, confidant, religious elder, or parental figure (Hernandez-Ramdwar, 2014, p. 108). Nonetheless, they often function as informal counselors who fulfill the demand for mental health services among diverse Latina/os (Rosario & De la Rosa, 2013; Viladrich & Abraido-Lanza, 2009). They are regarded as mental health providers because they are healers who share the language, culture, and worldview of their clients and as a person who describes and explains the problem and devises a course of action to address that problem. Thus, the consultation or *registro* is similar to a visit with a mental health provider, as the *santera/o* listens, attempts to understand the problem, and identifies appropriate solutions. A *santera/o* may use a divinatory system, such as *Diloggun* or seashell divination, through which the *orishas* speak to the *santera/o* and identify the source of the problem and appropriate solutions to restore harmony or avoid ancestral wrath (Martinez et al., 2014; Rosario & De la Rosa, 2013).

The etiology of a client's problem may include a supernatural causation, such as punishment by the *orishas* due to neglect, sorcery or *brujería* (witchcraft), or disruptions caused by sprits of dead ancestors who have been neglected in rituals (Martinez et al., 2014). A solution may include ritual cleansing (*despojo*), a Catholic mass for the dead, or an animal sacrifice. However, *santera/os* may also use their personal intuition and provide *consejos* (advice) from their insight and wisdom. Furthermore, rites and rituals are cathartic techniques that serve to also connect the living with the dead and establish a continuity of traditions, values, and family and community ties (Martinez et al., 2014).

Rosario and De la Rosa (2014) indicate that *Santería* is a culturally congruent informal mental health support for Latina/os who are coping with cancer, particularly with the added spiritual dimension that offers explanations for "why" health or illness occur. As with mental health professionals, *santeros* possess four common components of an effective mental health professional: (1) shared worldview with a client; (2) personal qualities of the healer; (3) patient expectations regarding the healer's capacities; and (4) training and the employment of specific techniques (McNeill & Cervantes, 2008). In addition, their healing practices share (a) an emotionally charged, confiding relationship with a healer, (b) a healing context in which the healer has the power and expertise to help by possessing a socially sanctioned role to provide these services, (c) a rational or conceptual schema to explain problems, and (d) a ritual or procedure that is consistent with the treatment's rationale (McNeil & Cervantes, 2008, p. xxvi).

Spirituality and Social Justice

Comas-Díaz (2006) suggests that "Western healing is not Latino-centered" and calls for the need for mind–body approaches that honor and address the mind–body connection and encourage healing and liberation (p. 440). In particular, she calls for the necessity to integrate *Latino ethnic psychology* into psychotherapy to capture spiritual traditions through contextualism, interconnectedness, and magical realism. The use of cultural values such as *familisimo* (family), *respeto* (respect), *simpatía* (social harmony), and *sabiduría* (a spiritually informed wisdom) also aid in understanding the implications of the well-being of Latina/os. She also proposes the use of language to create new meanings such as *plática* (social conversation), *cuentos* (storytelling), *testimonios* (testimonies), and *dichos* (Spanish proverbs), and other cultural practices (i.e., visualization, rituals, body movement, and massage) promote emotional and spiritual redemption. As a culturally resilient practice, Latino ethnic psychology aims to foster healing and liberation for Latina/os. Because of the collectivistic nature of Latina/os, these spiritual practices restore a sense of belonging and promote self-healing by maintaining a harmonious balance among Latina/o clients, their family, community, and the cosmos (Comas-Díaz, 2006, p. 446).

Indeed spirituality is a way of life for Latina/os and a coping strategy that emerged out of turmoil and cultural trauma. In the face of adversity and dislocation, many Latina/os reconnect with their indigenous beliefs through syncretism (Comas-Díaz, 2012a, p. 197); their syncretized and healing practices enable them to regain a sense of belonging to a community and gain relief from their experiences of oppression. Comas-Díaz (2012a) proposes the benefits of a *colored spirituality*, a culturally relevant syncretic practice that addresses the psychosocial needs of ethnic minorities and enables them to reconnect with their cultural and spiritual roots and to fight against oppression by focusing on cultural resilience, consciousness, and liberation. In addition to promoting resistance and affirmation, a colored spirituality fosters redemption among ethnic minorities by restoring their sense of belonging and through the promotion of self-healing and social justice. Aided by a set of guidelines, colored spirituality includes being resilient, syncretic, communal, relational, holistic, metaphysical, committed, and emancipatory (Comas-Díaz, 2012a).

Comas-Díaz (2014) also suggests that despite their diverse religious orientations and spiritual practices, Latinas share a "folk spirituality" that emerged out of their experiences of colonization and oppression. This spirituality is also relational, mutual and collectivistic, and female-inspired. She notes that because they are female-inspired, the spirituality of Latina feminists may focus on *La Diosa*—a syncrestic sacred feminine that enables them to manage the intersection of racism, sexism, elitism, xenophobia, and other forms of oppression (p. 217). *La Diosa* is an icon of feminine resistance, liberation, and transformation. Thus, folk spirituality for Latinas has healing, empowering, and transformative elements that entail a holistic worldview and *sanación*, emotional, physical, and spiritual healing. Syncretism also facilitates their spiritual development and spiritual activism. For instance, the most popular icon of *La Diosa* is the Virgin Mary. Latina feminists also syncretize the Aztec goddess *Tonantzin* into Our Lady of Guadalupe to transform her into a feminist icon and recognize her as a subversive warrior, emancipator, guerrilla combatant, and the most powerful freedom fighter. She also imparts dignity, provides sustenance, hope, and a sense of belonging (Comas-Díaz, 2006, 2014). The empowering legacy of the Latina sacred feminine transcends Catholicism, as syncretism also facilitates their spirituality as well as their social justice development through a commitment to social action. Anzaldúa (2002) suggests that spiritual activism, combined social activism and spiritual vision, enables Latinas to develop a global consciousness, embrace collective solidarity, and have a vision for worldwide peace (Comas-Díaz, 2014).

Similarly, Comas-Díaz (2008, 2016) posits that Latinas reconnect with original and cultural values to promote social action through womanist/*mujerista* spiritual development. Isasi-Díaz (1996) introduced the term *mujerismo* to designate a type of Latina feminism and to develop a new consciousness. *Mujerista* theology emerged out of the intersections of cultural theology, feminist theology, and liberation theology (Comas-Díaz, 2016). In critique of gender inequality within liberation theology, *mujerismo* fosters resistance, subversion, reconstruction, activism, and liberation among Latinas (Isasi-Díaz, 1996). However, Comas-Díaz (2016) advanced *mujerista* psychospirituality as a foundation for *mujerista* psychology. Accordingly, *mujerista* psychology is a type of Latina feminism that is infused with a spiritual-feminist liberation approach and a commitment to social justice. In this context, psychospirituality includes the belief in interconnections, holism, communality, solidarity, global liberation, and transformation. Comas-Díaz (2016) offers a case illustration of how a Mexican American woman retrieves her soul through a *mujerista* psychospirituality. As a *mujerista* psychologist, Comas-Díaz (2016) demonstrates cultural empathy and embraces a plurality of roles, including therapist, healer, mentor, guide, teacher, and fellow spiritual seeker. In doing so, Comas-Díaz helps her client reclaim her ancestral self, recover her voice, and empower herself through the use of *platica, testimonios* (testimonies), the incorporation of psychospiritual elements, and mind–body–soul healing.

These psychospiritual elements are also evident within Comas-Díaz' journey as a feminist psychotherapist. In a discussion of her development as a *mujerista*, special bonds with her cousin and *abuela* (grandmother), and her development as a psychotherapist, Comas-Díaz (2013) notes how her *mujerista abuela* (grandmother), was "a marianista by birth and a mujerista by choice" (p. 65). She remarks how her *abuela* taught her to honor herself as a mixed-raced person and how her *cuentos* (stories) carried the commandments of *mujerismo*. In particular, her abuela's 10 commandments include the following:

Honor your inner divinity.
Ask for help—she will respond.
Be aware of who you are, but be open to change.
Remember that your identity transcends your self.
Aim to empower others.
Encourage connectedness and solidarity.
Fight oppression.
Become resilient and learn to overcome adversity.
Transform low self-esteem into self-love.
Dance with life, when the music changes, choreograph new steps.

Treatment Considerations

Cervantes and Parham (2005) posit that although most mental health providers receive extensive training, this training is anchored within a European American psychological perspective, and its application to ethnic minorities is limited, particularly when considering the notion of spirituality. In order to embrace the concept of spirituality, mental health providers are encouraged to avoid the tendency to assume that spirituality is synonymous with religiosity. While the terms are often used interchangeably, religiosity is regarded as an organized belief system that characteristically includes shared, institutionalized views about a Higher Power and involvement in a faith community. However, spirituality is described as an overarching concept that includes transcendent beliefs and practices (Cervantes & Parham, 2005). Cervantes and Parham (2005) further suggest that as appropriate, mental health providers should integrate any related prayer content, religious imagery, and rituals that are salient to their clients. Doing so will allow for their clients' spirituality to unfold. For example, since prayer, ritual, and ceremony are essential ingredients in the healing of Latina/os and their communities, the recognition that prayer comes in many forms and that ceremonies are culturally sanctioned processes, can aid in therapeutic interventions. The understanding of prayer through spoken words, affirmations, song, poetry, and walking meditations help promote the ingredients that are meaningful (p. 76).

Given the limited attention to the notion of spirituality, it is not surprising that there are limited integrative therapeutic models that embrace indigenous and spiritual perspectives. Identified as *Mestizo Spirituality*, Cervantes (2008, 2010) offers a holistic and psychospiritual therapeutic model for clinical work that begins with the premise that traumas, emotional/physical insults, joys, and suffering are elements of one's journey toward wholeness. In addition, the model reinforces belief in the connectedness of life, the need for balance within relationships, the need to honor family and community responsibilities, and clarity in one's daily challenges. In particular, a *mestizo* spirituality emphasizes the following philosophical concepts:

- Awareness, respect, kindness, and inner responsibility for the sacredness of one's life journey and its interconnectedness to the larger cosmic reality;
- Review and renewal of one's religious/spiritual beliefs, rituals, and traditions;
- Rediscovering and re-remembering the lost traditions, ceremonies, and prayers of the ancient ones;
- Forgiveness of one's wrongdoings and reaffirmation of one's connection to a larger cosmic reality;
- Learning to become a person of knowledge/becoming impeccable;
- Realization that service to others is the natural order of things (Cervantes, 2008, p. 9).

Psychological problems and behavioral impairment are regarded as spiritual maladies. Thus, the mental health provider is regarded as guide and co-journeyer and the therapeutic relationship resembles the cultural practices of *curanderismo*. Mutual learning between the client and mental health provider is based on a healing process that fosters egalitarian interactions and a respectful relationship. Techniques are less important than the healing presence of the mental health provider because it enables clients to increase their awareness regarding their reactions, feelings, and behaviors and to understand distinctive cultural themes that are inherent within their experiences.

In Cervantes's (2010) case study, therapeutic work addresses symptoms of depression, anger at God, and client restoration. The instillation of hope, prayers to the Virgin of Guadalupe, recollection of her supportive mother and grandmother, and the use of sage contribute to her improved functioning, emotional resolution, and restored self-belief. Cervantes (2010) notes that because this model focuses on relevance of one's spiritual journey as the basis for the healing process, this approach is inappropriate for clients who are solely interested in symptom reduction and not social justice perspectives. This model requires existential dialogue toward understanding the human condition. (Cervantes, 2010). Nonetheless, while a Latina/o heritage is not required to effectively utilize this model, a crucial element of the model requires a mental health provider's developed spirituality, familiarity with Mexican/Mexican American populations, indigenous spirituality, and an a appreciation for the historical elements and social justice that underlie the approach.

Ortiz et al. (2008) also provide a conceptual model that integrates specific therapeutic competencies and practices for mental health providers (see Table 9.3). Their conceptual model is based on Sue, Arredondo, and McDavis's (1992) Multicultural Competencies Model and the conceptualization that competency includes self-awareness, knowledge, and skills. In particular, they apply these dimensions to integrate spiritual and religious aspects into counseling and also apply elements of mestizo and Mesoamerican indigenous worldviews. These elements include holistic, ritualistic, and sacramental (experiential) domains and religious experiences. They apply their model to a case study for a Zapotec woman who is experiencing *susto* and describe how her metaphorical narratives and indigenous lexical explanations of symptoms allow the mental health provider to connect with her frame of reference. In addition, they describe how the exploration of meanings associated with rituals and symbols enable her to relieve her anxiety and worry.

Baez and Hernandez (2001) echo similar sentiments and express that successful navigation of spiritual issues with Latina/os requires an understanding of clients' views regarding indigenous healing and how these forms of healing serve their needs (Yeh et al., 2004). Mental health providers who are aware of their own spiritual perspectives and the spiritual underpinnings of their therapeutic style are able to identify areas of spiritual convergence and dissonance with their clients. This awareness will also reduce the possibility that these underpinnings will adversely impact their work with Latina/os. Thus, openness to indigenous healing and an awareness of one's assumptions and beliefs regarding indigenous healers and alternative forms of healing are crucial (Yeh et al., 2004). Baez and Hernandez (2001) suggest that while mental health providers are not required to believe in their client's spiritual beliefs, such as *espiritismo* and *Santería*, a key element in

Table 9.3 Ortiz, Davis, and McNeill's Conceptual Framework for Spirituality and Religiously Oriented Psychotherapy

---

Self-Awareness
- Be aware and sensitive to your own beliefs and assumptions concerning health and disease, as well as value-alternative worldviews.
- Monitor how your own experiences, attitudes, values, and biases may influence the therapeutic process.
- Be comfortable with differences that exist between yourself and clients in terms of religious and spiritual experiences.
- Include issues of spirituality, religion, culture, and language during intake, assessment, diagnosis, and treatment.

Knowledge
- Recognize the limits of your knowledge of indigenous concepts and worldviews.
- Acquire specific knowledge of personal worldviews on disease processes in your own culture and in other cultures.
- Establish consultative relationships with folk healers, cultural consultants (interpreters), and religious and spiritual leaders.

Skills
- Learn metaphors and culture-specific or indigenous descriptors and use them in the proper context to connect with your client's frame of reference.
- Incorporate the use of indigenous therapeutic practices into your clinical practice and theoretical orientation.
- Role-play, consult, and receive feedback on the practice of ethically responsible therapeutic practices that use alternative methods of treatment.

Holism
- Use multidimensional conceptualization of issues that consider holistic approaches during assessment and treatment, with close consideration of multiple levels of human reality (body, mind, soul, and spirit) across multiple dimensions of existence (terrestrial, natural, and supernatural, etc.).
- Attend to the interplay of both internal and external factors contributing to the client's reported issues and determine the sense of balance and harmony in human reality and existence.
- Appreciate the overlap and interrelation between internal subjective constructions (cognitions, emotions, beliefs, perceptions, values, attitudes, orientations, epistemologies, consciousness levels, expectations, and personhood) and external constructions of reality (artifacts, roles, institutions, social structures, and lifestyles).

(continued)

Table 9.3 Ortiz, Davis, and McNeill's Conceptual Framework for Spirituality and Religiously Oriented Psychotherapy (*continued*)

Ritual
  • Discuss the use of symbols and ritual in the client's experience in both the domestic and organized/denominational spheres.
  • Explore the meanings attached to symbol and ritual and how these relate to other levels of human reality and areas of functioning in the client's life.
  • Encourage rituals that are practical and proportional when they address relationships—either human or spiritual—that are healing.

Experiential/Sacramental Practices
  • Be receptive and sensitive to the client's sacramental imagination and experience of the divine his his/her life.
  • Identify any transformational experience, spiritual experience, or sacramental moment and how this impacted the client.
  • Facilitate the description and expression of the client's participation in sensual, visual, and communal practices related to the transcendent and divine. This may include client use/demonstration of material religion.

Source: Ortiz, F., A., Davis, K.G., & McNeill, B.W. (2008). Curanderismo: Religious and spiritual worldviews and indigenous healing traditions. In B. W. McNeill & J. M. Cervantes (Eds.), *Latina/o healing practices: Mestizo and indigenous perspectives* (pp. 271–302). New York: Routledge.

the successful engagement and treatment strategies with Latina/o clients is a mental health provider's respectful attitude.

For instance, respectful interventions include a willingness to explore references to alternative spiritual beliefs but not dismissive or cynical attitudes toward a client's participation in *Santería* or *espiritismo*. Mental health providers should also express interest in the outcomes of any complementary consultation or intervention and not solely encourage participation in traditional mental health treatment. They should also attempt to make dignified references to spiritual practitioners who are consulted by their clients, such as a priest or rabbi, and avoid the use of pejorative terms. Lastly, mental health providers should welcome therapeutic input from spiritual sources and avoid excluding the spiritual world by solely focusing on the treatment of the material world (Baez & Hernandez, 2001, p. 413).

Mental health providers may experience difficulties determining which spiritual interventions are best for their clients. Thus, consultation with Latina/o clinicians and indigenous healers is also necessary. Unfortunately, Western practitioners experience difficulties identifying a qualified spiritual collaborator for purposes of collaboration. However, given their oppression, indigenous healers might display suspicion or distrust of

Western practitioners. Thus, building rapport is an essential step to any consultation, and mental health providers must demonstrate genuine respect, interest, and mutual concern for their client. While pragmatic issues such as confidentiality and ethical issues may emerge and pose challenges, these collaborative efforts are nonetheless important (Parks et al., 2014), as therapeutic alliances with healers are important for the creation of therapeutic alliances that involve both clients and indigenous healers (Yeh et al., 2004).

Collaborations and working relationships with a variety of spiritual practitioners are also important for purposes of referrals. For example, a joint effort such as the Therapist-Spiritist Training Project in Puerto Rico (Koss, 1980, 1987) included collaboration between *espiritistas* and various practitioners, such as psychologists, nurses, social workers, and physicians over a 10-month period. They exchanged information regarding their healing systems and attempted to synthesize the most effective techniques within each system. An outcome of the project included client referrals between the systems and on occasion, *espiritistas* and therapists consulted with one another regarding their own personal problems (Koss, 1980).

There are numerous benefits of addressing spirituality within traditional mental heath services, particularly as Latina/os often favor integrative, holistic, and syncrestic healing approaches (Comas-Díaz, 2012c). APA Multicultural Guidelines (American Psychological Association, 2003) encourage mental health providers to develop self-awareness of their spiritual perspectives and how they impact the therapeutic process. These guidelines encourage mental health providers to increase their understanding regarding helping practices and healing traditions that are used among multicultural populations that are suitable for clinical practice. Indeed mainstream mental health interventions can benefit from the integration of indigenous healing (Comas-Díaz, 2006). Also, noting the importance of integrating indigenous forms of healing, Yeh et al. (2004) build on the work of other scholars and provide the following suggestions for integrating indigenous forms of healing within the therapeutic process:

1. Be open to the idea of indigenous healing, because it may emerge within therapy.
2. Be aware of your own assumptions and beliefs, both positive and negative, about indigenous healers and alternative forms of healing.
3. Seek to understand clients' views on indigenous healing and how such forms of healing serve their needs.
4. Research and seek knowledge about the various forms of indigenous healing.
5. Acknowledge that it is impossible and unrealistic to be an expert on all forms of indigenous healing. However, openness to such healing practices is the key to more effective counseling.

6. Reach out to, and develop connections with, indigenous healers.
7. Discuss with indigenous healers their philosophies and recognize similarities and differences between traditional Western counseling and indigenous healing.
8. Form alliances with healers because they will become members of the therapeutic relationship.
9. Create therapeutic alliances that involve both clients and indigenous healers.
10. Understand that indigenous healing may not be scientific, measurable, or goal-oriented.
11. Define the benefits of your own work with clients as well as the benefits of indigenous healing.
12. Counselors often work within frameworks that are personally congruent; therefore, develop your spirituality and connection to others, the cosmos, and nature (p. 415).

CONCLUSION

To decrease the gap between Latina/o clients and mental health providers, it is important for mental health providers to understand and address the spiritual beliefs and practices of their Latina/o clients. For many Latina/os, these spiritual practices are important and provide strength, resilience, and comfort during challenging periods. In addition, they are a response to a history of colonization, displacement, class stratification, and other forms of oppression (Comas-Díaz, 2006; McNeill & Cervantes, 2008). Genuine respect and cultural empathy will demonstrate to clients that their worldviews are equally valid (Parks et al., 2014) and certainly aid in the therapeutic process. Along with recognizing and integrating their belief systems, mental health providers must incorporate indigenous forms of healing when appropriate (Yeh et al., 2004). These types of healing are particularly appealing for Latina/os, since they entail a holistic approach that includes cultural, physical, mental, spiritual, social, religious, and natural dimensions to achieve balance (Valdez, 2014). Furthermore, a collectivistic focus that also includes family, community, and society within treatment and healing rituals may increase treatment efficacy (Valdez, 2014). In addition to holistic approaches, emancipatory interventions that incorporate Latina/o cultural values, spirituality, and social justice are warranted in order to restore a sense of belonging and promote self-healing (Comas-Díaz, 2012a, b, c). Lastly, successful clinical navigation of clinical issues with Latina/os demands that mental health providers develop self-awareness of their own spiritual perspectives and how they impact the therapeutic process (Yeh et al., 2004).

Chapter 10

Future Considerations

From the founding of the United States to the present day, the right to good health and well-being has been a basic tenet the nation holds dear.
—David Satcher, 2006, p. 547

Given our nation's current political turmoil and sociopolitical landscape, vulnerable communities, including Latina/os, are in jeopardy for the basic human rights, such as good health. The Latina/o community, now more than ever, requires advocacy and social justice. Despite the current state of health and mental health care in the United States, the well-being of Latina/os can be protected, prioritized, and promoted through concerted efforts aimed at establishing culturally appropriate health and mental health care delivery, and identifying and increasing community resources that are accessible to Latina/os. Complex multifaceted issues require comprehensive multifaceted solutions. In the case of Latina/os, a comprehensive and informed understanding of the current state of Latina/o health is certainly ideal.

In this final chapter, we provide future directions for the physical and mental health promotion of Latina/os. Specifically, we outline opportunities to improve outreach and programs for Latina/os and address the need for increased policies and research to inform best practices. Special consideration is taken to explore how the current political landscape influences opportunities to conduct research for underserved and vulnerable groups such as Latina/os. More importantly, we address why conducting this research is more important now than ever before.

THE LATINA/O HEALTH PROFILE

As discussed in prior chapters, Latina/os are disproportionately burdened by a number of mental and physical health issues (American Cancer Society, 2015; Haile et al., 2012). Although the prevalence of certain mental health disorders is similar to the general population, their mental health is frequently exacerbated by their increased likelihood to delay seeking mental health treatment (Alegría et al., 2012; Cabassa et al., 2006). Additionally, Latina/os are more likely to experience comorbidities than White/European Americans (Alegría et al., 2012).

Increased research is needed regarding the comorbidities that impact Latina/os. As discussed, there are several similarities between the underlying contributors of their mental and physical health. The simultaneous examination of these conditions can certainly provide greater comprehensive explanatory models. For instance, Erving (2017) examined the co-occurrence of physical and psychiatric health problems among White/European Americans and Latina/o heritage groups. The use of data from the National Comorbidity Survey Replication and the National Latino and Asian American Study allows for the examination of specific trends among Mexican Americans, Cubans, Puerto Ricans, and Other Latina/os, and White/European Americans. Respondents self-report prior diagnosis of arthritis, asthma, cancer, chronic lung disease, diabetes, heart disease, high blood pressure, stroke, or ulcer. Participants' self-reported height and weight are used to calculate morbid obesity. The World Mental Health Survey Initiative version of the WHO Composite International Diagnostic Interview (WMH-CIDI) is also utilized to determine psychological disorders. Responses determine the presence of mood disorders (e.g., major depressive disorder, dysthymia), anxiety (e.g., agoraphobia, panic attack, social phobia, posttraumatic stress disorder), and substance use disorders (e.g., alcohol abuse, drug abuse).

Results suggest that foreign-born Mexican men are most likely to be "healthy," as 71% of Mexican men do not report either physical or mental illnesses. Foreign-born Cuban men are most likely to solely report physical health problems (52%). Island-born Puerto Rican men are more likely to demonstrate both physical and psychiatric illness than White/European American men. After controlling for sociodemographic characteristics, Mexican Americans and Other Latina/os have an unexpected health advantage over White/European Americans, providing support for the Latino paradox. These findings certainly highlight the increased need to simultaneously examine physical and psychiatric illness among Latina/os and across heritage groups.

The urgency to address the health issues of Latina/os is compounded by barriers to health care. As discussed within Chapters 3 and 7, several barriers to health care contribute to their decreased help-seeking behaviors and limited access to medical and psychological treatment (Alegría et al., 2002; Berdahl & Stone, 2009; Ransford, Carrillo, & Rivera, 2010). An ecological perspective allows us to contextualize the influence of individual, cultural, organizational, and societal factors (Bledsoe, 2008) and the significant overlap between medical and mental health barriers of Latina/os. Because these barriers interact and impact their physical health and mental health, immediate action and preventive measures are imperative (Valdez & de Posada, 2006). Thus, we begin this chapter by identifying opportunities for improving access to health care and mental health treatment for Latina/os, such as increasing the cultural competence of health care and mental health providers.

CULTURALLY APPROPRIATE CONSIDERATIONS FOR HEALTH CARE AND MENTAL HEALTH CARE DELIVERY

Culturally appropriate health care and mental health treatment are indeed important. Benefits of culturally appropriate health care and mental health treatment include increased patient satisfaction and increased utilization of health care services (Castro & Ruiz, 2009). Patient satisfaction is predictive of their likelihood to continue visits with their physicians and treatment adherence (Moore, Saywell, Thakker, & Jones, 2002). Conversely, low patient satisfaction is associated with an increased likelihood to change providers and subsequent emergency room visits (Ware & Davis, 1983). Similarly, while in treatment, Latina/os with limited English proficiency face the risk of misdiagnosis and inappropriate mental health treatment, as well as dissatisfaction and premature termination (Kouyoumdjian et al., 2003).

As discussed in earlier chapters, several factors directly impact access to health care and mental health treatment, including patients' ability to feel understood and comfortable disclosing information to their physicians (see Chapter 3). Culturally appropriate health care is frequently discussed in terms of cultural competence (Acevedo, 2008; Brown, Garcia, Kouzekanani, & Hanis, 2002; Hernandez et al., 2009; Sue, 2001). We begin this chapter by examining the concept of cultural competence in health care and mental health treatment. We specifically highlight two models and provide recommendations to further elucidate the concept; we then assess its association with patient health and mental health outcomes.

CULTURAL COMPETENCE

Cultural competence is generally defined as the condition in which a set of congruent behaviors, attitudes, and policies come together in a system, agency, or among professionals to enable effective cross-cultural work (Cross, 1989). Other definitions of cultural competence suggest that it is the process that occurs when culture care values, expressions, or patterns are known and used appropriately and meaningfully by the practitioner with individuals or groups (Leininger, 1991). Cultural competence is also defined as the ability to communicate between and among cultures while working within the cultural context of a client, be it an individual, family, or community (Campihna-Bacote, 1999). Researchers contend that these definitions lack sufficient operationalization, and are thus unhelpful in guiding health care providers and systems with directions or strategies to increase their cultural competence (Hernandez et al., 2009). However, three specific models can serve as frameworks for cultural competence and provide comprehensive examinations of cultural competence, such as the Hernandez Model (Hernandez et al., 2009), Multidimensional Model of Cultural Competence (Sue, 2001), and Purnell Model of Cultural Competence (Purnell, 2014).

Hernandez Model

Hernandez and colleagues (2009) conducted a literature review of 1,100 articles to identify common themes in how researchers operationalize cultural competence and how practitioners use cultural competence to inform practice in mental health treatment settings. The results of the review suggest that cultural competence is the condition in which four factors are compatible—community context, cultural characteristics of local populations, organizational infrastructure, and direct service support (Hernandez et al., 2009). Although Hernandez et al. (2009) specifically developed this model for application to mental health care, aspects of cultural competence can be applied to the general health care system as well.

Hernandez and colleagues (2009) suggest that all four factors are necessary and require alignment to achieve cultural competence. For instance, community context includes the sociopolitical context in which the care is provided. The history of a client's culture in the community directly impacts a provider's ability to engage with the client or patient in a manner that communicates cultural competence. Additionally, knowledge of how a provider's culture is perceived and treated in the context of the community allows for the provision of culturally responsive care. The community context can also impact perceptions of health care or mental health care delivery (Cauce et al., 2002). For example, African American youth are more likely than White/European American youth to enter into the mental health care system through involuntary methods such as the juvenile justice system. This context impacts patients' perceptions of health care and mental health care systems and warrant acknowledgement for cultural competence to exist.

Providers must understand and appreciate the cultural characteristics of local populations. These characteristics include, but are not limited to, a community's values, beliefs, and practices. This aspect of cultural competence is highlighted within other models and measures of cultural competence and includes the knowledge, attitudes, and skills needed to work with culturally diverse groups (Andrea, Daniels, & Heck, 1991; Sue et al., 1982). Training for health professionals is critical to ensure that both health care and mental health care providers increase their familiarity of culturally diverse groups and how their perspectives differ. Further, it is critical to recognize barriers to accessing health care, such as contradictions with existing value systems.

The organizational infrastructure is critical in establishing cultural competence as well. Organizational policies and practices either promote cultural competence by providing and promoting training of staff, encouraging community participation in the development of planning and data collection, specific directives to guide the provision of services, and establishing open communication with the community; the lack of these resources hinders cultural competence (Hernandez et al., 2009). One example of how organizations can impede the establishment of cultural competence is illustrated by a prior study in Texas (Dettlaff & Rycraft, 2009). A federally funded initiative was employed to train child welfare practitioners to provide culturally competent care for Latina/o children and their families through the use of an evidence-based framework—systems of care. The evaluation results illustrated that when the new framework was implemented, 100% of cases were not involved in substantiated reports of maltreatment by the six-month follow-up. However, multiple barriers were identified, including high workloads, staff shortages, and high turnover. The lack of organizational change to support and integrate this new framework indicated that only 40% of the training participants were able to sufficiently implement the new framework.

Direct service support includes the ways in which an organization increases the availability, accessibility, and utilization of its services and direct service support is critical to establishing cultural competence (Hernandez et al., 2009). There are simple ways to increase availability of services, such as ensuring that these services reflect community needs. Therefore, community feedback and input can help to ensure congruence between perceived community needs and direct services. Accessibility of services is important to achieve cultural competency. As discussed in Chapters 3 and 7, language is a significant barrier in accessing care, especially among foreign-born Latina/os with limited English proficiency. Services and information that are provided throughout health care or mental health care delivery systems must be available in Spanish to ensure accessibility among Latina/os with limited English proficiency. Finally, promoting utilization of these services can include providing services to alleviate barriers to utilization, such as reminder texts or telephone calls for appointments, providing transportation services and child care, and flexible hours of operation (Aguilar-Gaxiola et al., 2012; Friedmann, D'Aunno, Jin, & Alexander, 2000).

The Hernandez model provides a few key benefits over traditional views of cultural competence. In both mental health care and general health care settings, the individual health care provider's responsibility is emphasized for increasing cultural competence with little or no recognition of the context in which the cultural competence should occur (Hernandez et al., 2009). In other words, the idea of cultural competence focuses on the health care provider's knowledge and skills related to communicating with members of other cultures. This conceptual framework, however, takes into account the role of the community, organization, and direct service support as well as the characteristics of local populations.

Multidimensional Model of Cultural Competence

Another model helpful in understanding the comprehensive nature of cultural competence is the Multidimensional Model of Cultural Competence (MDCC) (Sue, 2001). The MDCC proposes a multidimensional approach to cultural competence that includes three overarching dimensions—racial and culture-specific attributes of competence, components of cultural competence, and foci of cultural competence. Similar to the Hernandez model, the MDCC illustrates a comprehensive perspective on cultural competence, and does not focus on the provider alone. Rather, the MDCC views cultural competence as a multidimensional and ecological perspective, including the provider, profession, organization, and society.

The MDCC is informed by a tripartite framework of personal identity, recognizing that individual, group and universal levels impact client/patient-perceived identity (Sue, 2001). The individual level of identity primarily focuses on how each person is unique and highlights the person's unique tendencies and traits. The group level of identity includes group identity in which individuals identify with a group based on shared characteristics. This is most closely related to ethnic identity and how a shared race or ethnic group identifies their commonalities with others from the same ethnic background. The universal level of personal identity includes an individual's shared characteristics with all other human beings, such as a drive for self-awareness and shared common life experiences. Sue (1998) contends that previous work in psychology overemphasized either the individual, focusing on personal traits and characteristics, or the universal level of identity, such as attempts to describe commonalities in the human psyche. Sue (1998) argues that the tendency to neglect group level identity is partially due to the need to avoid potentially controversial topics associated with race and the sociopolitical oppression of certain groups. These tendencies, however, underemphasize the group level of identity—a level critical to the understanding of cultural competence.

The MDCC model, alike the Hernandez model, recognizes the context in which cultural competence takes place. Whereas previous models acknowledge the need to address the practitioner's attitudes/beliefs, knowledge, and skills (Andrea et al., 1991; Sue et al., 1982), Sue (1998) includes these dimensions but asserts an overarching responsibility for a practitioner's skill development, as well as an overarching responsibility to pursue social justice. Sue explains that social justice underlies cultural competence and the goal of cultural competence. Counseling and psychotherapy can act as forms of cultural oppression when culturally diverse clients are viewed as deviant or abnormal because they differ from the majority culture (Sue & Sue, 1999). Additionally, when psychologists fail to recognize the impact of race and ethnicity and instead approach these systemic issues by solely targeting clients, they ignore and do not directly address unjust inequities (Sue, 2001).

Within the mental health care system, Sue (2001), like Hernandez et al. (2009), identifies the multiple levels of influence on cultural competence. Sue identifies these levels as individual, professional, organizational, and societal. Cultural competence occurs when all foci are addressed; however, each area includes barriers to change. The individual level includes the realization of personal biases. Barriers to this level include potential cognitive dissonance among practitioners if they value justice and equity, while acknowledging their personal prejudices. The professional level includes a change in the entire psychological profession, in which the field of psychology reevaluates its definition of itself and adopts multicultural codes of ethics and standards of practice (Sue, 2001).

Organizational change toward cultural competence includes a shift from being a monocultural organization, through nondiscriminatory practices, and ideally becoming a multicultural organization. Main changes that aid in the transition from being a monocultural organization to becoming a multicultural organization include the following: (1) the development of an organizational vision that reflects multiculturalism; (2) reflecting the contributions of diverse cultural and social groups; (3) valuing multiculturalism and viewing it as an asset; (4) actively engaging in problem-solving activities to allow for equal access and opportunities; (5) realizing that equal access and opportunities are not equal treatment; and (6) appreciating the diversity of the environment. Finally, the societal level aids in cultural competence when individuals from all segments of society act toward each other in ways that communicate cultural awareness, sensitivity, and respect.

The MDCC provides a much more comprehensive approach to cultural competence than traditional models. Additionally, the MDCC provides a means for assessing and increasing cultural competence in knowledge, attitudes, and skills and calls for a broad and integrated approach to cultural competence. The model highlights the need to intervene beyond the individual level and the need to address other levels of influence, such as the organizational and societal levels. As research in cultural competence moves forward, these models provide alternative areas for examination.

The Purnell Model for Cultural Competence

The Purnell Model for Cultural Competence (2014) provides a comprehensive framework for cultural competence in any health care setting. The model includes 12 cultural domains and their concepts that require attention when addressing patients and their families in various settings. In addition, no single domain stands alone, as they are all interconnected. Purnell (2014) notes that health care providers can also use these same concepts to increase their understanding of their own attitudes and behaviors. Nonetheless, these 12 domains include the following: overview and heritage, communications, family roles and organization, workforce issues, biocultural ecology, high-risk health behaviors, nutrition, pregnancy and childbearing practices, death rituals, spirituality, health care practices, and health care providers.

The Purnell Model also includes the concept of cultural consciousness and an unknown phenomenon. Because cultural competence is not an endpoint but a process, the model identifies four types of competence. For example, unconscious incompetence includes the inability to recognize that one lacks knowledge about another culture, while conscious incompetence includes being aware that one lacks knowledge about another culture. It is theorized that as health care providers increase their self-awareness, they progress into conscious competence and learn about their patient's culture, verify generalizations, and provide culturally specific interventions. Finally, unconscious competence includes automatically providing culturally congruent care to culturally diverse patients.

One advantage of the Purnell Model is the assessment guide that aligns with 12 cultural domains, as health care providers can use the model as a guide for assessing, planning, implementing, and evaluating their interventions. The assessment guide is extensive, and a health care provider can select questions that are the most appropriate in the cultural assessments of their patients. The answers to these questions can direct the health care provider to include their patient's cultural values and background in their assessment and treatment recommendations. Sample questions for each domain are provided in Table 10.1. Additionally, the Purnell Model includes an ecological framework that includes person, family, community, and global society. Similar to the Hernandez and MDCC models, the Purnell Model includes assumptions regarding the need for systemic changes to occur to achieve cultural competence—the practitioner as the only change agent is insufficient to truly create cultural competence.

IMPACT OF CULTURAL COMPETENCE

The lack of culturally competent care is costly to patients and clients. Low cultural competence is associated with inaccurate identification of health problems and limited recognition and treatment of disease (Smith, 2001; Walker & Jaranson, 1999). Lack of cultural competence can lead to decreased communication or less effective communication between physician and patient (Perez-Escamilla, 2009), whereas high cultural competence in health care and mental health care systems is associated with improved clinical outcomes and reduced health care disparities (Kripalani, Bussey-Jones, Katz, & Genao, 2006).

Cultural competence in health care delivery is not limited to the cultural competence of the physician. The cultural competence of nurse practitioners can also impact patient satisfaction. For example, a cross-sectional study of 15 nurse practitioners in Arizona and 218 of their Latina patients examined patient satisfaction and acculturation levels and their association with cultural competence (i.e., cultural proficiency, cultural competency, and cultural awareness) among nurse practitioners (Castro & Ruiz, 2009). Findings indicate diversity in levels of cultural competency among nurse practitioners, as two report cultural proficiency, seven report cultural competency, and six report cultural awareness. Patient satisfaction is associated with cultural competency, time spent with provider, an American orientation, and a Latina nurse practitioner. Conversely, patient satisfaction is negatively associated with patient waiting time, number of years since earning a RN degree, and patient health insurance status. Nurse practitioners' cultural competence is associated with being Latina, possessing certification, cultural competence training, speaking Spanish, and attending masters-level programs. While this study does not measure cultural competence beyond the nurse practitioner, it demonstrates the importance of cultural competency among all health care providers, such as nurses.

Table 10.1 Purnell Model for Cultural Competence and Sample Assessment Questions

Domain	Sample of Domain Features	Sample Questions
Overview/ Heritage	Origins, residence, topography, economics	Where do you currently live? What is your ancestry?
Communications	Dominant language, dialects, contextual use, volume/tone	What is your primary language? Are you usually on time for appointments?
Family Roles and Organization	Head of household, gender roles, developmental tasks, goals & priorities	Who makes the most decisions in your family? What are the duties of the women in the family?
Workforce Issues	Acculturation, autonomy, language barriers	Do you consider yourself a "loyal" employee? Do you consider yourself to be assertive in your job?
Biocultural Ecology	Biological variations, skin color, heredity, genetics	What are the major illnesses and disease in your family?
High-Risk Behaviors	Tobacco, alcohol, recreational drugs, physical activity	How many daily cigarettes do you smoke?
Nutrition	Meaning of food, common foods, rituals, deficiencies	Are you satisfied with your weight? Which foods do you eat every day?
Pregnancy	Fertility practices, pregnancy beliefs, views toward pregnancy	How many children do you have? What do you use for birth control?
Death Rituals	Death rituals, bereavement	How do men grieve? What does death mean to you?
Spirituality	Religious practices, use of prayer, meaning of life	Do you consider yourself deeply religious?
Health Care Practices	Focus on health care, traditional practices, responsibility for health	What herbal teas and folk medicines do you use?
Health Care Providers	Perceptions of providers, folk practitioners	What health care providers do you see when you are ill?

Source: Adapted from Purnell, L. D. (2014). *Guide to culturally competent health care*. Philadelphia: Davis.

Efforts to increase cultural competence also illustrate the importance of addressing community needs. In a report by the California Reducing Disparities Project, community members work in conjunction with various organizations to identify specific needs that are critical to improving health conditions of Latina/os (Aguilar-Gaxiola et al., 2012). These needs inform strategic directions to improve mental health care services. Cultural competence is addressed in two of the seven strategic directions. For example, Strategic Direction 4 addresses workforce development and Strategic Direction 5 addresses the need to provide culturally and linguistically appropriate treatments. Both strategies aim to increase cultural competence in the profession through workforce development. Workforce development encourages medical and mental health organizations to recruit and retain a diverse workforce that reflects their client population. Pipeline efforts to increase a diverse workforce, such as additional training and mentoring programs, and increased support for underrepresented groups to enter the workforce, are critical. Strategic Direction 5, such as the provision of culturally and linguistically appropriate treatments, is attainable by ensuring that culturally and linguistically appropriate treatments are available at all sites. Although health care and mental health treatment facilities are encouraged to provide translation services, the enforcement of these services is minimal and do not adequately address clients' cultural needs by themselves.

SUMMARY

Cultural competence can potentially increase patient and client satisfaction and the utilization of health care and mental health care services. New models of cultural competence can increase the rigor of assessing and increasing cultural competence beyond the practitioner level. When entire professions, organizations, and societies increase their cultural competence, cultural competence will truly exist, decreasing barriers to access and providing more equitable opportunities and social justice for all.

Community-Based Participatory Research among Latina/os

Community Based Participatory Research (CBPR) was briefly introduced in Chapter 4. We provide greater detail regarding the process of CBPR, the benefits of using community-based participatory approaches in health care and mental health treatment, and issues specific to the Latina/o community that warrant consideration when conducting CBPR.

CBPR is a framework for conducting research that is inclusive and informed by the target population (Minkler, 2005). Community members are active members in the research process, including the needs assessment through identifying priority issues and potential solutions, as well as conducting evaluation research and disseminating findings. This research framework differs from traditional research in which the researcher conducts a needs assessment, identifies goals and objectives, plans a project, and subsequently engages community members during recruitment of participants. Many researchers advocate for the use of CBPR because it yields better-informed research, higher participation rates and buy-in from community members, and increased sustainability (O'Toole et al., 2003).

CBPR research is extremely beneficial in conducting research on underrepresented groups, such as Latina/os. Despite their increased presence in the United States, Latina/os remain disproportionally underrepresented in research of health-related issues, such as cancer (Underwood, 2000). There is an urgent need to effectively recruit Latina/os into clinical trials and engage Latina/os in all aspects of the research. As mentioned earlier, CBPR is one method for engaging and collaborating with Latina/o communities to ensure that their most important health issues are prioritized, culturally appropriate interventions are developed, and to ensure that findings are disseminated among the groups that will benefit from such findings. Clinical trials will also benefit from this approach, as researchers largely engage Latina/o communities at the point of recruitment, rather than engaging and collaborating with these communities. Unfortunately, the lack of cultural sensitivity and engagement also decreases the likelihood that Latina/os will participate in clinical trials.

The Hispanic Community Health Study/Study of Latinos (HCHS/SOL) serves as an excellent example of a clinical study that uses a community-based approach to engage community members in the research process. The HCHS/SOL study is described in detail in Chapter 2. As a prospective, population-based, and cohort study, the HCHS/SOL aims to identify risk factors associated with cardiovascular disease risk among different Latina/o heritage groups (Sorlie et al., 2010). HCHS/SOL includes four different recruitment sites and researchers established a Community Advisory Board at each site to contribute their knowledge regarding their local communities. Researchers presented study procedures, including recruitment, to Community Advisory Boards and Board members in return provided feedback and suggestions to ensure the cultural appropriateness of all methods. Community Advisory Board members were also asked to review recruitment materials and provide feedback on translations (Sorlie et al., 2010).

To address the increased need for Latinas to engage in cancer prevention, Larkey and colleagues (2009) also used CBPR strategies. They involved community members in the networking and recruitment of sites and participants, project development, and gathered community feedback throughout the project. Consequently, Larkey and colleagues (2009) were able to increase their potential recruitment list from 42 to 110 sites, and succeeded in enrolling a significant number Latinas to form 144 randomized groups. They credit their robust recruitment to leader support and community buy-in. *Promotoras* and an advisory board assisted in securing buy-in, support, and subsequent recruitment of participants.

The Increased Need to Empirically Examine Latina/o Heritage Groups

As discussed in Chapter 1, Latina/os are a diverse and heterogeneous group and originate from more than 25 countries in the Northern and Southern hemispheres, Central America, as well as the Caribbean (Arredondo et al., 2014; Borrell & Crawford, 2009). In addition to differences in their countries of origin, Latina/os differ in their geographic regions, immigration patterns, sociopolitical histories, socioeconomic status, English profanely (Betancourt & Flynn, 2009), and other salient factors such as beliefs and cultural practices that shape their health and mental health. Consequently, it is crucial for researchers, providers, and policymakers to consider the varied demographic characteristics that exist among Latina/o heritage groups. However, most health and mental health research largely examines Mexican Americans perhaps because they comprise 63% of Latina/os in the United States (Ennis et al., 2011). While certain national data sets may include a small number of Puerto Ricans and Cubans, other Latina/o heritage groups are rarely included within these studies or aggregated to form an "Other" category. In addition to variations in country of origin, Latina/o heritage groups also reside within different geographic regions of the United States. As discussed in Chapter 1, a large proportion of Mexicans reside in the West (51.8%) and South (34.4%). This differs from the large proportion of Cubans (77%) and Dominicans (78%), who tend to reside in the South and Northeast (Ennis et al., 2011).

As discussed throughout this text, the inability to distinguish among country of origin as well as nativity status prevents researchers, health providers, and policy makers from truly understanding the protective and risk factors that are associated with Latina/o heritage groups, geographic region, social conditions, and health outcomes. The inability to distinguish among Latina/o heritage groups also leads to the homogenization of a highly heterogeneous ethnic group (Elder et al., 2009). Treating Latina/os as a monolithic group negatively impacts research findings, the delivery of care, and ultimately, health outcomes.

Another promising area of research is investigation of protective factors and strengths-based approaches to health. In contrast to deficit models, which primarily focus on identifying needs and deficits to create a risk profile, strengths-based approaches aim to assess capacity and resilience (Weick, Rapp, Sullivan, & Kisthardt, 1989). Strengths-based approaches rest on the assumption that all individuals have strengths and thus aim to identify those strengths (Epstein & Sharma, 1998). Resilience is also a relevant focus of research among Latina/os. Resilience is defined as the process of encountering and coping with life experiences and the ability to prosper despite the encounter (Brownlee et al., 2013). Identifying the factors that contribute to Latina/o resilience can inform intervention work to develop similar or increased resilience in future generations. In addition, increased research regarding Latina/os and coping mechanisms can inform future interventions.

The Continued Need to Focus upon LGBTQIA Latina/os

There is a significant need for concerted efforts to address the health and mental health needs of LGBTQIA Latina/os. As overlapping members of sexual minority and ethnic minority groups, they are impacted by multifaceted stressors, such as homophobia, discrimination, and poverty. Unfortunately, these stressors jeopardize their full participation in family life and the LBTQ community, limit educational and professional opportunities (Díaz et al., 2001), as well as increase their vulnerability to violence and persecution (Cerezo et al., 2014). Indeed, these stressors can compromise their health and well being. Special efforts to include LGBTQIA Latina/os in programmatic and outreach efforts are also necessary. However, these programs should build upon their resilience due to family and peer support, personal empowerment, community involvement, and social activism that help buffer against their multiple forms of discrimination (Díaz et al., 2001; Espín, 2012; Pastrana et al., 2017).

In addition to programmatic and outreach efforts, increased research regarding LGBTQIA Latina/os is also imperative. The limited collection of data related to LGBTQIA status reflects insufficient responses to the needs of this group (Cahill & Makadon, 2014), and thus limits our ability to examine health and mental health trends among LGBTQIA Latina/os. Encouraging researchers to collect data on sexual orientation and identity across research topics will help build the foundation of knowledge that is necessary to direct future research, legislation, health and mental heath care, and other programmatic efforts for LGBTQIA Latina/os. However, research approaches that examine their intersectionality are also important to identify how the experiences of LGBTQIA Latina/os entail a complex interplay of both potential conflicts and resilience.

The Increased Need for Health and Mental Promotion among Latino Men

Latino men are traditionally underrepresented in health promotion and research and utilize mental health care less frequently compared to their Latina counterparts. For example, Latino men with LEP are less likely to report colorectal cancer screening than non-Latino men, English proficient Latino men, and even Latinas with LEP (Diaz, Roberts, Clarke, Simmons, Goldman, & Rakowski, 2013). In addition to language, men's masculinity also shapes their screening behaviors. For example, Mexican men's limited colorectal cancer screening behaviors are shaped by low health literacy, medical jargon, and limited knowledge of screening behaviors and procedures, as well as masculinity, including stigma, fears, and embarrassment (Getrich et al., 2012). Masculinity also influences Latino men's mental heath care, as they are less likely to seek mental health treatment because of perceptions that therapy is emasculating for men (Bledsoe, 2008; Echeverry, 1997; Rastogi et al., 2012).

Given these disparities, health and mental health providers are tasked with increasing the engagement of Latino men. Aguilar-Gaxiola et al. (2012) offer strategic recommendations to reduce Latina/o mental health care disparities that can inform efforts to better serve Latina/os. Below we present modified recommendations to guide practitioners in the increased engagement of Latino men in health promotion, research, and mental health services.

- Strategic direction 1: Use media to raise awareness of Latino health issues, reduce stigma associated with mental health disorders among men, and promote information and resources about early intervention and the importance of Latino men's involvement in research.
  - Recommended actions:
    - Engage Latina/o news and social media and the entertainment industry to promote balanced and informed portrayals of physical and mental health problems.
    - Engage Latina/o news and social media and the entertainment industry to promote positive portrayals of Latino men utilizing health and mental health-care services.
    - Collaborate with news media and social media to promote Latino men's involvement in research
    - Create and disseminate *fotonovelas* (stories told with photos and dialogue) to promote greater awareness of the prevalence of health and mental health issues among Latino men and promote service utilization.

- Strategic direction 2: Develop and sustain a culturally and linguistically competent workforce consistent with the culture, language, and values of Latino men.
  - Recommended actions:
    - Support career pathway activities that lead to certification programs and advanced degrees with a focus on bicultural and bilingual training and other population-specific subject matter, including courses related to geriatrics and addiction treatment.
    - Establish a certificate course of study at the community college level through which Latino men interested in the health, mental health field, and health research can be certified as Latino health or mental health specialists.
    - Increase the priority of offering loan forgiveness programs for Latinos pursuing a career in the health or mental health field or research and for current Latino and non-Latino providers looking for retraining opportunities.
- Strategic direction 3: Provide culturally and linguistically appropriate treatment for Latino men
  - Recommended actions:
    - Develop and implement training guidelines that adequately assess the ability of the current and future workforce to effectively conduct culturally and linguistically appropriate care for Latino men.
    - Create an inventory of resources to address the unique issues faced by Latino men with regard to accessing health or mental health services or participating in research.

The Increased Need to Empirically Examine Acculturation among Latina/os

Acculturation is a key variable in most health outcomes and mental health research among Latina/os. *Acculturation* is defined as the process by which individuals adapt to a new living environment and potentially adopt the norms, values, and practices of their new host society (Abraido-Lanza, Echeverria, & Florez, 2016). However, researchers criticize the measurement and operationalization of acculturation (Thomson & Hoffman-Goetz, 2009) and the lack of consistency by which acculturation is measured. These issues contribute to debates surrounding its utility (Hunt, Schneider, & Comer, 2004). The debate regarding issues of validity may partially explain why several studies report that acculturation is associated with positive health outcomes whereas other studies report that it is associated with negative health outcomes (Ayala, Baquero, & Klinger, 2008; Berrigan et al., 2006; Bethel & Schenker, 2005).

Limitations of acculturation research include differing definitions of acculturation, limited research on the ecological contexts in which acculturation takes place, imperfect proxy measures, and limited research across Latina/o heritage groups (Lopez-Class, Castro, & Ramirez, 2011).

Differing definitions of acculturation might be due, in part, to the various fields of study that examine acculturation (Thomson & Hoffman-Goetz, 2009). The concept of acculturation was formulated in anthropology and described a group dynamic. However, the subsequent adaptation by psychologists to an individual-level phenomenon contributed to new approaches to the measurement and conceptualization of acculturation, but these adaptations also introduced limitations (Lopez-Class et al., 2011). Since then, public health and other fields have adopted various definitions for research purposes. While *acculturation* is generally defined as a process, debate remains regarding what aspects of the complex adaptation process should be included in its definition.

The examination of acculturation as an individual-level phenomenon has partially contributed to an overemphasis on individual-level factors and an underappreciation of environmental factors that influence the acculturation process (Lopez-Class et al., 2011). Research suggests that family relationships and group acceptance of an individual's assimilation can impact the likelihood that the individual will acculturate to the host society and therefore increase acculturative stress among adolescents (Bacallao & Smokowski, 2009). When researchers solely examine individual-level changes, they miss important opportunities to understand the acculturation process and its impact on other health and mental health outcomes. Thankfully, researchers are increasingly recognizing that the acculturation process emerges from and is reinforced by broader social determinants (Abraido-Lanza, Armbrister, Flórez, & Aguirre, 2006).

Proxy measures are often used to assess acculturation. Common proxy measures include language, years of U.S. residence, and generational status. Language is often used as a proxy for acculturation. Questionnaire language (English or Spanish) is often used to make conclusions regarding acculturation; however, this view of acculturation is extremely limited and does not capture the complex process of acculturation that underlies the theoretical construct of acculturation (Lara et al., 2005).

The proxy measure of years of U.S. residence and generational status are also used to measure acculturation despite inherent issues (Abraído-Lanza et al., 2006). For example, the use of years of U.S. residence may lead researchers to erroneously assume that all members of an ethnic minority group experience exposure in a uniform manner simply based on their years of U.S. residence. For example, use of the proxy years of U.S. residence will result in the assumption that the acculturation experiences are uniform among individuals who reside in the United States for a similar time period. Some researchers suggest that these measures may perhaps assess exposure to discrimination in the United States (Viruell-Fuentes, 2007). However, if this is the case, specific measures to assess perceived discrimination would serve as a more appropriate metric. Research suggests that perceived discrimination is associated with mental health issues (Chou, Asnaani, & Hofmann, 2012; Lee & Ahn, 2012), substance abuse (Otiniano Verissimo, Grella, Amaro, & Gee, 2014) and physical health issues among Latina/os (Molina & Simon, 2014). Understanding the underlying mechanisms that impact perceptions of discrimination and its impact on health, as well as how these relationships differ by Latina/o heritage group would provide interesting new directions.

Emerging research suggests that discrimination is associated with health outcomes. For example, Molina and Simon (2014) used data from the National Latino and Asian American Study (NLAAS) to assess daily discrimination and the presence of chronic health conditions among Latina/os. They examined scores on the Everyday Discrimination Scale (Williams, Yu, Jackson, & Anderson, 1997) to assess the frequency of routine experiences of unfair treatment. They also examined data on socioeconomic position through the use of variables on education level and data on subjective social position using the MacArthur Scale of Subjective Social Status (Adler, Epel, Castellazzo, & Ickovics, 2000). Finally, they examined data regarding the total count of chronic health conditions. Findings indicated that discrimination was associated with an increased number of chronic conditions (Molina & Simon, 2014). Household income modified the association between discrimination and chronic health issues. However, this association was not observed among Latina/os who perceived low levels of discrimination.

Suggestions for Advancing Research on Acculturation   Abraido-Lanza et al. (2016) identified key directions for advancing acculturation research. Among these key directions is the need to examine acculturation across levels, including intrapersonal, interpersonal, social environment, community, and global context. While most acculturation studies focus on individuals, understanding how families and groups acculturate may certainly yield valuable information. Exploratory studies are needed to examine the underlying processes that groups experience through the acculturation process (Castro, Kellison, Boyd, & Kopak, 2010), and these studies may elucidate processes of cultural adaptation and potentially lead to more informed and improved acculturation models (Chirkov, 2009).

Abraido-Lanza et al. (2016) also suggest that researchers examine acculturation through approaches that enable cross-disciplinary research to contribute to public health and population health research on acculturation. Life course approaches, developmental approaches, and segmented assimilation are possible areas of examination through the use of cross-disciplinary research. In addition, increased research that identities which specific cultural values change during the acculturation process can also inform the field. For example, researchers have focused on specific values such as *marianismo* (see Chapter 1) and their relationship to health behaviors (Castillo, Perez, Castillo, & Ghosheh 2010). Increased research on specific values and their relationship to health behaviors and outcomes can certainly inform how to best serve Latina/os during the immigration and acculturation process.

Insurance

As of this writing, the possible repeal of the Affordable Care Act is looming. Now more than ever, we must consider how to provide access to health care for the uninsured, particularly Latina/os, since they demonstrate lower access to health care than their White/European American counterparts (see Chapters 1 and 3). The implications of lower access were extensively addressed throughout the current text to highlight how limited access to health care contributes to significant health and mental health disparities among Latina/os as compared with other groups. Despite their employment, many Latina/o workers do not receive health insurance through their employers. For instance, while employer-provided insurance is a common source of health insurance for working-age adults and their families, Latina/os are less likely than White/European Americans to receive health insurance benefits from their employers. If the Affordable Care Act is repealed, the replacement program must provide insurance to lower-income populations, such as Latina/os that reflects quality care, including no-cost preventive care, no annual or lifetime limits, and culturally competent providers and services.

Anti-Latina/o Sentiments

Anti-Latina/o sentiments also jeopardize Latina/o health and well-being. Unfortunately, the increased political rhetoric regarding illegal immigration contributes to increased violence and hate crimes toward Latina/os, immigration raids, criminalization, and other forms of discrimination. Policies that allow for the racial profiling of Latina/os if they "look illegal" also contributes to the increased tolerance of discrimination against this vulnerable group (Otiniano Verissimo, Grella, Amaro, & Gee, 2014). There is significant evidence suggesting that these additional stressors exacerbate mental health and physical health risks. For example, a study of 27 recent Latino immigrants assessed the health, work and living conditions of day laborers and apartment-complex dwellers (Fernandez-Esquer, Agoff, & Leal, 2017). Through focus groups Latino men describe how their immigration status contributes to the elimination of their legal and social protections and exposes them to significant stress and subsequent health consequences. Further, the constant fear of deportation also impacts them on a daily basis, as they report living spoiled identities. For instance, they are restricted to jobs that are often rejected by others and experience exploitation and instability because of their immigration status.

Policies that provide a pathway to citizenship are necessary to protect the health and well-being of Latina/os. Unfortunately, President Trump ordered the repeal of DACA and urged Congress to pass a replacement before phasing out its protections to 750,000 Dreamers in March 2018. A majority of Dreamers are Latina/os, but all Dreamers face the potential threat of deportation. The uncertainty of their status has taken a toll on their physical and mental health, as well as others. The recent onslaught of discriminatory legislation, increased fear and intimidation from federal authorities, and political rhetoric necessitate the need for increased political representation on all governmental levels, as well as and organizations that serve Latina/o communities, such as schools, health and mental health facilities, etc., to advance the basic rights of Latina/os and other vulnerable groups. Increased diversity among politicians who embrace social justice is long overdue. Equally important, health care providers and mental health practitioners must also engage in advocacy and social justice to protect the vulnerable. Advocacy should include collaborations with community organizations, as well as collaborations with lawmakers to oppose discriminatory policies. This representation can help create positive changes by increasing awareness of the numerous issues that impact Latina/os. Informed politicians must also increase their cultural competence, inform policy, and provide more insightful solutions to immigration reform and the removal of discriminatory legislation. Comprehensive, informed, evidence-based solutions are needed to protect the safety of all persons, regardless of their immigration status and other social identities.

CONCLUSION

The Latina/o population is rapidly increasing. The emerging presence of Latina/os in new communities and their ongoing presence in communities throughout the United States warrant attention to their health profile to improve their health and mental health outcomes. Clearly, there is an urgent need to address the substantial health and mental health issues that impact Latina/o communities. Positive changes within Latina/o community will depend on rigorous research, advocacy and social justice, cultural competence, an increased understanding of the various Latina/o heritage groups, and federal policies to support equitable access to health-conducive environments, as well as equitable health and mental health care.

Suggested Readings

LATINA/O HEALTH

Aguirre-Molina, M., Molina, C. W., & Zambrana, R. E. (2002). *Health issues in the Latino community* (Vol. 7). New York: Wiley.

Arcury, T. A., & Quandt, S. A. (Eds.). (2009). *Latino farmworkers in the eastern United States: Health, safety and justice.* New York: Springer Science & Business Media.

Benuto, L. T., & Donohue, W. O. (Eds.). (2016). *Enhancing behavioral health in Latino populations.* Geneva, Switzerland: Springer International.

Chong, N. (Ed.). (2002). *The Latino patient: A cultural guide for the health care providers.* Boston: Intercultural Press.

Díaz, R. M. (1998). *Latino gay men and HIV: Culture, sexuality, and risk behavior.* New York: Routledge.

Guendelman, S. (1998). Health and disease among Hispanics. In S. Loue (Ed.), *Handbook of immigrant health* (pp. 277–301). New York: Springer.

Organista, K. C. (2007). *Solving Latino psychosocial and health problems: Theory, practice, and populations.* Hoboken, NJ: Wiley.

Torres, M. I., & Cernada, G. P. (2003). *Sexual and reproductive health promotion in Latino populations: Parteras, promotoras y poetas: Case studies across the Americas.* Amityville, NY: Baywood.

LATINA/O MENTAL HEALTH

Adames, H. Y., & Chavez-Dueñas, N. Y. (2017). *Cultural formulations and interventions in Latino/a mental health: History, theory and within group differences.* New York: Routledge.

Aguilar-Gaxiola, S. A., & Gullota, T. P. (Eds.). (2008). *Depression in Latinos: Assessment, treatment, and prevention.* New York: Springer.

Akhtar, S., & Bertoglia, S. M. (Eds.). (2015). *The American Latino: Psychodynamic perspectives on culture and mental health.* Lanham, MD: Rowman & Littlefield.

Arredondo, P., Gallardo-Cooper, M., Delgado-Romero, E. A., & Zapata, A. L. (Eds.). (2014). *Culturally responsive counseling with Latinas/os.* Alexandria, VA: American Counseling Association.

Buki, L. P., & Piedra, L. M. (Eds.). (2011). *Creating infrastructures for Latino mental health.* New York: Springer.

Cabrera, N. J., Villarruel, F. A., & Fitzgerald, H. E. (Eds.). (2011). *Latina and Latino children's mental health, Volume 1, Development and context.* Santa Barbara, CA: Praeger.

Cabrera, N. J., Villarruel, F. A., & Fitzgerald, H. E. (Eds.). (2011). *Latina and Latino children's mental health, Volume 2, Prevention and treatment.* Santa Barbara, CA: Praeger.

Falicov, C. J. (2014). *Latino families in therapy: A guide to multicultural practices* (2nd ed.). New York: Guilford.

Flores, Y. G. (2013). *Chicana and Chicano mental health: Alma, mente y corazón.* Tucson: University of Arizona Press.

Garcia, J. G., & Zea, M. C. (Eds.). (1997). *Psychological interventions and research with Latino populations.* Boston: Allyn and Bacon.

Grey, H., & Hall-Clark, B. N. (Eds.). (2015). *Cultural considerations in Latino American mental health.* New York: Oxford University Press.

Kawahara, D. M., & Espín, O. M. (Eds.). (2013). *Feminist therapy with Latina women: Personal and social voices.* New York: Routledge.

Lewis-Fernández, R., Aggarwal, N. K., Hinton, L., Hinton, D. E., & Kirmayer L. K. (2016). *DSM-5 handbook on the Cultural Formulation Interview.* Washington, DC: American Psychiatric Publishing.

López, A. G., & Carrillo, E. (Eds.). (2001). *The Latino psychiatric patient: Assessment and treatment.* Washington, DC: American Psychiatric Publishing.

McNeill, B. M., & Cervantes, J. M. (Eds.). (2008). *Latina/o healing practices: Mestizo and indigenous perspectives* (pp. 271–302). New York: Routledge.

Organista, K. C. (2007). *Solving Latino psychosocial and health problems: Theory, practice, and populations.* Hoboken, NJ: Wiley.

Ramírez, M. (1998). *Multicultural/multiracial psychology: Mestizo perspectives in personality and mental health.* Northvale, NJ: Aronson.

Santiago-Rivera, A. L., Arredondo, P., & Gallardo-Cooper, M. (Eds.). (2002). *Counseling Latinas/os and la familia: A practical guide.* Thousand Oaks, CA: Sage.

Smith, R. L., & Montilla, E. (Eds.). (2006). *Counseling and family therapy with Latino populations: Strategies that work.* New York: Routledge.

Velasquez, R. Arellano, L. M., & McNeill, B. W. (Eds.). (2004). *The handbook of Chicana/o psychology and mental health.* Mahwah, NJ: Routledge

Villarruel, F. A., Carlo, G., Grau, J. A., Azmitia, M., Cabrera, N. J., & Chahin, T. J. (Eds.). (2009). *Handbook of U.S. Latino psychology: Developmental and community-based perspectives.* Thousand Oaks, CA: Sage.

RELATED RESOURCES

American Psychological Association. (2012). *Crossroads: The psychology of immigration in the new century.* Washington, DC: Author.

Bernal, G., & Domenech Rodríguez, M. M. (Eds.). (2011). *Cultural adaptations: Tools for evidence-based practice with diverse populations.* Washington, DC: American Psychological Association.

Bryant-Davis, T., Austria, A. M., Kawahara, D. M., & Willis, D. J. (Eds.). (2014). *Religion and spirituality for diverse women. Foundations of strength and resilience.* Santa Barbara, CA: Praeger.

Bryant-Davis, T., & Comas-Díaz, L. (Eds.). (2016). *Womanist and mujerista psychologies: Voices of fire, acts of courage.* Washington, DC: American Psychological Association.

Comas-Díaz, L. (2011). *Multicultural care: A clinician's guide to cultural competence.* Washington, DC: American Psychological Association.

Comas-Díaz, L., & Greene, B. (Eds.). (2013). *Psychological health of women of color: Intersections, challenges, and opportunities.* New York: Praeger.

Englar-Carlson, M., & Stevens, M. A (Eds.). (2006). *In the room with men: A casebook of therapeutic change.* Washington, DC: American Psychological Association.

Gallardo, M. E., & McNeill, B. W. (Eds.). (2009). *Intersections of multiple identities: A casebook of evidence-based practices with diverse populations.* New York: Routledge.

Gallardo, M. E., Yeh, C. A., Trimble, J. E., & Parham, T. A. (Eds.). (2012). *Culturally adaptive counseling skills: Demonstrations of evidence-based practices* (pp. 77–112). Thousand Oaks, CA: Sage.

Geisinger, K. F. (Ed.). (2015). *Psychological testing of Hispanics: Clinical, cultural, and intellectual issues* (2nd ed.). Washington, DC: American Psychological Association.

Hays, P. A., & Iwamasa G. Y. (2006). *Culturally responsive cognitive-behavioral therapy: Assessment, practice and supervision.* Washington, DC: American Psychological Association.

Huff, R. M., Kline, M. V., & Peterson, D. V. (Eds.). (2014). *Health promotion in multicultural populations: A handbook for practitioners and students.* Thousand Oaks, CA: Sage.

Miville, M. L. (Ed.). (2013). *Multicultural gender roles: Applications for mental health and education.* Hoboken, NJ: Wiley.

Paniagua, F. A., & Yamada, A. (Ed.). (2013). *Handbook of multicultural mental health: Assessment and treatment of diverse populations* (2nd ed.). San Diego: Academic Press.

Satcher, D., & Paimies, R. J. *Multicultural medicine and health disparities.* New York: McGraw Hill.

Sue, D. W., & Sue, D. (2015). *Counseling the culturally diverse: Theory and practice* (7th ed.). Hoboken, NJ: Wiley.

Sutherland, P., Moodley, R., & Chevannes (Eds.). (2014). *Caribbean healing traditions: Implications for health and mental health.* New York: Routledge.

References

Abraído-Lanza, A. F., Armbrister, A. N., Flórez, K. R., & Aguirre, A. N. (2006). Toward a theory-driven model of acculturation in public health research. *American Journal of Public Health, 96*(8), 1342–1346.

Abraido-Lanza, A. F., Dohrenwend, B. P., Ng-Mak, D. S., & Turner, J. B. (1999). The Latino mortality paradox: A test of the "salmon bias" and healthy migrant hypotheses. *American Journal of Public Health, 89*(10), 1543–1548.

Abraido-Lanza, A. F., Echeverria, S. E., & Florez, K. R. (2016). Latino immigrants, acculturation, and health: Promising new directions in research. *Annual Reviews in Public Health, 37*, 219–236. doi:10.1146/annurev-publhealth -032315-021545

Abraído-Lanza, A. F., Vásquez, E., & Echeverría, S. E. (2004). En las manos de Dios [in God's hands]: Religious and other forms of coping among Latinos with arthritis. *Journal of Consulting and Clinical Psychology, 72*(1), 91.

Acevedo, V. (2008). Cultural competence in a group. *Health and Social Work, 33*(2), 111–120.

Acevedo-Garcia, D., Soobader, M.-J., & Berkman, L. F. (2007). Low birthweight among US Hispanic/Latino subgroups: The effect of maternal foreign-born status and education. *Social Science & Medicine, 65*(12), 2503–2516.

Adames, H. Y., & Chavez-Dueñas, N. Y. (Eds.). (2017). *Cultural foundations and interventions in Latino/a mental health: History, theory and within group differences*. New York: Routledge.

Adler, N. E., Epel, E. S., Castellazzo, G., & Ickovics, J. R. (2000). Relationship of subjective and objective social status with psychological and physiological functioning: Preliminary data in healthy, White women. *Health Psychology, 19*(6), 586.

Aguilar-Gaxiola, S. A., Kramer, E. J., Resendez, C., & Magaña, C. G. (2008). The context of depression in Latinos in the United States. In S. A. Aguilar-Gaxiola & T. P. Gullota (Eds.), *Depression in Latinos: Assessment, treatment, and prevention* (pp. 29–52). New York: Springer.

Aguilar-Gaxiola, S. A., Loera, G., Mendez, L., Sala, M., & Nakamoto, J. (2012). *Community-defined solutions for Latino mental health care disparities: California reducing disparities project, Latino Strategic Planning Workgroup Population Report*. Sacramento, CA: UC Davis.

Aguilar-Gaxiola, S. A., Zelezny, L., Garcia, B., Edmondson, C., Alejo-Garcia, C., & Vega, W. A. (2002). Translating research into action: Reducing disparities in mental health care for Mexican Americans. *Psychiatric Services, 53*, 1563–1568. doi:10.1176/appi.ps.53.12.1563

Ai, A. L., Aisenberg, E., Weiss, S. I., & Salazar, D. (2014). Racial/ethnic identity and subjective physical and mental health of Latino Americans: An asset within? *American Journal of Community Psychology, 53*(1–2), 173–184.

Aklin, W. M., & Turner, S. M. (2006). Toward understanding ethnic and cultural factors in the interviewing process. *Psychotherapy: Theory, Research, Practice, Training, 43*, 50–64. doi:10.1037/0033-3204.43.1.50

Alcalá, H. E., Chen, J., Langellier, B. A., Roby, D. H., & Ortega, A. N. (2017). Impact of the Affordable Care Act on health care access and utilization among Latinos. *Journal of the American Board of Family Medicine, 30*(1), 52–62.

Alcoff, L. M. (2005). Latino vs. Hispanic: The politics of ethnic names. *Philosophy & Social Criticism, 31*(4), 395–407.

Alegría, M., Canino, G., Ríos, R., Vera, M., Calderón, J., Rusch, D., & Ortega, A. N. (2002). Mental health care for Latinos: Inequalities in use of specialty mental health services among Latinos, African Americans, and non-Latino Whites. *Psychiatric Services, 53*(12), 1547–1555.

Alegría, M., Canino, G., Shrout, P. E., Woo, M., Duan, N., Vila, D., . . . & Meng, X.-L. (2008). Prevalence of mental illness in immigrant and non-immigrant US Latino groups. *American Journal of Psychiatry, 165*(3), 359–369.

Alegría, M., Canino, G. Stinson, F. S., & Grant, B. F. (2006). Nativity and DSM-IV psychiatric disorders among Puerto Ricans, Cuban Americans, and non-Latino whites in the United States: Results from the National Epidemiologic Survey on Alcohol and Related Conditions. *Journal of Clinical Psychiatry, 67*, 56–65.

Alegría, M., Chatterji, P., Wells, K., Cao, Z., Chen, C.-N., Takeuchi, D., . . . & Meng, X.-L. (2008). Disparity in depression treatment among racial and ethnic minority populations in the United States. *Psychiatric Services, 59*(11), 1264–1272.

Alegría, M., Mulvaney-Day, N., Torres, M., Gao, S., Oddo, V., & Woo, M. (2007a). Correlates of past-year mental health service use among Latinos: Results from the National Latino and Asian American Study. *American Journal of Public Health, 97*, 76–83.

Alegría, M., Mulvaney-Day, N., Torres, M., & Polo, A. (2007b). Prevalence of psychiatric disorders across Latino subgroups in the United States. *American Journal of Public Health, 97*, 68–75.

Alegría, M., Mulvaney-Day, N., Woo, M., & Viruell-Fuentes, E. A. (2012). Psychology of Latino adults: Challenges and an agenda for action. In E. Chang & C. A. Downey (Eds.), *Handbook of race and development in mental health* (pp. 279–306). New York: Springer.

Alegría, M., Shrout, P. E., Wood, M., Guarnaccia, P., Sribney, W., Vil, D., . . . & Canino, G. (2007c). Understanding differences in past year psychiatric disorders for Latinos living in the US. *Social Science & Medicine, 65*, 214–230.

Alegría, M., Sribney, W., Woo, M., Torres, M., & Guarnaccia, P. (2007d). Looking beyond nativity: The relation of age of immigration, length of residence, and birth cohorts to the risk of onset of psychiatric disorders for Latinos. *Research in Human Development, 4*, 19–47. doi:10.1080/15427600701480980

Alegría, M., Takeuchi, D., Canino, G., Duan, N., Shrout, P., Meng, X. L., . . . & Woo, M. (2004). Considering context, place and culture: The National Latino and Asian American Study. *International Journal of Methods in Psychiatric Research, 13*, 208–220.

Alegría, M., & Woo, M. (2009). Conceptual issues in Latino mental health. In F. A. Villarruel, G. Carlo, J. M. Grau, M. Azmitia, N. J. Cabrera, & T. J. Chahin (Eds.), *Handbook of U.S. Latino psychology: Developmental and community-based perspectives* (pp. 15–30). Thousand Oaks, CA: Sage.

Alegría, M., Woo, M., Cao, Z., Torres, M., Meng, X., & Striegel-Moore, R. (2007e). Prevalence and correlates of eating disorders in Latinos in the United States. *International Journal of Eating Disorders, 40*, S15–S21. doi:10.1002/eat.20406

Allen, B., Cisneros, E. M., & Tellez, A. (2015). The children left behind: The impact of parental deportation on mental health. *Journal of Child and Family Studies, 24*(2), 386–392.

Allen, J., Leyva, B., Torres, M. I., Ospino, H., Tom, L., Rustan, S., & Bartholomew, A. (2012). Religious beliefs and cancer screening behaviors among Catholic Latinos: Implications for faith-based interventions. *Journal of Health Care for the Poor & Underserved, 25*(2), 503–526.

Allen, J. D., Pérez, J. E., Tom, L., Leyva, B., Diaz, D., & Torres, M. I. (2014). A pilot test of a church-based intervention to promote multiple cancer-screening behaviors among Latinas. *Journal of Cancer Education, 29*(1), 136–143.

Allison, M. A., Budoff, M. J., Wong, N. D., Blumenthal, R. S., Schreiner, P. J., & Criqui, M. H. (2008). Prevalence of and risk factors for subclinical cardiovascular disease in selected US Hispanic ethnic groups: The multiethnic study of atherosclerosis. *American Journal of Epidemiology, 167*(8), 962–969.

Altman, R., Nunez de Ybarra, J., & Villablanca, A. C. (2014). Community-based cardiovascular disease prevention to reduce cardiometabolic risk in Latina women: A pilot program. *Journal of Women's Health, 23*(4), 350–357.

American Cancer Society. (2015). Cancer facts & figures for Hispanics/Latinos 2015–2017. Atlanta, GA: American Cancer Society.

American Diabetes Association (2017). Diabetes basics. Retrieved from http://www.diabetes.org/diabetes-basics/?loc=db-slabnav

American Psychiatric Association. (2013). *Diagnostic and statistical manual of mental disorders* (5th ed.). Washington, DC: Author.

American Psychological Association. (2003). Guidelines on multicultural education, training, research, practice, and organizational change for psychologists. *American Psychologist, 58*, 377–402.

American Psychological Association. (2012). *Crossroads: The psychology of immigration in the new century*. Report of the APA Presidential Task Force on Immigration. Washington, DC: Author.

Amirehsani, K. A., & Wallace, D. C. (2013). Tes, licuados, and capsulas: Herbal self-care remedies of Latino/Hispanic immigrants for type 2 diabetes. *Diabetes Educator, 39*(6), 828–840. doi:10.1177/0145721713504004

Anderson, R. N., & Smith, B. L. (2003). Death: Leading causes for 2001. *National Vital Statistics Reports, 52*(9), 1–86.

Andrade, F. C., & Viruell-Fuentes, E. A. (2011). Latinos and the changing demographic landscape: Key dimensions for infrastructure building. In L. P. Buki & L. M. Piedra (Eds.), *Creating infrastructures for Latino mental health* (pp. 3–30). New York: Springer.

Andrea, M. D., Daniels, J., & Heck, R. (1991). Evaluating the impact of multicultural counseling training. *Journal of Counseling and Development, 70*(1), 143.

Andrews, A., Jobe-Shields, L., López, C., Metzger, I., de Arellano, M., Saunders, B., & Kilpatrick, D. (2015). Polyvictimization, income, and ethnic differences in trauma-related mental health during adolescence. *Social Psychiatry & Psychiatric Epidemiology, 50*, 1223–1234. doi:10.1007/s00127-015-1077-3

Andrews, T. J., Ybarra, V., & Matthews, L. L. (2013). For the sake of our children: Hispanic immigrant and migrant families' use of folk healing and biomedicine. *Medical Anthropology Quarterly, 27*(3), 385–413. doi:10.1111/maq.12048

Añez, L. M., Paris, M., Jr., Bedregal, L. E., Davidson, L., & Grilo, C. M. (2005). Application of cultural constructs in the care of first generation Latino clients in a community mental health setting. *Journal of Psychiatric Practice, 11*(4), 221–230.

Añez, L. M., Silva, M. A., Paris, M. J., & Bedregal, L. E. (2008). Engaging Latinos through the integration of cultural values and motivational interviewing principles. *Professional Psychology: Research and Practice, 39*, 153–159.

Anzaldúa, G. (2002). Now let us shift . . . the path of conocimiento . . . inner work, public acts. In G. E. Anzaldúa & A. L. Keating (Eds.), *This bridge we call home: Radical visions for transformation* (pp. 540–570). New York: Routledge.

Applewhite, S. L. (1995). Curanderismo: Demystifying the health beliefs and practices of elderly Mexican Americans. *Health & Social Work, 20*, 247–253.

Araújo, B. Y., & Borrell, L. N. (2006). Understanding the link between discrimination, mental health outcomes, and life chances among Latinos. *Hispanic Journal of Behavioral Sciences, 28*(2), 245–266.

Arbona, C., Olvera, N., Rodriguez, N., Hagan, J., Linares, A., & Wiesner, M. (2010). Acculturative stress among documented and undocumented Latino immigrants in the United States. *Hispanic Journal of Behavioral Sciences, 32,* 362–384. doi:10.1177/0739986310373210

Archive of Indigenous Languages of Latin America. (n.d.). The indigenous languages of Latin America. Retrieved from http://www.ailla.utexas.org/site/lg_about .html.

Arcia, E., Castillo, H., & Fernandez, M. C. (2004). Maternal cognitions about distress and anxiety in young Latino children with disruptive behaviors. *Transcultural Psychiatry, 41,* 99–119. doi:10.1177/1363461504041356.

Arciniega, G. M., Anderson, T. C., Tovar-Blank, Z. G., & Tracey, T. J. (2008). Toward a fuller conception of Machismo: Development of a traditional Machismo and Caballerismo Scale. *Journal of Counseling Psychology, 55*(1), 19.

Arellano, L. M., & Ayala-Alcantar, C. (2004). Multiracial feminism for Chicana/o psychology. In R. J. Velasquez, L. M. Arellano, & B. W. Mc Neill (Eds.), *The handbook of Chicana/o psychology and mental health* (pp. 215–230). Mahwah, NJ: Erlbaum.

Arellano-Morales, L., Elder, J. P., Sosa, E. T., Baquero, B., & Alcántara, C. (2016). Health promotion among Latino adults: Conceptual frameworks, relevant pathways, and future directions. *Journal of Latina/o Psychology, 4,* 83–97. doi. org/10.1037/lat0000051

Arellano-Morales, L., Roesch, S. C., Gallo, L. C., Emory, K. T., Molina, K. M., Gonzalez, P., . . . & Deng, Y. (2015). Prevalence and correlates of perceived ethnic discrimination in the Hispanic Community Health Study/Study of Latinos Sociocultural Ancillary Study. *Journal of Latina/o Psychology, 3,* 160–176. doi.org/10.1037/lat0000040

Arredondo, P., Gallardo-Cooper, M., Delgado-Romero, E. A., & Zapata, A. L. (Eds.). (2014). *Culturally responsive counseling with Latinas/os.* Alexandria, VA: American Counseling Association.

Aviera, A. (1996). "Dichos" therapy group: A therapeutic use of Spanish language proverbs with hospitalized Spanish-speaking psychiatric patients. *Cultural Diversity and Mental Health, 2,* 73–87.

Avila, E., & Parker, J. (1999). *Woman who glows in the dark: A curandera reveals traditional Aztec secrets of physical and spiritual health.* New York: Tarcher/Putnam.

Avila, R. M., & Bramlett, M. D. (2013). Language and immigrant status effects on disparities in Hispanic children's health status and access to health care. *Maternal Child Health Journal, 17*(3), 415–423. doi:10.1007/s10995-012 -0988-9

Ayala, G. X., Baquero, B., & Klinger, S. (2008). A systematic review of the relationship between acculturation and diet among Latinos in the United States:

Implications for future research. *Journal of the American Dietetic Association*, *108*, 133–44.

Ayala, G. X., Vaz, L., Earp, J. A., Elder, J. P., & Cherrington, A. (2010). Outcome effectiveness of the lay health advisor model among Latinos in the United States: An examination by role. *Health Education Research*, *25*(5), 815–840.

Ayón, C., & Becerra, D. (2013). Mexican immigrant families under siege: The impact of anti-immigrant policies, discrimination, and the economic crisis. *Advances in Social Work*, *14*, 206–228.

Ayón, C., Peña, V., & Naddy, M. B. G. (2014). Promotoras' efforts to reduce alcohol use among Latino youths: Engaging Latino parents in prevention efforts. *Journal of Ethnic & Cultural Diversity in Social Work*, *23*, 129–147. doi:10.10 80/15313204.2014.903137

Babamoto, K. S., Sey, K. A., Camilleri, A. J., Karlan, V. J., Catalasan, J., & Morisky, D. E. (2009). Improving diabetes care and health measures among Hispanics using community health workers: Results from a randomized controlled trial. *Health Education & Behavior*, *36*(1), 113–126. doi:10.1177/1090198108325911

Baca Zinn, M., & Dill, B. T. (1996). Theorizing difference from multiracial feminism. *Feminist Studies*, *22*, 321–331.

Bacallao, M. L., & Smokowski, P. R. (2009). Entre dos mundos/between two worlds: Bicultural development in context. *Journal of Primary Prevention*, *30*, 421–451. doi:10.1007/s10935-009-0176-x

Baer, R. D., Weller, S. C., de Alba Garcia, J. G., Glazer, M., Trotter, R., Pachter, L., & Klein, R. E. (2003). A cross-cultural approach to the study of the folk illness nervios. *Culture, Medicine and Psychiatry*, *27*, 315–337.

Baez, A., & Hernandez, D. (2001). Complementary spiritual beliefs in the Latino community: The interface with psychotherapy. *American Journal of Orthopsychiatry*, *71*, 408–415.

Baig, A. A., Lockin, C. A., Wiles, A. E., Oborski, D. D., Acevedo, J. C., Gorawara-Bhat, R., . . . & Chin, M. H. (2014). Integrating diabetes self-management interventions for Mexican-Americans into the Catholic church setting. *Journal of Religion and Health*, *53*, 105–118.

Baker, S. P., Braver, E. R., & Chen, L. H. (1998). Motor vehicle occupant deaths among Hispanic and black children and teenagers. *Archives of Pediatric and Adolescent Medicine*, *152*(12), 1209–1212.

Balcazar, A. J., Grineski, S. E., & Collins, T. W. (2015). The Hispanic health paradox across generations: The relationship of child generational status and citizenship with health outcomes. *Public Health*, *129*(6), 691–697.

Balcazar, et al. (2000). Su corazon su vida: manual del promotor y promotora de salud. National Institutes of Health: National Heart, Lung, and Blood Institute, Washington, D.C.

Balcázar, H., Alvarado, M., Fulwood, R., Pedregon, V., & Cantu, F. (2009). A promotora de salud model for addressing cardiovascular disease risk factors in the US-Mexico border region. *Preventing Chronic Disease*, *6*(1), 1–8.

Balcazar, H., Alvarado, M., Hollen, M. L., Gonzalez-Cruz, Y., Hughes, O., Vazquez, E., & Lykens, K. (2006). Salud Para Su Corazon-NCLR: A comprehensive Promotora outreach program to promote heart-healthy behaviors among Hispanics. *Health Promotion Practice, 7*(1), 68–77.

Balcazar, H. G., Byrd, T. L., Ortiz, M., Tondapu, S. R., & Chavez, M. (2009). A randomized community intervention to improve hypertension control among Mexican Americans: Using the promotoras de salud community outreach model. *Journal of Health Care for the Poor & Underserved, 20*(4), 1079–1094.

Balderrama, F. E., & Rodríguez, R. (1995). *Decade of betrayal. Mexican repatriation in the 1930s.* Albuquerque: University of New Mexico Press.

Balfour, P. C., Jr., Ruiz, J. M., Talavera, G. A., Allison, M. A., & Rodriguez, C. J. (2016). Cardiovascular disease in Hispanics/Latinos in the United States. *Journal of Latina/o Psychology, 4*(2), 98–113.

Bámaca-Colbert, M. Y., Plunkett, S. W., & Espinosa-Hernández, G. (2011). Cultural and interpersonal contexts in adolescent depression among Latina females. In N. Cabrera, F. Villarruel, & H. E. Fitzgerald (Eds.), *Latina and Latino children and mental health: Volume 2: Prevention and treatment* (pp. 35–62). Santa Barbara, CA: Praeger.

Banegas, M. P., Leng, M., Graubard, B. I., & Morales, L. S. (2013). The risk of developing invasive breast cancer in Hispanic women. *Cancer, 119*(7), 1373–1380.

Barnes, P. M., Bloom, B., & Nahin, R. L. (2008). *Complementary and alternative medicine use among adults and children: United States, 2007.* Hyattsville, MD: US Department of Health and Human Services, Centers for Disease Control and Prevention, National Center for Health Statistics.

Barnes, P. M., Powell-Griner, E., McFann, K., & Nahin, R. L. (2004). Complementary and alternative medicine use among adults: United States, 2002. *Seminars in Integrative Medicine, 2,* 54–71.

Barranco, R. (2016). Suicide, religion, and Latinos: A macrolevel study of U.S. Latino suicide rates. *Sociological Quarterly, 57,* 256–281. doi:10.1111/tsq .12110

Barrera, M., & Castro, F. (2006). A heuristic framework for the cultural adaptation of interventions. *Clinical Psychology: Science and Practice, 13,* 311–316.

Barrera, M., Castro, F. G., Strycker, L. A., & Toobert, D. J. (2013). Cultural adaptations of behavioral health interventions: A progress report. *Journal of Consulting and Clinical Psychology, 81,* 196–205. doi:10.1037/ a0027085

Barrio, C., Hernández, M., & Barragán, A. (2011). Serving Latino families caring for a person with serious mental illness. In L. P. Buki & L. M. Piedra (Eds.), *Creating infrastructures for Latino mental health* (pp. 159–176). New York: Springer.

Barrio, C., Palinkas, L. A., Yamada, A.-M., Fuentes, D., Criado, V., Garcia, P., & Jeste, D. V. (2008). Unmet needs for mental health services for Latino older adults: Perspectives from consumers, family members, advocates, and service providers. *Community Mental Health Journal, 44*(1), 57–74.

Barrio, C., & Yamada, A. M. (2010). Culturally based intervention development: The case of Latino families dealing with schizophrenia. *Research on Social Work Practice, 20*, 483–492. doi:10.1177/1049731510361613

Battle, J., Pastrana, A., & Daniels, J. (2013). Social Justice Sexuality Survey: The executive summary for the Latina/o population. Retrieved from http://socialjusticesexuality.com/files/2014/09/Latino_ExecutiveSummary_062013.pdf

Bauer, I., & Guerra, J. J. (2014). *Physicians' knowledge and communication about traditional, complementary and alternative medicine use among Latino patients at Kaiser Permanente, Oakland CA.* Retrieved from https://factsreports.revues.org/3221

Baum, J., Jones, R., & Berry, C. (2010). *In the child's best interest? The consequences of losing a lawful immigrant parent to deportation.* Collingdale, PA: Diane Publishing.

Bayles, B., & Katerndahl, D. (2009). Culture-bound syndromes in Hispanic primary care patients. *International Journal of Psychiatry in Medicine, 39*, 15–31. doi:10.2190/PM.39.1.b

Beehler, S., Birman, D., & Campbell, R. (2012). The effectiveness of cultural adjustment and trauma services (CATS): Generating practice-based evidence on a comprehensive, school-based mental health intervention for immigrant youth. *American Journal of Community Psychology, 50*(1–2), 155–168.

Benuto, L. T. (Ed.). (2016). *Guide to psychological assessment with Hispanics.* New York: Springer.

Benuto, L. T., & O'Donohue, W. (2015). Is culturally sensitive cognitive behavioral therapy an empirically supported treatment? The case for Hispanics. *International Journal of Psychology & Psychological Therapy, 15*, 405–421.

Benuto, L. T., & O'Donohue, W. (2016). Integrative care: A potential solution to behavioral health disparities among Latinos. In L. T. Benuto & W. O'Donohue (Eds.), *Enhancing behavioral health in Latino populations: Reducing disparities through integrated behavioral and primary care* (pp. 1–10). New York: Springer.

Berdahl, T. A., & Stone, R. A. T. (2009). Examining Latino differences in mental healthcare use: The roles of acculturation and attitudes towards healthcare. *Community Mental Health Journal, 45*(5), 393–403.

Bernal, G., Bonilla, J., & Bellido, C. (1995). Ecological validity and cultural sensitivity for outcome research: Issues for the cultural adaptation and development of psychosocial treatments with Hispanics. *Journal of Abnormal Child Psychology, 23*, 67–82. doi:10.1007/bf01447045

Bernal, G., Jiménez-Chafey, M. I., & Domenech-Rodríguez, M. M. (2009). Cultural adaptation of treatments: A resource for considering culture in evidence-based practice. *Professional Psychology: Research and Practice, 40*, 361–368.

Bernal, G., & Saéz-Santiago, E. (2006). Culturally centered psychosocial interventions. *Journal of Community Psychology, 34*, 121–132. doi:10.1002/jcop.20096

Berrigan, D., Dodd, K., Troiano, R. P., Reeve, B. B., & Ballard-Barbash, R. (2006). Physical activity and acculturation among adult Hispanics in the United States. *Research Quarterly for Exercise and Sport, 77,* 147–57.

Bersamin, M., Garbers, S., Gold, M. A., Heitel, J., Martin, K., Fisher, D. A., & Santelli, J. (2016). Measuring success: Evaluation designs and approaches to assessing the impact of school-based health centers. *Journal of Adolescent Health, 58*(1), 3–10.

Betancourt, H., & Flynn, P. (2009). The psychology of health: Physical health and the role of culture in behavior. In F. A. Villarruel, G. Carlo, J. M. Grau, M. Azmitia, N. J. Cabrera, & T. J. Chahin (Eds.), *Handbook of U.S. Latino psychology: Developmental and community-based perspectives* (pp. 347–361). Thousand Oaks, CA: Sage.

Betancourt, J. R., Carrillo, J. E., Green, A. R., & Maina, A. (2004). Barriers to health promotion and disease prevention in the Latino population. *Clinical Cornerstone, 6*(3), 16–29.

Bethel, J., & Schenker, M. (2005). Acculturation and smoking patterns among Hispanics: A review. *American Journal of Preventive Medicine, 29,* 143–148.

Bickel, G., Nord, M., Price, C., Hamilton, W., & Cook, J. (2000). *Guide to measuring household food insecurity.* Alexandria, VA: Food and Nutrition Service.

Black, D. S., Lam, C. N., Nguyen, N. T., Ihenacho, U., & Figueiredo, J. C. (2016). Complementary and integrative health practices among Hispanics diagnosed with colorectal cancer: Utilization and communication with physicians. *Journal of Alternative & Complementary Medicine, 22*(6), 473–479. doi:10.1089/acm.2015.0332

Bledsoe, S. E. (2008). Barriers and promoters of mental health services utilization in a Latino context: A literature review and recommendations from an ecosystems perspective. *Journal of Human Behavior in the Social Environment, 18*(2), 151–183.

Bogart, L. M., Derose, K. P., Kanouse, D. E., Grifin, B. A., Haas, A. C., & Williams, M. V. (2015). Correlates of HIV testing among African American and Latino church congregants: The role of HIV stigmatizing attitudes and discussions about HIV. *Journal of Urban Health, 92*(1), 93–107.

Borrell, L. N., & Crawford, N. D. (2009). All-cause mortality among Hispanics in the United States: Exploring heterogeneity by nativity status, country of origin, and race in the National Health Interview Survey–linked mortality files. *Annals of Epidemiology, 19*(5), 336–343.

Bostean, G. (2013). Does selective migration explain the Hispanic paradox? A comparative analysis of Mexicans in the US and Mexico. *Journal of Immigrant and Minority Health, 15*(3), 624–635.

Brabeck, K., & Xu, Q. (2010). The impact of detention and deportation on Latino immigrant children and families: A quantitative exploration. *Hispanic Journal of Behavioral Sciences, 32*(3), 341–361.

Brazil, N. (2017). Spatial variation in the Hispanic paradox: Mortality rates in new and established Hispanic US destinations. *Population, Space, and Health, 23,* 1–17.

Brenner, H., Rothenbacher, D., & Arndt, V. (2009). Epidemiology of stomach cancer. *Cancer Epidemiology: Modifiable Factors, 472,* 467–477.

Brewster, A. B., & Bowen, G. L. (2004). Teacher support and the school engagement of Latino middle and high school students at risk of school failure. *Child & Adolescent Social Work Journal, 21,* 47–67.

Bronfenbrenner, U. (1977). Toward an experimental ecology of human development. *American Psychologist, 32,* 513–531.

Brown, S. A., Garcia, A. A., Kouzekanani, K., & Hanis, C. L. (2002). Culturally competent diabetes self-management education for Mexican Americans. *Diabetes Care, 25*(2), 259–268.

Brownlee, K., Rawana, J., Franks, J., Harper, J., Bajwa, J., O'Brien, E., & Clarkson, A. (2013). A systematic review of strengths and resilience outcome literature relevant to children and adolescents. *Child and Adolescent Social Work Journal, 30*(5), 435–459.

Buki, L. P., & Piedra, L. M. (2011). *Creating infrastructures for Latino mental health.* New York: Springer.

Buki, L. P., Salazar, S. I., & Pitton, V. O. (2009). Design elements for the development of cancer education print materials for a Latina/o audience. *Health Promotion Practice, 10*(4), 564–572.

Burnam, M. A., Hough, R. L., Karno, M., Escobar, J. I., & Telles, C. A. (1987). Acculturation and lifetime prevalence of psychiatric disorders among Mexican Americans in Los Angeles. *Journal of Health and Social Behavior, 21*(1), 89–102.

Burrow-Sánchez, J. J., Minami, T., & Hops, H. (2015). Cultural accommodation of group substance abuse treatment for Latino adolescents: Results of an RCT. *Cultural Diversity & Ethnic Minority Psychology, 21,* 571–583. doi:10.1037/cdp0000023

Bustamante, A. V., Fang, H., Rizzo, J. A., & Ortega, A. N. (2009a). Heterogeneity in health insurance coverage among US Latino adults. *Journal of General Internal Medicine, 24*(Suppl 3), 561–566. doi:10.1007/s11606-009-1069-7

Bustamante, A. V., Fang, H., Rizzo, J. A., & Ortega, A. N. (2009b). Understanding observed and unobserved health care access and utilization disparities among U.S. Latino adults. *Medical Care Research and Review, 66*(5), 561–577.

Cabassa, L. J. (2007). Latino immigrant men's perceptions of depression and attitudes toward help seeking. *Hispanic Journal of Behavioral Sciences, 29*(4), 492–509.

Cabassa, L. J., & Hansen, M. C. (2007). A systematic review of depression treatments in primary care for Latino adults. *Research on Social Work Practice, 17*(4), 494–503.

Cabassa, L. J., Zayas, L. H., & Hansen, M. C. (2006). Latino adults' access to mental health care: A review of epidemiological studies. *Administration and Policy in Mental Health and Mental Health Services Research, 33*, 316–330.

Cahill, S., & Makadon, H. (2014). Sexual orientation and gender identity data collection in clinical settings and in electronic health records: A key to ending LGBT health disparities. *LGBT Health, 1*(1), 34–41.

Caldwell, A., Couture, A., & Nowotny, H. (2008). *Closing the mental health gap: Eliminating disparities in treatment for Latinos.* Kansas City, MO: Mattie Rhodes Center.

Camacho, A., Ng, B., Bejarano, A., Simmons, A., & Chavira, D. (2012). Crisis visits and psychiatric hospitalizations among patients attending a community clinic in rural Southern California. *Community Mental Health Journal, 48*(2), 133–137.

Campinha-Bacote, J. (1999). A model and instrument for addressing cultural competence in health care. *Journal of Nursing Education, 38*(5), 203–207.

Canino, G., & Alegría, M. (2009). Understanding psychopathology among the adult and child Latino population from the United States and Puerto Rico. In F. A. Villarruel, G. Carlo, J. M. Grau, M. Azmitia, N. J. Cabrera, & T. J. Chahin (Eds.), *Handbook of U.S. Latino psychology: Developmental and community-based perspectives* (pp. 31–44). Thousand Oaks, CA: Sage.

Canino, G. J., Bird, H. R., Shrout, P. E., Rubio-Stipec, M., Bravo, M., Martinez, R., . . . & Guevara, L. M. (1987). The prevalence of specific psychiatric disorders in Puerto Rico. *Archives of General Psychiatry, 44*(8), 727–735.

Canino, I. A., & Stolberg, G.C. (2001). Puerto Ricans. In A. G. López & E. Carrillo (Eds.), *The Latino psychiatric patient: Assessment and treatment.* Washington, DC: American Psychiatric Publishing.

Cano, M. Á., Schwartz, S. J., Castillo, L. G., Romero, A. J., Huang, S., Lorenzo-Blanco, E. I., . . . & Szapocznik, J. (2015). Depressive symptoms and externalizing behaviors among Hispanic immigrant adolescents: Examining longitudinal effects of cultural stress. *Journal of Adolescence, 42*, 31–39. doi.org/10.1016/j .adolescence.2015.03.017

Caplan, S., & Cordero, C. (2015). Development of a faith-based mental health literacy program to improve treatment engagement among Caribbean Latinos in the northeastern United States of America. *International Quarterly of Community Health Education, 35*, 199–214. doi:10.1177/0272684X15581347

Capps, R., Castañeda, R. M., Chaudry, A., & Santos, R. (2007). *Paying the price: The impact of immigration raids on America's children.* Retrieved from http:// publications.nclr.org/handle/123456789/1163

Cardemil, E. V., Adams, S. T., Calista, J. L., Connell, J., Encarnacion, J., Esparza, N. K., . . . & Wang, E. (2007). The Latino Mental Health Project: A local mental health needs assessment. *Administration and Policy in Mental Health and Mental Health Services Research, 34*, 331–341. doi:10.1007/s10488-007 -0113-3

Cardemil, E. V., Kim, S., Pinedo, T. M., & Miller, I. W. (2005). Developing a culturally appropriate depression prevention program: The Family Coping Skills Program. *Cultural Diversity and Ethnic Minority Psychology, 11,* 99–112. doi:10.1037/1099-9809.11.2.99

Cardemil, E. V., & Sarmiento, I. A. (2009). Clinical approaches to working with Latino adults. In F. A. Villarruel, G. Carlo, J. M. Grau, M. Azmitia, N. J. Cabrera, & T. J. Chahin (Eds.), *Handbook of U.S. Latino psychology developmental and community-based perspectives* (pp. 329–345). Thousand Oaks, CA: Sage.

Carvajal, S. C., Hanson, C. E., Romero, A. J., & Coyle, K. K. (2002). Behavioural risk factors and protective factors in adolescents: A comparison of Latinos and non-Latino whites. *Ethnicity & Health, 7,* 181–193.

Casas, J. M., Alamilla, S. G., Cabrera, A. P., & Ortega, S. (2015). The browning of the United States from generalizations to specifics: A mental health perspective. In H. Grey & B. N. Hall-Clark (Eds.), *Cultural considerations in Latino American mental health* (pp. 1–30). New York: Oxford University Press.

Castañeda, S. F., Buelna, C., Giacinto, R. E., Gallo, L. C., Sotres-Alvarez, D., Gonzalez, P., . . . & Giachello, A. L. (2016). Cardiovascular disease risk factors and psychological distress among Hispanics/Latinos: The Hispanic Community Health Study/Study of Latinos (HCHS/SOL). *Preventive Medicine, 87,* 144–150.

Castillo, L. G., Perez, F. V., Castillo, R., & Ghosheh, M. R. (2010). Construction and initial validation of the Marianismo Beliefs Scale. *Counseling Psychology Quarterly, 23*(2), 163–175.

Castro, A., & Ruiz, E. (2009). The effects of nurse practitioner cultural competence on Latina patient satisfaction. *Journal of the American Academy of Nurse Practitioners, 21*(5), 278–286. doi:10.1111/j.1745-7599.2009.00406.x

Castro, F. G., Balcazar, H., & Cota, M. (2008). Health promotion in Latino populations. Program planning, development, and evaluation. In M. V. Kine & R. M. Huff (Eds.), *Health promotion in multicultural populations: A handbook for practitioners and students* (2nd ed., pp. 222–258). Thousand Oaks, CA: Sage.

Castro, F. G., Barrera, M., & Holleran Steiker, L. K. (2010). Issues and challenges in the design of culturally adapted evidence-based interventions. *Annual Review of Clinical Psychology, 6,* 213–239. doi:10.1146/annurev-clinpsy-033109-132032.

Castro, F. G., Barrera, M., & Martinez, C. R. (2004). The cultural adaptation of prevention interventions: Resolving tensions between fidelity and fit. *Prevention Science, 5,* 41–45. doi:10.1023/b: prev.0000013980.12412.cd

Castro, F. G., Kellison, J. G., Boyd, S. J., & Kopak, A. (2010). A methodology for conducting integrative mixed methods research and data analyses. *Journal of Mixed Methods Research, 4*(4), 342–360.

Castro, F. G., Stein, J. A., & Bentler, P. M. (2009). Ethnic pride, traditional family values, and acculturation in early cigarette and alcohol use among Latino adolescents. *Journal of Primary Prevention, 30*(3–4), 265–292.

Catalano, R. F., Haggerty, K. P., Hawkins, J. D., & Elgin, J. (2011). Prevention of substance use and substance use disorders: Role of risk and protective factors. In Y. Kaminer & K. C. Winters (Eds.), *Clinical manual of adolescent substance abuse treatment* (pp. 25–63). Arlington, VA: American Psychiatric Publishing.

Cauce, A. M., Domenech-Rodríguez, M., Paradise, M., Cochran, B. N., Shea, J. M., Srebnik, D., & Baydar, N. (2002). Cultural and contextual influences in mental health help seeking: A focus on ethnic minority youth. *Journal of Consulting and Clinical Psychology, 70*(1), 44–55.

Cavazos-Rehg, P. A., Zayas, L. H., & Spitznagel, E. L. (2007). Legal status, emotional well-being and subjective health status of Latino immigrants. *Journal of the National Medical Association, 99*, 1126–1131.

Cavender, A., Gladson, V. G., Cummings, J., & Hammet, M. (2011). Curanderismo in Appalachia: The use of remedios caseros among Latinos in Northeastern Tennessee. *Journal of Appalachian Studies, 17*(1/2), 144–167.

Centers for Disease Control and Prevention (2013). Mental health surveillance among children—United States, 2005–2011. *Morbidity and Mortality Weekly Report (MMWR) Supplement, 62*, 1–35.

Centers for Disease Control and Prevention. (2014a). Summary health statistics: National Health Interview Survey, 2014—Table C-5a. Retrieved from https://ftp.cdc.gov/pub/Health_Statistics/NCHS/NHIS/SHS/2014_SHS _Table_C-5.pdf

Centers for Disease Control and Prevention. (2014b). Summary health statistics: National Health Interview Survey, 2014—Table C-6a. Retrieved from https://ftp.cdc.gov/pub/Health_Statistics/NCHS/NHIS/SHS/2014_SHS_Table _C-6.pdf

Centers for Disease Control and Prevention. (2017). About diabetes. Retrieved from https://www.cdc.gov/diabetes/basics/diabetes.html

Centers for Disease Control and Prevention. (2015a, June). National Health Interview Survey Early Release Program. Health insurance coverage: Early release of estimates from the National Health Interview Survey, 2014. Retrieved from https://www.cdc.gov/nchs/data/nhis/earlyrelease/insur201506.pdf

Centers for Disease Control and Prevention. (2015b). Summary of health statistics tables for U.S. children: National Health Interview Survey, 2014. Table C-5c. Retrieved from http://ftp.cdc.gov/pub/Health_Statistics/NCHS/NHIS /SHS/2014_SHS_Table_C-5.pdf

Centers for Disease Control and Prevention. (2015c). HHS report shows more American children with health coverage. Retrieved from https://www.cdc .gov/nchs/pressroom/02news/release200207.htm

Centers for Disease Control and Prevention. (2017a). About diabetes. Retrieved from https://www.cdc.gov/diabetes/basics/diabetes.html

Centers for Disease Control and Prevention. (2017b). Social determinants of health: Know what affects health. Retrieved from https://www.cdc.gov/socialdetermi nants

Cerezo, A., Morales, A., Quintero, D., & Rothman, S. (2014). Trans migrations: Exploring life at the intersection of transgender identity and immigration. *Psychology of Sexual Orientation and Gender Diversity, 1*(2), 170–180.

Cervantes, J. M. (2008). What is indigenous about being indigenous? The mestizo/o experience. In B. W. McNeill & J. M. Cervantes (Eds.), *Latina/o healing practices. Mestizo and indigenous perspectives* (pp. 3–28). New York: Routledge.

Cervantes, J. M. (2010). Mestizo spirituality: Toward an integrated approach to psychotherapy for Latina/os. *Psychotherapy: Theory, Research & Practice, 47*, 527–539. doi:10.1037/a0022078

Cervantes, J. M., & McNeill, B.W. (2008). Summary and future research and practice. In B. W. McNeill & J. M. Cervantes (Eds.), *Latina/o healing practices. Mestizo and indigenous perspectives* (pp. 303–314). New York: Routledge.

Cervantes, J. M., & Parham, T. A. (2005). Toward a meaningful spirituality for people of color: Lessons for the counseling practitioner. *Cultural Diversity and Ethnic Minority Psychology, 11*, 69–81. doi:10.1037/1099-9809.11.1.69

Cervantes, R., Goldbach, J., & Santos, S. M. (2011). Familia Adelante: A multi-risk prevention intervention for Latino families. *Journal of Primary Prevention, 32*, 225–234. doi:10.1007/s10935-011-0251-y

Chaudry, A., Capps, R., Pedroza, J., Castaneda, R., Santos, R., & Scott, M. (2010). *Facing our future: Children in the aftermath of immigration enforcement.* Washington, DC: The Urban Institute. Retrieved from http://www.urban.org /sites/default/files/publication/28331/412020-Facing-Our-Future.PDF

Chávez, T. A. (2016). Humanistic values in traditional healing practices of curanderismo. *Journal of Humanistic Counseling, 55*(2), 129–135. doi:10.1002/johc .12029

Chavez-Korell, S., Beer, J., Rendón, A. D., Rodriguez, N., Garr, A. D., Pine, C. A., . . . & Malcolm, E. (2012). Improving access and reducing barriers to depression treatment for Latino elders: Un Nuevo Amanecer (A New Dawn). *Professional Psychology: Research & Practice, 43*, 217–226. doi:10.1037/a002 6695

Chirkov, V. (2009). Critical psychology of acculturation: What do we study and how do we study it, when we investigate acculturation? *International Journal of Intercultural Relations, 33*(2), 94–105.

Cho, H., Kim, I., & Velez-Ortiz, D. (2014). Factors associated with mental health service use among Latino and Asian Americans. *Community Mental Health Journal, 50*(8), 960–967.

Cho, H., Velez-Ortiz, D., & Parra-Cardona, J. R. (2014). Prevalence of intimate partner violence and associated risk factors among Latinos/as: An exploratory study with three Latino subpopulations. *Violence against Women, 20*(9), 1041–1058.

Chou, T., Asnaani, A., & Hofmann, S. (2012). Perception of racial discrimination and psychopathology across three U.S. ethnic minority groups. *Cultural Diversity & Ethnic Minority Psychology, 18*, 74–81. doi:10.1037/a0025432

Chung, G. Y., Brown, G., & Gibson, D. (2015). Increasing melanoma screening among Hispanic/Latino Americans: A community-based educational intervention. *Health Education and Behavior, 42*(5), 627–632. doi:10.1177/109019 8115578748

Clair, C., Rigotti, N. A., Porneala, B., Fox, C. S., D'Agostino, R. B., Pencina, M. J., & Meigs, J. B. (2013). Association of smoking cessation and weight change with cardiovascular disease among adults with and without diabetes. *Journal of American Medical Association, 309*(10), 1014–1021.

Clark, L., Bunik, M., & Johnson, S. L. (2010). Research opportunities with curanderos to address childhood overweight in Latino families. *Qualitative Health Research, 20*(1), 4–14. doi:10.1177/1049732309355285

Cochran, S. D., Mays, V. M., Alegría, M., Ortega, A. N., & Takeuchi, D. (2007). Mental health and substance use disorders among Latino and Asian American lesbian, gay, and bisexual adults. *Journal of Consulting and Clinical Psychology, 75*, 785–794.

Coffin-Romig, N. (2015). Ending intimate partner violence among Latinas: Aguantando no mas. *Hispanic Health Care International, 13*(4), 186–196.

Coffman, M. J., Shobe, M. A., & O'Connell, B. (2008). Self-prescription practices in recent Latino immigrants. *Public Health Nursing, 25*(3), 203–211. doi:10 .1111/j.1525-1446.2008.00697.x

Cohn, D., Patten, E., & Lopez, M. H. (2014). *Puerto Rican population declines on island, grows on US mainland.* Washington, DC: Pew Research Center.

Cokkinides, V. E., Bandi, P., Siegel, R. L., & Jemal, A. (2012). Cancer-related risk factors and preventive measures in US Hispanics/Latinos. *CA: A Cancer Journal for Clinicians, 62*(6), 353–363.

Colby, S. L., & Ortman, J. M. (2015). *Projections of the size and composition of the U.S. population: 2014 to 2060, Current Population Reports, P25-1143.* Washington, DC: U.S. Census Bureau.

Comas-Díaz, L. (1981). Puerto Rican espiritismo and psychotherapy. *American Journal of Orthopsychiatry, 51*, 636–645. doi:10.1111/j.1939-0025.1981 .tb01410.x

Comas-Díaz, L. (1997). Mental health needs of Latinos with professional status. In J. M. Garcia & M. C. Zea (Eds.), *Psychological interventions and research with Latino populations* (pp. 142–165). Needham Heights, MA: Allyn & Bacon.

Comas-Díaz, L. (2006). Latino healing: The integration of ethnic psychology into psychotherapy. *Psychotherapy: Theory, Research, Practice, Training, 43*, 436–453. doi:10.1037/0033-3204.43.4.436

Comas-Díaz, L. (2008). Spirita: Reclaiming womanist sacredness into feminism. *Psychology of Women Quarterly, 32*, 13–21. doi.org/10.1111/ j.1471-6402 .2007.00403.x

Comas-Díaz, L. (2012a). Colored spirituality: The centrality of spirit among ethnic minorities. In L. J. Miller (Ed.), *The Oxford handbook of psychology and spirituality* (pp. 197–206). New York: Oxford University Press.

Comas-Díaz, L. (2012b). Humanism and multiculturalism: An evolutionary alliance. *Psychotherapy, 49,* 437–441. doi:10.1037/a0027126

Comas-Díaz, L. (2012c). *Multicultural care: A clinician's guide to cultural competence.* Washington, DC: American Psychological Association.

Comas-Díaz, L. (2013). Comadres: The healing power of a female bond. *Women & Therapy, 36,* 62–75. doi:10.1080/02703149.2012.720213

Comas-Díaz, L. (2014). La diosa: Syncretistic folk spirituality among Latinas. In T. Bryant-Davis, A. M. Austria, D. M. Kawahara, & D. J. Willis (Eds.), *Religion and spirituality for diverse women: Foundations of strength and resilience* (pp. 215–234). Santa Barbara, CA: Praeger.

Comas-Díaz, L. (2016). In T. Bryant-Davis & L. Comas-Díaz. L. (Eds.), *Womanist and mujerista psychologies: Voices of fire, acts of courage* (pp. 149–169). Washington, DC: American Psychological Association.

Constantine, M. G., Myers, L. J., Kindaichi, M., & Moore, J. L. (2004). Exploring indigenous mental health practices: The roles of healers and helpers in promoting well-being in people of color. *Counseling and Values, 48,* 110–125. doi:10.1002/j.2161-007X.2004.tb00238.x

Cook, B., Alegría, M., Lin, J. Y., & Guo, J. (2009). Pathways and correlates connecting Latinos' mental health with exposure to the United States. *American Journal of Public Health, 99,* 2247–2254.

Cook, B. L., McGuire, T., & Miranda, J. (2007). Measuring trends in mental health care disparities, 2000–2004. *Psychiatric Services, 58,* 1533–1540.

Corona, R., Rodríguez, V. M., McDonald, S. E., Velazquez, E., Rodríguez, A., & Fuentes, V. E. (2017). Associations between cultural stressors, cultural values, and Latina/o college students' mental health. *Journal of Youth and Adolescence, 46,* 63–77. doi:10.1007/s10964-016-0600-5

Coronado, G. D., Golovaty, I., Longton, G., Levy, L., & Jimenez, R. (2011). Effectiveness of a clinic-based colorectal cancer screening promotion program for underserved Hispanics. *Cancer, 117*(8), 1745–1754. doi:10.1002/cncr.25730

Costantino, G., Malgady, R. G., & Primavera, L. H. (2009). Congruence between culturally competent treatment and cultural needs of older Latinos. *Journal of Consulting & Clinical Psychology, 77,* 941–949.

Costantino, G., Malgady, R. G., & Rogler, L. H. (1986). Cuento therapy: A culturally sensitive modality for Puerto Rican children. *Journal of Consulting and Clinical Psychology, 54,* 639–645.

Coughlin, S. S., Richards, T. B., Nasseri, K., Weiss, N. S., Wiggins, C. L., Saraiya, M., et al. (2008). Cervical cancer incidence in the United States in the US-Mexico border region, 1998–2003. *Cancer, 113*(Suppl 10), 2964–2973.

Cross, T. L., Bazron, B. J., Dennis, K. W., & Isaacs, M. R. (1989). *Toward a culturally competent system of care: A monograph on effective services for minority children who are severely emotionally disturbed.* Washington, DC: Georgetown University Child Development Center. Retrieved from http://files.eric.ed.gov/fulltext/ED330171.pdf

Crowley, M., & Lichter, D. T. (2009). Social disorganization in new Latino destinations? *Rural Sociology, 74,* 573–604. doi:10.1111/j.1549-0831.2009.tb00705.x

Daniel, M. (2010). Strategies for targeting health care disparities among Hispanics. *Family & Community Health, 33,* 329–342.

Daviglus, M. L., Pirzada, A., Durazo-Arvizu, R., Chen, J., Allison, M., Avilés-Santa, L., . . . & Schneiderman, N. (2016). Prevalence of low cardiovascular risk profile among diverse Hispanic/Latino adults in the United States by age, sex, and level of acculturation: The Hispanic Community Health Study/Study of Latinos. *Journal of the American Heart Association, 5*(8), e003929.

Daviglus, M. L., Pirzada, A., & Talavera, G. A. (2014). Cardiovascular disease risk factors in the Hispanic/Latino population: Lessons from the Hispanic Community Health Study/Study of Latinos (HCHS/SOL). *Progress in Cardiovascular Diseases, 57*(3), 230–236.

Daviglus, M. L., Talavera, G. A., Avilés-Santa, M. L., Allison, M., Cai, J., Criqui, M. H., . . . & Kaplan, R. C. (2012). Prevalence of major cardiovascular risk factors and cardiovascular diseases among Hispanic/Latino individuals of diverse backgrounds in the United States. *Journal of American Medical Association, 308*(17), 1775–1784.

de Heer, H. D., Balcazar, H. G., Wise, S., Redelfs, A. H., Rosenthal, E. L., & Duarte, M. O. (2015). Improved cardiovascular risk among Hispanic border participants of the Mi Corazón Mi Comunidad Promotores De Salud Model: The HEART II Cohort Intervention Study 2009–2013. *Frontiers in Public Health, 3,* 149.

De Jesus, M., & Xiao, C. (2014). Predicting health care utilization among Latinos: Health locus of control beliefs or access factors? *Health Education and Behavior, 41*(4), 423–430. doi:10.1177/1090198114529130

De la Cancela, V., Guarnaccia, P. J., & Carrillo, E. (1986). Psychosocial distress among Latinos: A critical analysis of ataques de nervios. *Humanity and Society, 10*(4), 431–447.

DeHaven, M. J., Hunter, I. B., Wilder, L., Walton, J. W., & Berry, J. (2004). Health programs in faith-based organizations: Are they effective? *American Journal of Public Health, 94*(6), 1030–1036.

Delgado, M., & Humm-Delgado, D. (1982). Natural support systems: Source of strength in Hispanic communities. *Social Work, 27,* 83–89.

Delgado-Romero, E. A., Espino, M. M., Werther, E., & González, M. J. (2011). Building infrastructure through training and interdisciplinary collaboration. In L. P. Buki & L. M. Piedra (Eds.), *Creating infrastructures for Latino mental health* (pp. 99–116). New York: Springer.

Delgado-Romero, E. A., Galván, N., Hunter, M. R., Torres, V., & McAuliffe, G. (2008). Latino/Latina Americans. In G. McAuliffe (Ed.), *Culturally alert counseling: A comprehensive introduction* (pp. 323–352). Thousand Oaks, CA: Sage.

Derose, K. P., Kanouse, D. E., Bogart, L. M., Griffin, B. A., Haas, A., Stucky, B. D., . . . & Flórez, K. R. (2016). Predictors of HIV-related stigmas among African

American and Latino religious congregants. *Cultural Diversity and Ethnic Minority Psychology, 22*(2), 185–195.

Dettlaff, A. J., & Rycraft, J. R. (2009). Culturally competent systems of care with Latino children and families. *Child Welfare, 88*(6), 109–126.

Diaz, J., Roberts, M., Clarke, J., Simmons, E., Goldman, R., & Rakowski, W. (2013). Colorectal cancer screening: Language is a greater barrier for Latino men than Latino women. *Journal of Immigrant and Minority Health/Center for Minority Public Health, 15,* 472–475. doi:10.1007/s10903-012-9667-6

Diaz, M. A., Miville, M. L., & Gil, N. (2013). Latino male gender roles. In M. L. Miville (Ed.), *Multicultural gender roles: Applications for mental health and education* (pp. 97–132). Hoboken, NJ: Wiley.

Diaz, R. M., Ayala, G., Bein, E., Henne, J., & Marin, B. V. (2001). The impact of homophobia, poverty, and racism on the mental health of gay and bisexual Latino men: Findings from 3 US cities. *American Journal of Public Health, 91*(6), 927–932.

Díaz-Lázaro, C. M., Verdinelli, S., & Cohen, B. B. (2012). Empowerment feminist therapy with Latina immigrants: Honoring the complexity and socio-cultural contexts of clients' lives. *Women & Therapy, 35,* 80–92. doi:10.1080/02703149.2012.634730

Dietz, W. H. (1998). Health consequences of obesity in youth: Childhood predictors of adult disease. *Pediatrics, 101*(Suppl 2), 518–525.

Dixon, L. B., Sundquist, J., & Winkleby, M. (2000). Differences in energy, nutrient, and food intakes in a US sample of Mexican-American women and men: Findings from the Third National Health and Nutrition Examination Survey, 1988–1994. *American Journal of Epidemiology, 152*(6), 548–557.

Domenech Rodríguez, M. M., Baumann, A., & Schwartz, A. (2011). Cultural adaptation of an empirically supported intervention: From theory to practice in a Latino/a community context. *American Journal of Community Psychology, 47,* 170–186.

Domenech Rodríguez, M. M., & Bernal, G. (2012). Frameworks, models, and guidelines for cultural adaptation. In G. Bernal & M. M. Domenech Rodríguez (Eds.), *Cultural adaptations: Tools for evidence-based practice with diverse populations* (pp. 23–44). Washington, DC: American Psychological Association.

Domenech Rodríguez, M. M., & Weiling, E. (2004). Developing culturally appropriate, evidence-based treatments for interventions with ethnic minority populations. In M. Rastogin & E. Weiling (Eds.), *Voices of color: First person accounts of ethnic minority therapists* (pp. 313–333). Thousand Oaks, CA: Sage.

Dominguez, K., Penman-Aguilar, A., Chang, M.-H., Moonesinghe, R., Castellanos, T., Rodriguez-Lainz, A., & Schieber, R. (2015). Vital signs: Leading causes of death, prevalence of diseases and risk factors, and use of health services among Hispanics in the United States—2009–2013. *MMWR: Morbidity and Mortality Weekly Report, 64*(17), 469–478.

Donlan, W., & Lee, J. (2010). Screening for depression among indigenous Mexican migrant farmworkers using the patient health questionnaire–9. *Psychological Reports, 106*, 419–432. doi:10.2466/pr0.106.2.419-432

Dreby, J. (2012). The burden of deportation on children in Mexican immigrant families. *Journal of Marriage and Family, 74*, 829–845.

Dunn, M. G., & O'Brien, K. M. (2009). Psychological health and meaning in life: Stress, social support, and religious coping in Latina/Latino immigrants. *Hispanic Journal of Behavioral Sciences, 31*, 204–227.

Dupree, L. W., Herrera, J. R., Tyson, D. M., Jang, Y., & King-Kallimanis, B. L. (2010). Age group differences in mental health care preferences and barriers among Latinos. *Best Practices in Mental Health, 6*, 47–59.

Durà-Vilà, G., & Hodes, M. (2012). Cross-cultural study of idioms of distress among Spanish nationals and Hispanic American migrants: Susto, nervios and ataque de nervios. *Social Psychiatry and Psychiatric Epidemiology, 47*, 1627–1637.

Eamranond, P. P., Legedza, A. T., Diez-Roux, A. V., Kandula, N. R., Palmas, W., Siscovick, D. S., & Mukamal, K. J. (2009). Association between language and risk factor levels among Hispanic adults with hypertension, hypercholesterolemia, or diabetes. *American Heart Journal, 157*(1), 53–59.

Echeverry, J. L. (1997). Treatment barriers: Accessing and accepting professional help. In J. G. Garcia & M. C. Zea (Eds.), *Psychological interventions and research with Latino populations* (pp. 94–107). Boston: Allyn and Bacon.

Eggerth, D., DeLaney, S., Flynn, M., & Jacobson, C. (2012). Work experiences of Latina immigrants: A qualitative study. *Journal of Career Development, 39*, 13–30. doi:10.1177/0894845311417130

Elder, J. P., Ayala, G. X., Parra-Medina, D., & Talavera, G. A. (2009). Health communication in the Latino community: Issues and approaches. *Annual Review of Public Health, 30*, 227–251. doi:10.1146/annurev.publhealth.031308 .100300

Ell, K., Aranda, M., Wu, S., Oh, H., Lee, P., & Guterman, J. (2017). Promotora assisted depression and self-care management among predominantly Latinos with concurrent chronic illness: Safety net care system clinical trial results. *Contemporary Clinical Trials, 61*, 1–9. doi:10.1016/j.cct.2017.07.001

Engstrom, D. W., & Piedra, L. M. (2005). Central American survivors of political violence: An examination of contextual factors and practice issues. *Journal of Immigrant & Refugee Services, 3*(1–2), 171–190.

Ennis, S. R., Rios-Vargas, M., & Albert, N. G. (2011). *The Hispanic population: 2010.* Retrieved from https://www.census.gov/prod/cen2010/briefs/c2010br-04.pdf

Enriquez, L. E. (2015). Multigenerational punishment: Shared experiences of undocumented immigration status within mixed-status families. *Journal of Marriage & Family, 77*, 939–953. doi:10.1111/jomf.12196

Epstein, M., & Sharma, J. (1998). *Emotional and Behavioural Rating Scale: A strengths based approach to assessment.* Austin, TX: Pro-Ed.

Erving, C. L. (2017). Physical-psychiatric comorbidity: Implications for health measurement and the Hispanic epidemiological paradox. *Social Science Research, 64,* 197–213.

Eschbach, K., Ostir, G. V., Patel, K. V., Markides, K. S., & Goodwin, J. S. (2004). Neighborhood context and mortality among older Mexican Americans: Is there a barrio advantage? *American Journal of Public Health, 94*(10), 1807–1812.

Espín, O. M. (2012). "An illness we catch from American Women"? The multiple identities of Latina lesbians. *Women & Therapy, 35,* 45–56.

Evans, S., Tsao, J. C. I., & Zelter, L. K. (2008). Complementary and alternative medicine for acute procedural pain in children. *Alternative Therapies in Health and Medicine, 14*(5), 52–56.

Falbe, J., Cadiz, A. A., Tantoco, N. K., Thompson, H. R., & Madsen, K. A. (2015). Active and healthy families: A randomized controlled trial of a culturally tailored obesity intervention for Latino children. *Academic Pediatrics, 15*(4), 386–395.

Falicov, C. J. (1998). *Latino families in therapy: A guide to multicultural practice.* New York: Guilford.

Falicov, C. J. (1999). The value of religion and spirituality in immigrant Latinos. In. T. Walsh (Ed.), *Spirituality and family therapy* (pp. 104–120). New York: Guilford.

Falicov, C. J. (2009a). Commentary: On the wisdom and challenges of culturally attuned treatments for Latinos. *Family Process, 48,* 292–309. doi:10.1111/j.1545-5300.2009.01282.x

Falicov, C. J. (2009b). Religion and spiritual traditions in immigrant families: Significance for Latino health and mental health. In T. Walsh (Ed.), *Spiritual resources in family therapy* (2nd ed., pp. 156–173). New York: Guilford.

Falicov, C. J. (2014). *Latino families in therapy: A guide to multicultural practices* (2nd ed.). New York: Guilford.

Fallon, A., & Bauza, P. (2015). Latino gender roles. In S. Akhtar & S. M. Bertoglia (Eds.), *The American Latino: Psychodynamic perspectives on culture and mental health* (pp. 63–82). Lanham, MD: Rowman & Littlefield.

Faulkner, S. L. (2003). Good girl or flirt girl: Latinas' definitions of sex and sexual relationships. *Hispanic Journal of Behavioral Sciences, 25,* 174–200. doi:10.1177/0739986303025002003

Federico, S. G., Abrams, L., Everhart, R. M., Melinkovich, P., & Hambidge, S. J. (2010). Addressing adolescent immunization disparities: A retrospective analysis of school-based health center immunization delivery. *American Journal of Public Health, 100*(9), 1630–1634.

Feldmann, J. M., Wiemann, C. M., Sever, L., & Hergenroeder, A. C. (2008). Folk and traditional medicine use by a subset of Hispanic adolescents. *International Journal of Adolescent Medicine and Health, 20*(1), 41–51.

Fernández-Esquer, M. E., Agoff, M. C., & Leal, I. M. (2017). Living sin papeles: Undocumented Latino workers negotiating life in "Illegality." *Hispanic Journal of Behavioral Sciences, 39*(1), 3–18.

Fernandez, O. M., Murphy, J. M., & Paravisini-Gebert, L. (2011). *Religion, race, & ethnicity: Creole religions of the Caribbean: An introduction from vodou and santeria to obeah and espiritismo* (2nd ed.). New York: New York University Press.

Findley, S. E., Irigoyen, M., Schulman, A. (1999). Children on the move and vaccination coverage in a low-income, urban Latino population. *American Journal of Public Health, 89*(11), 1728–1731.

Flores, G., Abreu, M., & Tomany-Korman, S. C. (2006). Why are Latinos the most uninsured racial/ethnic group of US children? A community-based study of risk factors for and consequences of being an uninsured Latino child. *Pediatrics, 118*(3), e730–e740.

Flores, G., Fuentes-Afflick, E., Barbot, O., Carter-Pokras, O., Claudio, L., Lara, M., . . . & Mendoza, F. (2002). The health of Latino children: Urgent priorities, unanswered questions, and a research agenda. *Journal of the American Medical Association, 288*(1), 82–90.

Flores, Y. G. (2013). *Chicana and Chicano mental health: Alma, mente y corazón.* Tucson: University of Arizona Press.

Flores-Ortiz, Y. G. (2004). Domestic violence in Chicana/o families. In R. Velásquez, L. Arellano, & B. W. McNeill (Eds.), *The handbook of Chicana/o psychology and mental health* (pp. 267–284). Mahwah, NJ: Erlbaum.

Folsom, D. P., Gilmer, T., Barrio, C., Moore, D. J., Bucardo, J., Lindamer, L. A., . . . & Patterson, T. (2007). A longitudinal study of the use of mental health services by persons with serious mental illness: Do Spanish-speaking Latinos differ from English-speaking Latinos and Caucasians? *American Journal of Psychiatry, 164*(8), 1173–1180.

Fonseca-Becker, F., Perez-Patron, M. J., Munoz, B., O'Leary, M., Rosario, E., & West, S. K. (2010). Health competence as predictor of access to care among Latinos in Baltimore. *Journal of Immigrant & Minority Health, 12*(3), 354–360. doi:10.1007/s10903-007-9101-7

Fortier, M. A., Gillis, S., Gomez, S. H., Wang, S. M., Tan, E. T., & Kain, Z. N. (2014). Attitudes toward and use of complementary and alternative medicine among Hispanic and White mothers. *Alternative Therapies in Health and Medicine, 20*(1), 13–19.

Fortuna, L. R., Perez, D. J., Canino, G., Sribney, W., & Alegría, M. (2007). Prevalence and correlates of lifetime suicidal ideation and attempts among Latino subgroups in the United States. *Journal of Clinical Psychiatry, 68*, 572–581.

Foxen, P. (2016). *Mental health services for Latino youth: Bridging culture and evidence.* Washington, DC: National Council of La Raza.

Freeman, H. P. (2004). A model patient navigation program: Breaking down barriers to ensure that all individuals with cancer receive timely diagnosis and treatment. *Oncology Issues, 19*(5), 44–46

Friedmann, P. D., D'Aunno, T. A., Jin, L., & Alexander, J. A. (2000). Medical and psychosocial services in drug abuse treatment: Do stronger linkages promote client utilization? *Health Services Research, 35*(2), 443.

Fry, R. (2014). Latino youth finishing college: The role of selective pathways. Washington, DC: Pew Hispanic Center. Retrieved from http://www.pewhispanic .org/2004/06/23/latino-youth-finishing-college/

Fung, M. P., & Fox, R. A. (2014). The culturally-adapted Early Pathways program for young Latino children in poverty: A randomized controlled trial. *Journal of Latina/o Psychology, 2*, 131–145. doi:10.1037/lat0000019

Furness, B. W., Simon, P. A., Wold, C. M., & Asarian-Anderson, J. (2004). Prevalence and predictors of food insecurity among low-income households in Los Angeles County. *Public Health Nutrition, 7*(6), 791–794.

Fussell, E. (2011). The deportation threat dynamic and victimization of Latino immigrants: Wage theft and robbery. *Sociological Quarterly, 52*, 593–615. doi:10.1111/j.1533–8525.2011.01221.x

Galarraga, J. (2007). *Hispanic-American culture and health.* Cleveland, OH: Case Western Reserve University.

Gallardo, M. E. (2012). Therapists as cultural architects and systemic advocates: Latina/o skills identification stage model. In M. E. Gallardo, C. J. Yeh, J. E. Trimble, & T. A. Parham (Eds.), *Culturally adaptive counseling skills: Demonstrations of evidence-based practices* (pp. 77–112). Thousand Oaks, CA: Sage.

Gallo, L. C., Fortmann, A. L., McCurley, J. L., Isasi, C. R., Penedo, F. J., Daviglus, M. L., . . . & Gonzalez, F. II. (2015). Associations of structural and functional social support with diabetes prevalence in US Hispanics/Latinos: Results from the HCHS/SOL Sociocultural Ancillary Study. *Journal of Behavioral Medicine, 38*(1), 160–170.

Gans, K. M., Burkholder, G. J., Upegui, D. I., Risica, P. M., Lasater, T. M., & Fortunet, R. (2002). Comparison of baseline fat-related eating behaviors of Puerto Rican, Dominican, Colombian, and Guatemalan participants who joined a cholesterol education project. *Journal of Nutrition Education and Behavior, 34*(4), 202–210.

Garcia, A. (2013). The facts on immigration today. Retrieved from https://www. americanprogress.org/issues/immigration/reports/2014/10/23/59040/the -facts-on-immigration-today-3/

Garcia-Dominic, O., Wray, L. A., Treviño, R. P., Hernandez, A. E., Yin, Z., & Ulbrecht, J. S. (2010). Identifying barriers that hinder onsite parental involvement in a school-based health promotion program. *Health Promotion Practice, 11*(5), 703–713.

Garza, Y., & Watts, R. (2010). Filial therapy and Hispanic values: Common ground for culturally sensitive helping. *Journal of Counseling & Development, 88*, 108–113. doi:10.1002/j.1556-6678.2010.tb00157.x

Geisinger, K. F. (2015). Introduction. In K. R. Geisinger (Ed.), *Psychological testing of Hispanics. Clinical, cultural, and intellectual issues* (2nd ed., pp. 3–10). Washington, DC: American Psychological Association.

Getrich, C., Sussman, A., Helitzer, D., Hoffman, R., Warner, T., Sánchez, V., . . . & Rhyne, R. (2012). Expressions of machismo in colorectal cancer screening among New Mexico Hispanic subpopulations. *Qualitative Health Research, 22*, 546–546.

Giuliano, A. R., Papenfuss, M., Schneider, A., Nour, M., & Hatch, K. (1999). Risk factors for high-risk type human papillomavirus infection among Mexican-American women. *Cancer Epidemiology and Prevention Biomarkers, 8*(7), 615–620.

Giuntella, O. (2016). The Hispanic health paradox: New evidence from longitudinal data on second and third-generation birth outcomes. *SSM-Population Health, 2*, 84–89.

Glazer, M., Baer, R. D., Weller, S. C., Garcia de Alba, J. E., & Liebowitz, S. W. (2004). Susto and soul loss in Mexicans and Mexican Americans. *Cross-Cultural Research, 38*, 270–288. doi:10.1177/1069397104264277

Gloria, A., & Peregoy, J. J. (1996). Counseling Latino alcohol and other substance users/abusers cultural considerations for counselors. *Journal of Substance Abuse Treatment, 13*, 119–126. doi:10.1016/0740-5472(96)00035-9

Gloria, A., & Segura-Herrera, T. (2004). ¡Somos! Latinas and Latinos in the United States. *Counseling American Minorities, 6*, 279–299.

Glover, N. M., & Blankenship, C. J. (2007). Mexican and Mexican Americans' beliefs about God in relation to disability. *Journal of Rehabilitation, 73*(4), 41.

Goldman, D. P., Smith, J. P., & Sood, N. (2006). Immigrants and the cost of medical care. *Health Affairs, 25*(6), 1700–1711.

Gonzalez-Mercado, V. J., Williams, P. D., Williams, A. R., Pedro, E., & Colon, G. (2017). The symptom experiences of Puerto Rican children undergoing cancer treatments and alleviation practices as reported by their mothers. *International Journal of Nursing Practice, 23*(1).

Gonzales, N. A., Knight, G. P., Morgan-Lopez, A., Saenz, D., & Sirolli, A. (2002). Acculturation and the mental health of Latino youth: An integration and critique of the literature. In J. Contreras, A. Neal-Barnett, & K. Kerns (Eds.), *Latino children and families in the United States: Current research and future directions* (pp. 45–74). Westport, CT: Praeger.

González, H. M., Vega, W. A., Williams, D. R., Tarraf, W., West, B. T., & Neighbors, H. W. (2010). Depression care in the United States: Too little for too few. *Archives of General Psychiatry, 67*, 37–46. doi.org/10.1001/archgenpsychiatry.2009.168

González-Whippler, M. (2002). *Santería: The religion* (2nd ed.). St. Paul, MN: Llewellyn.

Goodkind, J. R., Gonzales, M., Malcoe, L. H., & Espinosa, J. (2008). The Hispanic Women's Social Stressor Scale: Understanding the multiple social stressors of US-and Mexico-born Hispanic women. *Hispanic Journal of Behavioral Sciences, 30*(2), 200–229.

Grad, Y. H., Lipsitch, M., & Aiello, A. E. (2012). Secular trends in Helicobacter pylori seroprevalence in adults in the United States: Evidence for sustained race/ethnic disparities. *American Journal of Epidemiology, 175*(1), 54–59.

Grafford, K. M., Nieto, M. J., & Santanello, C. D. (2016). Perceptions of medicinal plant use amongst the Hispanic population in the St. Louis metropolitan area. *Innovations in Pharmacy, 7*(3), 11.

Grant, B. F. (1996). Prevalence and correlates of drug use and DSM-IV drug dependence in the United States: Results of the National Longitudinal Alcohol Epidemiologic Survey. *Journal of Substance Abuse, 8*(2), 195–210.

Gray, N. G., Mendelsohn, D. M., & Omoto, A. M. (2015). Community connectedness: Challenges, and resilience among gay Latino immigrants. *American Journal of Community Psychology, 55*, 202–214. doi:10.1007/s10464-014-9697-4

Grey, H., & Hall-Clark, B. N. (2015). *Cultural considerations in Latino American mental health.* New York: Oxford University Press.

Guarnaccia, P. J., Canino, G., Rubio-Stipec, M., & Bravo, M. (1993). The prevalence of ataques de nervios in the Puerto Rico Disaster Study: The role of culture in psychiatric epidemiology. *Journal of Nervous and Mental Disease, 181*, 157–165.

Guarnaccia, P. J., Lewis-Fernández, J., & Marano, M. R. (2003). Toward a Puerto Rican popular nosology: Nervios and ataque de nervios. *Culture, Medicine, and Psychiatry, 27*, 339–366. doi:10.1023/A:1025303315932

Guarnaccia, P. J., Lewis-Fernández, R., Martinez Pincay, I., Shrout, P., Guo, J., Torres, M., . . . & Alegria, M. (2010). Ataque de nervios as a marker of social and psychiatric vulnerability: Results from the NLAAS. *International Journal of Social Psychiatry, 56*(3), 298–309.

Guarnaccia, P. J., Martinez, I., & Acosta, H. (2002). *Comprehensive in-depth literature review and analysis of Hispanic mental health issues.* Changing Minds, Advancing Mental Health for Hispanics. Mercerville: New Jersey Mental Health Institute. Retrieved from http://www.nrchmh.org/attachments /litreview.pdf

Guarnaccia, P. J., Martinez, I., & Acosta, H. (2005a). Chapter 2. Mental health in the Hispanic immigrant community. *Journal of Immigrant & Refugee Services, 3*, 21–46.

Guarnaccia, P. J., Martinez, I., Ramirez, R., & Canino, G. (2005b). Are ataques de nervios in Puerto Rican children associated with psychiatric disorder? *Journal of the American Academy of Child & Adolescent Psychiatry, 44*(11), 1184–1192.

Guarnaccia, P. J., Martínez Pincay, I., Alegría, M., Shrout, P. E., Lewis-Fernandez, R., & Canino, G. J. (2007). Assessing diversity among Latinos: Results from the NLAAS. *Hispanic Journal of Behavioral Sciences, 29*(4), 510–534.

Guarnaccia, P. J., Rivera, M., Franco, F., & Neighbors, C. (1996). The experiences of Ataques de nervios: Towards an anthropology of emotions in Puerto Rico. *Culture, Medicine and Psychiatry, 20*(3), 343–367.

Gulbas, L., Zayas, L., Yoon, H., Szlyk, H., Aguilar-Gaxiola, S., & Natera, G. (2016). Deportation experiences and depression among U.S. citizen-children with undocumented Mexican parents. *Child: Care, Health and Development, 42*, 220–230. doi:10.1111/cch.12307

Gutierrez, J., Devia, C., Weiss, L., Chantarat, T., Ruddock, C., Linnell, J., . . . & Calman, N. (2014). Health, community, and spirituality: Evaluation of a multicultural faith-based diabetes prevention program. *Diabetes Educator, 40*(2), 214–222.

Guzmán, M. R., & Carrasco, N. (2011). *Counseling & diversity, Counseling Latino/a Americans.* Belmont, CA: Brooks/Cole.

Haile, R. W., John, E. M., Levine, A. J., Cortessis, V. K., Unger, J. B., Gonzales, M., . . . & Tucker, K. L. (2012). A review of cancer in US Hispanic populations. *Cancer Prevention Research, 5*(2), 150–163.

Hall, H. I., Song, R., Rhodes, P., Prejean, J., An, Q., Lee, L. M., . . . & McKenna, M. T. (2008). Estimation of HIV incidence in the United States. *Journal of the American Medical Association, 300*(5), 520–529.

Harris, M., Velásquez, R. J., White, J., & Renteria, T. (2004). Folk healing and curanderismo within the contemporary Chicana/o community: Current status. In R. Velásquez, L. Arellano, & B. W. McNeill (Eds.), *The handbook of Chicana/o psychology and mental health* (pp. 111–126). Mahwah, NJ: Erlbaum.

Harwood, A. R. (1977). *Rx spiritist as needed: A study of a Puerto Rican community mental health resource.* New York: Wiley.

Hass, G. A., Dutton, M. A., & Orloff, L. E. (2000). Lifetime prevalence of violence against Latina immigrants: Legal and policy implications. *International Review of Victimology, 7*, 93–113. doi:10.1177/026975800000700306

Hayat, M. J., Howlader, N., Reichman, M. E., & Edwards, B. K. (2007). Epidemiology and Population Studies: SEERSeries. *The Oncologist, 12*, 20–37.

Hayes-Bautista, D. E. (2002). The Latino health research agenda. In M. M. Suarez-Orozco & M. M. Paez (Eds.), *Latinos: Remaking America.* Los Angeles: University of California Press.

He, M., Wilmoth, S., Bustos, D., Jones, T., Leeds, J., & Yin, Z. (2013). Latino church leaders' perspectives on childhood obesity prevention. *American Journal of Preventive Medicine, 44*(3), S232–S239.

Heathcote, J. D., West, J. H., Cougar Hall, P., & Trinidad, D. R. (2011). Religiosity and utilization of complementary and alternative medicine among foreign-born Hispanics in the United States. *Hispanic Journal of Behavioral Sciences, 33*(3), 398–408. doi:10.1177/0739986311410019

Hendrickson, B. (2014). Restoring the people: Reclaiming indigenous spirituality in contemporary curanderismo. *Spiritus: A Journal of Christian Spirituality, 14*(1), 76–83. doi:10.1353/scs.2014.0010

Hernandez, M., Nesman, T., Mowery, D., Acevedo-Polakovich, I. D., & Callejas, L. M. (2009). Cultural competence: A literature review and conceptual model for mental health services. *Psychiatric Services, 60*(8), 1046–1050.

Hernandez, M. Y., & Organista, K. C. (2013). Entertainment-Education? A foto-novela? A new strategy to improve depression literacy and help-seeking behaviors in at-risk immigrant Latinas. *American Journal of Community Psychology, 52*, 224–235. doi:10.1007/s10464-013-9587-1

Hernandez-Ramdwar, C. (2014). La regla de ocha (Santeria): Afro-Cuban healing in Cuba and the diaspora. In P. Sutherland, R. Moodley, & B. Chevannes (Eds.), *Caribbean healing traditions. Implications for health and mental health* (pp. 101–112). New York: Routledge.

Higginbotham, J. C., Trevino, F. M., & Ray, L. A. (1990). Utilization of curanderos by Mexican Americans: Prevalence and predictors. Findings from HHANES 1982–84. *American Journal of Public Health, 80*(Suppl), 32–35.

Higgins Neyland, M. K., & Bardone-Cone, A. M. (2016). Tests of escape theory of binge eating among Latinas. *Cultural Diversity and Ethnic Minority Psychology*. Advanced online publication. doi.org/10.1037/cdp0000130

Hill, I., Dubay, L., Kenney, G. M., Howell, E. M., Courtot, B., & Palmer, L. (2008). Improving coverage and access for immigrant Latino children: The Los Angeles Healthy Kids Program. *Health Affairs, 27*(2), 550–559.

Hinojosa, S. (2008). The Mexican American sobador, convergent disease discourse, and pain validation in south Texas. *Human Organization, 67*(2), 194–206.

Ho, D. V., Nguyen, J., Liu, M. A., Nguyen, A. L., & Kilgore, D. B. (2015). Use of and interests in complementary and alternative medicine by Hispanic patients of a community health center. *Journal of the American Board of Family Medicine, 28*(2), 175–183. doi:10.3122/jabfm.2015.02.140210

Holden, K., McGregor, B., Thandi, P., Fresh, E., Sheats, K., Belton, A., ... & Satcher, D. (2014). Toward culturally centered integrative care for addressing mental health disparities among ethnic minorities. *Psychological Services, 11*(4), 357.

Holliday, K. V. (2008). Religious healing and biomedicine in comparative context. In B. W. McNeill & J. M. Cervantes (Eds.), *Latina/o healing practices: Mestizo and indigenous perspectives* (pp. 249–270). New York: Routledge.

Holub, C. K., Lobelo, F., Mehta, S. M., Sánchez Romero, L. M., Arredondo, E. M., & Elder, J. P. (2014). School-wide programs aimed at obesity among Latino youth in the United States: A review of the evidence. *Journal of School Health, 84*(4), 239–246.

Hoogasian, R., & Gloria, A. M. (2015). The healing powers of a patrón espiritual: Latina/o clinicians' understanding and use of spirituality and ceremony in psychotherapy. *Journal of Latina/o Psychology, 3*, 177–192. doi:10.1037/lat0000045

Hoogasian, R., & Lijtmaer, R. (2010). Integrating Curanderismo into counselling and psychotherapy. *Counselling Psychology Quarterly, 23*, 297–307. doi:10.1080/09515070.2010.505752

Horigian, V. E., Anderson, A. R., & Szapocznik, J. (2016). Taking Brief Strategic Family Therapy from bench to trench: Evidence generation across translational phases. *Family Process, 55*, 529–542. doi:10.1111/famp.12233

Horneber, M., Bueschel, G., Dennert, G., Less, D., Ritter, E., & Zwahlen, M. (2012). How many cancer patients use complementary and alternative medicine: A systematic review and metaanalysis. *Integrative Cancer Therapies, 11*(3), 187–203.

Hough, R. L., Hazen, A. L., Soriano, F. I., Wood, P., McCabe, K., & Yeh, M. (2002). Mental health care for Latinos: Mental health services for Latino adolescents with psychiatric disorders. *Psychiatric Services, 53*(12), 1556–1562.

Hovey, J. D., Hurtado, G., & Seligman, L. D. (2014). Findings for a CBT support group for Latina migrant farmworkers in western Colorado. *Current Psychology: A Journal For Diverse Perspectives on Diverse Psychological Issues, 33,* 271–281. doi:10.1007/s12144-014-9212-y

Howell, L., Kochhar, K., Saywell, R., Zollinger, T., Koehler, J., Mandzuk, C., . . . & Allen, D. (2006). Use of herbal remedies by Hispanic patients: Do they inform their physician? *The Journal of the American Board of Family Medicine, 19*(6), 566–578.

Hu, R., Shi, L., Rane, S., Zhu, J., & Chen, C.-C. (2014). Insurance, racial/ethnic, SES-related disparities in quality of care among US adults with diabetes. *Journal of Immigrant and Minority Health, 16*(4), 565–575.

Humensky, J. L., Gil, R., Coronel, B., Cifre, R., Mazzula, S., & Lewis-Fernández, R. (2013). Life is precious: Reducing suicidal behavior in Latinas. *Ethnicity and Inequalities in Health and Social Care, 6,* 54–61. doi:10.1108/EIHSC-10 -2013-0027

Hummer, R. A., & Hayward, M. D. (2015). Hispanic older adult health & longevity in the United States: Current patterns & concerns for the future. *Daedalus, 144*(2), 20–30.

Hunt, L. M., Schneider, S., & Comer, B. (2004). Should "acculturation" be a variable in health research? A critical review of research on US Hispanics. *Social Science & Medicine, 59*(5), 973–986. doi:10.1016/j.socscimed.2003.12.009

Ibañez, G. E., Van Oss Marin, B., Flores, S. A., Millett, G., & Diaz, R. M. (2012). General and gay-related racism experienced by Latino gay men. *Journal of Latina/o Psychology, 1*(S), 66–77. doi:10.1037/2168-1678.1.S.66

Iniguez, E., & Palinkas, L. A. (2003). Varieties of health services utilization by underserved Mexican American women. *Journal of Health Care for the Poor & Underserved, 14*(1), 52–69.

Insaf, T. Z., Jurkowski, J., & Alomar, L. (2010). Sociocultural factors influencing delay in seeking routine health care among Latinas: Community-based participatory research study. *Ethnicity and Disease, 20,* 148–154.

Institute of Medicine. (2002). *Unequal Treatment: Confronting Ethnic and Racial Disparities in Healthcare.* Editors: Smeadley, B. D., Stith, A. Y., & Nelson, A. R.

Interian, A., Allen, L., Gara, M., & Escobar, J. (2008). A pilot study of culturally adapted cognitive behavior therapy for Hispanics with major depression. *Cognitive and Behavioral Practice, 15,* 67–75.

Interian, A., & Diaz-Martinez, A. M. (2007). Considerations for culturally competent cognitive-behavioral therapy for depression with Hispanic patients. *Cognitive and Behavioral Practice, 14,* 84–97.

Interian, A., Martinez, I. E., Guarnaccia, P. J., Vega, W. A., & Escobar, J. I. (2007). A qualitative analysis of the perception of stigma among Latinos receiving antidepressants. *Psychiatric Services, 58*(12), 1591–1594.

Isasi, C. R., Parrinello, C. M., Ayala, G. X., Delamater, A. M., Perreira, K. M., Daviglus, M. L., . . . & Van Horn, L. (2016). Sex differences in cardiometabolic risk factors among Hispanic/Latino youth. *The Journal of Pediatrics, 176,* 121–127.

Isasi-Díaz, A. M. (1996). *Mujerista theology: A theology for the twenty-first century.* Maryknoll, NY: Orbis Books.

Isong, U., & Weintraub, J. A. (2005). Determinants of dental service utilization among 2- to 11-year-old California children. *Journal of Public Health Dentistry, 63*(3).

Jacquez, F., Vaughn, L., Zhen-Duan, J., & Graham, C. (2016). Health care use and barriers to care among Latino immigrants in a new migration area. *Journal of Health Care for the Poor & Underserved, 27*(4), 1761–1778.

Jemal, A., Siegel, R., Ward, E., Hao, Y., Xu, J., Murray, T., & Thun, M. J. (2008). Cancer statistics, 2008. *CA: A Cancer Journal for Clinicians, 58*(2), 71–96.

Johnson, R. L., Saha, S., Arbelaez, J. J., Beach, M. C., & Cooper, L. A. (2004). Racial and ethnic differences in patient perceptions of bias and cultural competence in health care. *Journal of General Internal Medicine, 19,* 101–110.

Jones, M. O., & Hernández, C. J. (2009). Latina/o traditional medicine in Los Angeles: Asking about, archiving, and advocating cultural resources. *InterActions: UCLA Journal of Education and Information Studies, 5*(1), 1–17.

Kaiser Family Foundation. (2004). Immigrants' health care coverage and access. Menlo Park, CA: Kaiser Commission on Medicaid and Uninsured. Retrieved from https://kaiserfamilyfoundation.files.wordpress.com/2013/01/immigrants-health-care-coverage-and-access-fact-sheet.pdf

Kaiser Foundation. (2008). Eliminating racial/ethnic disparities in health care: What are the options? Retrieved from https://www.kff.org/disparities-policy/issue-brief/eliminating-racialethnic-disparities-in-health-care-what/

Kalenderian, E., Pegus, C., Francis, C., Goodwin, N., Saint Jacques, H., Lasa, D., & Members of the American Heart Association Health Disparities Committee (2009). Cardiovascular disease urban intervention: Baseline activities and findings. *Journal of Community Health, 34*(4), 282–287.

Kann, H., McManus, T., Harris, W. A., Shanklin, S. L., Flint, K. H., Hawkins, J., . . . & Zaza, S. (2016). Youth risk behavior surveillance—United States, 2015. *MMWR: Morbidity & Mortality Weekly Report, 65,* 1–174.

Kaplan, S. A., Ruddock, C., Golub, M., Davis, J., Foley, R., Sr., Devia, C., . . . & Carter, T. (2009). Stirring up the mud: Using a community-based participatory approach to address health disparities through a faith-based initiative. *Journal of Health Care for the Poor & Underserved, 20*(4), 1111.

Kardec, A. (1957). *El evangelio según el espiritismo* [The Gospel According to Spiritism]. México: Diana.

Kardec, A. (1975). *Colección de oraciones escogidas* [Collection of Selected Prayers]. Bronx, NY: De Pablo International.

Kataoka, S. H., Stein, B. D., Jaycox, L. H., Wong, M., Escudero, P., Tu, W., . . . & Fink, A. (2003). A school-based mental health program for traumatized Latino immigrant children. *Journal of the American Academy of Child & Adolescent Psychiatry, 42*(3), 311–318.

Kataoka, S. H., Zhang, L., & Wells, K. B. (2002). Unmet need for mental health care among US children: Variation by ethnicity and insurance status. *American Journal of Psychiatry, 159,* 1548–1555.

Katz, V. S., Ang, A., & Suro, R. (2012). An ecological perspective on U.S. Latinos' health communication behaviors, access, and outcomes. *Hispanic Journal of Behavioral Sciences, 34*(3), 437–456. doi:10.1177/0739986312445566

Kessler, R. C., McGonagle, K. A., Zhao, S., Nelson, C. B., Hughes, M., Eshleman, S., . . . & Kendler, K. S. (1994). Lifetime and 12-month prevalence of DSM-III-R psychiatric disorders in the United States: Results from the National Comorbidity Study. *Archives of General Psychiatry, 51,* 8–19.

Kessler, R. C., & Merikangas, K. R. (2004). The National Comorbidity Survey Replication (NCS-R): Background and aims. *International Journal of Methods in Psychiatric Research, 13*(2), 60–68.

Kiefer, D., Bradbury, E. J., & Tellez-Giron, P. (2014). A pilot study of herbal medicine use in a Midwest Latino population. *World Medical Journal, 113*(2), 64–71.

Kim, G., Loi, C. X. A., Chiriboga, D. A., Jang, Y., Parmelee, P., & Allen, R. S. (2011). Limited English proficiency as a barrier to mental health service use: A study of Latino and Asian immigrants with psychiatric disorders. *Journal of Psychiatric Research, 45*(1), 104–110.

Kopak, A. M. (2013). The relative importance of immigrant generation for Mexican Americans' alcohol and tobacco use from adolescence to early adulthood. *Journal of Immigrant & Minority Health, 15,* 569–576.

Koss, J. D. (1980). The therapist-spiritist training project in Puerto Rico: An experiment to relate the traditional healing system to the public health system. *Social Science & Medicine, 14,* 255–266. doi:10.1016/0160-7987(80)90051-4

Koss, J. D. (1987). Expectations and outcomes for patients given mental health care or spiritist healing in Puerto Rico. *American Journal of Psychiatry, 144,* 56–61.

Koss-Chioino, J. D. (2013). Religion and spirituality in Latino life in the United States. In K. I. Pargament, J. J. Exline, & J. W. Jones (Eds.), *APA handbook of psychology: Religion, and spirituality: Volume 1. Context, theory, and research* (pp. 599–615). Washington, DC: American Psychological Association.

Kouyoumdjian, H., Zamboanga, B. L., & Hansen, D. J. (2003). Barriers to community mental health services for Latinos: Treatment considerations. *Clinical Psychology: Science and Practice, 10*(4), 394–422.

Kreuter, M. W., Lukwago, S. N., Bucholtz, D. C., Clark, E. M., & Sanders-Thompson, V. (2003). Achieving cultural appropriateness in health promotion programs: Targeted and tailored approaches. *Health Education & Behavior, 30*(2), 133–146.

Kripalani, S., Bussey-Jones, J., Katz, M. G., & Genao, I. (2006). A prescription for cultural competence in medical education. *Journal of General Internal Medicine, 21*(10), 1116–1120.

Krogstad, J. M. (2016). Five facts about Latinos and education. Retrieved from http://www.pewresearch.org/fact-tank/2016/07/28/5-facts-about-latinos-and-education/

Krogstad, J. M. (2017a). *Surge in Cuban immigration to U.S. continued through 2016.* Washington, DC: Pew Research Center. Retrieved from http://www.pewresearch.org/fact-tank/2017/01/13/cuban-immigration-to-u-s-surges-as-relations-warm/

Krogstad, J. M. (2017b). *Unauthorized immigrants covered by DACA face uncertain future.* Washington, DC: Pew Research Center. Retrieved from http://www.pewresearch.org/fact-tank/2017/01/05/unauthorized-immigrants-covered-by-daca-face-uncertain-future/

Krogstad, J. M., Passel, J. S., & Cohn, D. (2017). *Five facts about illegal immigration in the U.S.* Washington, DC: Pew Research Center. Retrieved from http://www.pewresearch.org/fact-tank/2017/04/27/5-facts-about-illegal-immigration-in-the-u-s

Kuczmarski, R. J., Ogden, C. L., Guo, S. S., Grummer-Strawn, L. M., Flegal, K. M., Mei, Z., . . . & Johnson, C. L. (2002). 2000 CDC growth charts for the United States: Methods and development. *Vital and Health Statistics, 11, 246,* 1–190.

Kumpfer, K., Pinyuchon, M., Melo, A., & Whiteside, H. (2008). Cultural adaptation process for international dissemination of the strengthening families program. *Evaluation & the Health Professions, 31,* 226–226. doi:10.1177/0163278708708315926

Kuperminc, G. P., Wilkins, N. J., Roche, C., & Alvarez-Jimenez, A. (2009). Risk, resilience, and positive development among Latino youth. In F. A. Villarruel, G. Carlo, J. M. Grau, M. Azmitia, N. J. Cabrera, & T. J. Chahin (Eds.), *Handbook of U.S. Latino psychology developmental and community-based perspectives* (pp. 213–233). Thousand Oaks, CA: Sage.

Lancaster, K., Carter-Edwards, L., Grilo, S., Shen, C., & Schoenthaler, A. (2014). Obesity interventions in African American faith-based organizations: A systematic review. *Obesity Reviews, 15*(S4), 159–176.

Lanouette, N. M., Folsom, D. P., Sciolla, A., & Jeste, D. V. (2009). Psychotropic medication nonadherence among United States Latinos: A comprehensive literature review. *Psychiatric Services, 60*(2), 157–174.

Lara, M., Gamboa, C., Kahramanian, M. I., Morales, L. S., & Bautista, D. E. (2005). Acculturation and Latino health in the United States: A review of the literature and its sociopolitical context. *Annual Review of Public Health*, 26, 367–397. doi:10.1146/annurev.publhealth.26.021304.144615

Lariscy, J. T., Hummer, R. A., & Hayward, M. D. (2015). Hispanic older adult mortality in the United States: New estimates and an assessment of factors shaping the Hispanic paradox. *Demography, 52*(1), 1–14.

Larkey, L. K., Gonzalez, J. A., Mar, L. E., & Glantz, N. (2009). Latina recruitment for cancer prevention education via Community Based Participatory Research strategies. *Contemporary Clinical Trials*, 30, 47–54.

Larson, E. L., Dilone, J., Garcia, M., & Smolowitz, J. (2006). Factors which influence Latino community members to self-prescribe antibiotics. *Nursing Research, 55*(2), 94–102.

LaVange, L. M., Kalsbeek, W. D., Sorlie, P. D., Avilés-Santa, L. M., Kaplan, R. C., Barnhart, J., . . . & Ryan, J. (2010). Sample design and cohort selection in the Hispanic Community Health Study/Study of Latinos. *Annals of Epidemiology, 20*(8), 642–649.

Lawton, K. E., & Gerdes, A. C. (2014). Acculturation and Latino adolescent mental health: Integration of individual, environmental, and family influences. *Clinical Child and Family Psychology Review, 17*(4), 385–398.

Lee, D. L., & Ahn, S. (2012). Discrimination against Latina/os: A meta-analysis of individual-level resources and outcomes. *Counseling Psychologist, 40*, 28–65. doi:10.1177/0011000011403326

Leininger, M. (1991). Transcultural care principles, human rights, and ethical considerations. *Journal of Transcultural Nursing, 3*(1), 21–23.

Levin, J. (2014). Faith-based partnerships for population health: Challenges, initiatives, and prospects. *Public Health Reports, 129*(2), 127–131.

Lewis-Fernández, R., Aggarwal, N. K., Hinton, L., Hinton, D. E., & Kirmayer, L. J. (Eds.). (2016). *DSM-5® handbook on the cultural formulation interview*. Arlington, VA: American Psychiatric Publishing.

Lewis-Fernández, R., & Díaz, N. (2002). The cultural formulation: A method for assessing cultural factors affecting the clinical encounter. *Psychiatric Quarterly, 73*(4), 271–295.

Lewis-Fernández, R., Gorritz, M., Raggio, G. A., Peláez, C., Chen, H., & Guarnaccia, P. J. (2010). Association of trauma-related disorders and dissociation with four idioms of distress among Latino psychiatric outpatients. *Culture, Medicine, and Psychiatry, 34*(2), 219–243.

Lewis-Fernández, R., Horvitz-Lennon, M., Blanco, C., Guarnaccia, P. J., Cao, Z., & Alegría, M. (2009). Significance of endorsement of psychotic symptoms by US Latinos. *Journal of Nervous and Mental Disease, 197*(5), 337.

Lin, L., Nigrinis, A., Christidis, P., & Stamm, K. (2015). *Demographics of the U.S. psychology workforce: Findings from the American Community Survey*. Washington, DC: American Psychological Association.

Livingston, G., & Cohn, D. (2012). US birth rate falls to a record low: Decline is greatest among immigrants. Washington, DC: Pew Research Center, Social and

Demographic Trends. Retrieved from http://www. pewsocialtrends. org/2012/11/ 29/us-birth-rate-falls-to-a-record-low-decline-is-greatest-among-immigrants

Livingston, G., Minushkin, S., & Cohn, D. (2008). *Hispanics and health care in the United States*. Retrieved from http://www.pewhispanic.org/2008/08/13 /hispanics-and-health-care-in-the-united-states-access-information-and -knowledge/

Loera, J. A., Reyes-Ortiz, C., & Kuo, Y. F. (2007). Predictors of complementary and alternative medicine use among older Mexican Americans. *Complementary Therapies in Clinical Practice, 13*(4), 224–231.

Long, J., Sowell, R., Bairan, A., Holtz, C., Curtis, A., & Fogarty, K. (2012). Exploration of commonalities and variations in health related beliefs across four Latino subgroups using focus group methodology: Implications in care for Latinos with type 2 diabetes. *Journal of Cultural Diversity, 19*, 133–142.

Lopez, C., Bergren, M. D., & Painter, S. G. (2008). Latino disparities in child mental health services. *Journal of Child and Adolescent Psychiatric Nursing, 21*(3), 137–145.

López, G., & Patten, E. (2015). *The impact of slowing immigration: Foreign-born share falls among 14 largest U.S. Hispanic origin groups*. Washington, DC: Pew Hispanic Research Center. Retrieved from http://www.pewhispanic. org/2015/09/15/the-impact-of-slowing-immigration-foreign-born-share -falls-among-14-largest-us-hispanic-origin-groups/

López, I., Ramirez, R., Guarnaccia, P., Canino, G., & Bird, H. (2011). Ataques de nervios and somatic complaints among Island and mainland Puerto Rican children. *CNS Neuroscience & Therapeutics, 17*, 158–166. doi:10.1111/j.1755 -5949.2010.00137.x

López, I., Rivera, F., Ramirez, R., Guarnaccia, P. J., Canino, G., & Bird, H. (2009). Ataques de nervios and their psychiatric correlates in Puerto Rican children from two different contexts. *Journal of Nervous and Mental Disease, 197*, 923–929. doi:10.1097/NMD.0b013e3181c2997d

Lopez, M. H., & Velasco, G. (2011). *Childhood poverty among Hispanics sets record, leads nation*. Washington, DC: Pew Hispanic Center.

Lopez, R. (2005). Use of alternative folk medicine by Mexican American women. *Journal of Immigrant Health, 7*, 23–31. doi:10.1007/s10903-005-1387-8

López, S. R., Lara, M. C., Kopelowicz, A., Solano, S., Foncerrada, H., & Aguilera, A. (2009). La CLAve to increase psychosis literacy of Spanish-speaking community residents and family caregivers. *Journal of Consulting and Clinical Psychology, 77*, 763–774. doi:10.1037/a0016031

Lopez-Class, M., Castro, F. G., & Ramirez, A. G. (2011). Conceptions of acculturation: A review and statement of critical issues. *Social Science Medicine, 72*(9), 1555–1562.

Lopez-Class, M., & Hosler, A. S. (2010). Assessment of community food resources: A Latino neighborhood study in upstate New York. *Journal of Poverty, 14*(4), 369–381.

Lopez-Quintero, C., Shtarkshall, R., & Neumark, Y. D. (2005). Barriers to HIV-testing among Hispanics in the United States: Analysis of the National Health Interview Survey, 2000. *AIDS Patient Care & STDs, 19*(10), 672–683.

Lopez-Tamayo, R., Seda, A., & Jason, L. A. (2016). The role of familismo and acculturation as moderators of the association between family conflict and substance abuse on Latino adult males. *Public Health (Fairfax, Va.), 1*(2), 48.

Lujan, J., & Campbell, H. B. (2006). The role of religion on the health practices of Mexican Americans. *Journal of Religion and Health, 45*(2), 183–195.

Lujan, J., Ostwald, S. K., & Ortiz, M. (2007). Promotora diabetes intervention for Mexican Americans. *Diabetes Educator, 33*(4), 660–670.

Mackenzie, E. R., Taylor, L., Bloom, B. S., Hufford, D. J., & Johnson, J. C. (2003). Ethnic minority use of complementary and alternative medicine (CAM): A national probability survey of CAM utilizers. *Alternative Therapies in Health and Medicine, 9*(4), 50.

Magaña, S., Parish, S., Rose, R., Timberlake, M., & Swaine, J. (2012). Racial and ethnic disparities in quality of health care among children with autism and other developmental disabilities. *Intellectual and Developmental Disabilities, 50*, 287–299. doi:10.1352/1934-9556-50.4.287

Magaña, S., Lopez, K., & Machalicek, W. (2017). Parents taking action: A psychoeducational intervention for Latino parents of children with autism spectrum disorder. *Family Process, 56*, 59–74.

Markides, K. S., & Coreil, J. (1986). The health of Hispanics in the southwestern United States: An epidemiologic paradox. *Public Health Reports, 101*(3), 253.

Markides, K. S., & Eschbach, K. (2005). Aging, migration, and mortality: Current status of research on the Hispanic paradox. *Journals of Gerontology Series B: Psychological Sciences and Social Sciences, 60*(Special Issue 2), S68–S75.

Marques, L., Alegría, M., Becker, A., Chen, C., Fang, A., Chosak, A., & Diniz, J. (2011). Comparative prevalence, correlates of impairment, and service utilization for eating disorders across US ethnic groups: Implications for reducing ethnic disparities in health care access for eating disorders. *International Journal of Eating Disorders, 44*, 412–420.

Marsella, J. J., & Yamada, A. M. (2007). Culture and psychopathology/foundations, issues, and directions. In S. Kitamaya & D. Cohen (Eds.), *Handbook of cultural psychology* (pp. 787–818). New York: Guilford.

Martinez, I. L., & Carter-Pokras, O. (2006). Assessing health concerns and barriers in a heterogeneous Latino community. *Journal of Health Care for the Poor & Underserved, 17*(4), 899–909.

Martinez, L. N. (2009). South Texas Mexican American use of traditional folk and mainstream alternative therapies. *Hispanic Journal of Behavioral Sciences, 31*(1), 128–143.

Martinez, R., Taylor, M. J., Calvert, W. J., Hirsch, J. L., & Webster, C. K. (2014). Santería as a culturally responsive healing practice. In R. Gurung (Ed.), *Multicultural approaches to health and wellness in America* (Vol. 1, pp. 329–348). Santa Barbara, CA: Praeger.

Matos, M., Torres, R., Santiago, R., Jurado, M., & Rodriguez, I. (2006). Adaptation of parent-child interaction therapy for Puerto Rican families: A preliminary study. *Family Process, 45*, 205–222.

Mattesich, P. W., & Monsey, B. R. (1992). *Collaboration: What makes it work?* St. Paul, MN: Amherst H. Wilder Foundation.

Mauer, M., & King, R. S. (2007). Uneven justice: State rates of incarceration by race and ethnicity. Retrieved from http://www.sentencingproject.org/wp-content/uploads/2016/01/Uneven-Justice-State-Rates-of-Incarceration-by-Race-and-Ethnicity.pdf

McCabe, S. E., Bostwick, W. B., Hughes, T. L., West, B. T., & Boyd, C. J. (2010). The relationship between discrimination and substance use disorders among lesbian, gay, and bisexual adults in the United States. *American Journal of Public Health, 100*, 1946–1952. doi:10.2105/AJPH.2009.163147

McCloskey, J. (2009). Promotores as partners in a community-based diabetes intervention program targeting Hispanics. *Family & Community Health, 32*(1), 48–57.

McCollister, K. E., Arheart, K. L., Lee, D. J., Fleming, L. E., Davila, E. P., LeBlanc, W. G., . . . & Erard, M. J. (2010). Declining health insurance access among US Hispanic workers: Not all jobs are created equal. *American Journal of Indian Medicine, 53*(2), 163–170. doi:10.1002/ajim.20720

McLaughlin, K. A., Hilt, L. M., & Nolen-Hoeksema, S. (2007). Racial/ethnic differences in internalizing and externalizing symptoms in adolescents. *Journal of Abnormal Child Psychology, 35*, 801–816. doi:10.1007/s10802-007-9128-1

McNeill, B. W., & Cervantes, J. M. (2008). Introduction: Counselors and curanderas/os-parallels in the healing process. In B. W. McNeill & J. M. Cervantes (Eds.), *Latina/o healing practices: Mestizo and indigenous perspectives* (pp. xvii–xxxi). New York: Routledge.

McNeill, B. W., Esquivel, E., Carrasco, A., & Mendoza, R. (2008). Santeria and the healing process in Cuba and the United States. In B. W. McNeill & J. M. Cervantes (Eds.), *Latina/o healing practices: Mestizo and indigenous perspectives* (pp. 63–82). New York: Routledge.

Medina-Inojosa, J., Jean, N., Cortes-Bergoderi, M., & Lopez-Jimenez, F. (2014). The Hispanic paradox in cardiovascular disease and total mortality. *Progress in Cardiovascular Diseases, 57*(3), 286–292.

Meigs, J. M., Wilson, P. W. F., Nathan, D. M., D'Agostino, R. B., Williams, K. & Haffner, S. M. (2003). Prevalence and characteristics of the metabolic syndrome in the San Antonio Heart and Framingham Offspring Studies. *Diabetes, 52*, 2160–2167.

Mekkodathil, A., El-Menyar, A., & Al-Thani, H. (2016). Occupational injuries in workers from different ethnicities. *International Journal of Critical Illness and Injury Science, 6*(1), 25.

Mercado-Crespo, M. C., Bartolomei, C., Hacker, T., Gianfortoni, E., & Arroyo, L. E. (2010). *Latino mental health in the United States: A community-based approach.* Washington, DC: National Council of La Raza. Retrieved from http://publications.nclr.org/handle/123456789/1143

Mikhail, N., Wali, S., & Ziment, I. (2004). Use of alternative medicine among Hispanics. *Journal of Alternative & Complementary Medicine, 10*(5), 851–859.

Minkler, M. (2005). Community-based research partnerships: Challenges and opportunities. *Journal of Urban Health, 82*(2 Suppl 2), ii3–ii12.

Minkler, M., Blackwell, A. G., Thompson, M., & Tamir, H. (2003). Community-based participatory research: Implications for public health funding. *American Journal of Public Health, 93*(8), 1210–1213.

Miranda, J., Azocar, F., Organista, K. C., Dwyer, E., & Arean, P. (2003). Treatment of depression among impoverished primary care patients from ethnic minority groups. *Psychiatric Services, 54,* 219–225.

Mirandé, A., Pitones, J. M., & Diaz, J. (2011). Quien es el mas macho? A comparison of day laborers and Chicano men. *Men and Masculinities, 14,* 309–334. doi:10.1177/1097184X10371288

Mizuno, Y., Borkowf, C. B., Ayala, G., Carballo-Diéguez, A., & Millett, G. A. (2015). Correlates of sexual risk for HIV among US-born and foreign-born Latino men who have sex with men (MSM): An analysis from the Brothers y Hermanos Study. *Journal of Immigrant & Minority Health, 17*(1), 47–55. doi:10.1007/s10903-013-9894-5

Molina, K. M., Jackson, B., & Rivera-Olmedo, N. (2016). Discrimination, racial/ethnic identity, and substance use among Latina/os: Are they gendered? *Annals of Behavioral Medicine, 50,* 119–129.

Molina, K. M., & Simon, Y. (2014). Everyday discrimination and chronic health conditions among Latinos: The moderating role of socioeconomic position. *Journal of Behavioral Medicine, 37*(5), 868–880.

Molina, M. N. (1996). Archetypes and spirits: A Jungian analysis of Puerto Rican espiritismo. *Journal of Analytical Psychology, 41,* 227–244.

Moore, A. A., Karno, M. P., Ray, L., Ramirez, K., Barenstein, V., Portillo, M. J., . . . & Barry, K. L. (2016). Development and preliminary testing of a Promotora-delivered, Spanish language, counseling intervention for heavy drinking among male, Latino day laborers. *Journal of Substance Abuse Treatment, 62,* 96–101. doi:10.1016/j.jsat.2015.11.003

Moore, J. D., Saywell, R. M., Thakker, N., & Jones, T. A. (2002). An analysis of patient compliance with nurse recommendations from an after-hours call center. *American Journal of Managed Care, 8*(4), 343–351.

Morales, E. (2013). Latino lesbian, gay, bisexual, and transgender immigrants in the United States. *Journal of LGBT Issues in Counseling, 7*, 172–184. doi:10.1 080/15538605.2013.785467

Morales, L. S., Lara, M., Kington, R. S., Valdez, R. O., & Escarce, J. J. (2002). Socio-economic, cultural, and behavioral factors affecting Hispanic health out-comes. *Journal of Health Care for the Poor & Underserved, 13*(4), 477.

Moralez, E. A., Rao, S. P., Livaudais, J. C., & Thompson, B. (2012). Improving knowledge and screening for colorectal cancer among Hispanics: Over-coming barriers through a Promotora-led home-based educational inter-vention. *Journal of Cancer Education, 27*(3), 533–539. doi:10.1007/s13187 -012-0357-9

Moreira-Almeida, A., & Koss-Chioino, J. D. (2009). Recognition and treatment of psychotic symptoms: Spiritists compared to mental health professionals in Puerto Rico and Brazil. *Psychiatry, 72*, 268–283.

Morgan, P. L., Staff, J., Hillemeier, M. M., Farkas, G., & Maczuga, S. (2013). Racial and ethnic disparities in ADHD diagnosis from kindergarten to eighth grade. *Pediatrics, 132*, 85–93. doi:10.1542/peds.2012-2390

Mulvaney-Day, N. E., Alegría, M., & Sribney, W. (2007). Social cohesion, social sup-port, and health among Latinos in the United States. *Social Science & Medi-cine, 64*(2), 477–495.

Muñoz, F. A., Servin, A. E., Kozo, J., Lam, M., & Zúñiga, M. L. (2013). A binational comparison of HIV provider attitudes towards the use of complementary and alternative medicine among HIV-positive Latino patients receiving care in the US–Mexico border region. *AIDS care, 25*(8), 990–997.

Murguia, A., Peterson, R. A., & Zea, M. C. (2003). Use and implications of ethno-medical health care approaches among Central American immigrants. *Health & Social Work, 28*(1), 43–51.

Naimi, T. S., Nelson, D. E., & Brewer, R. D. (2010). The intensity of binge alcohol consumption among US adults. *American Journal of Preventive Medicine, 38*(2), 201–207.

Nandi, A., Galea, S., Lopez, G., Nandi, V., Strongarone, S., & Ompad, D. C. (2008). Access to and use of health services among undocumented Mexican immigrants in a US urban area. *American Journal of Public Health, 98*(11), 2011–2020.

National Center for Complementary and Integrative Health. (2011). Complemen-tary, alternative, or integrative health: What's in a name? Retrieved from https://nccih.nih.gov/health/integrative-health

National Center for Health Statistics. (1985). *Plan and operation of the Hispanic Health and Nutrition Examination Survey, 1982–1984* (Vol. 19). Washington, DC: U.S. Public Health Service.

National Center for Health Statistics. (1999). National Health Interview Survey: Research for the 1995–2004 redesign (Vol. 126). Washington, DC: National Center for Health Statistics.

National Center for Health Statistics. (2014, February 3). About the National Health and Nutrition Examination Survey. Retrieved from https://www.cdc.gov/nchs/nhanes/about_nhanes.htm

National Center for Health Statistics. (2015). National Health and Examination Survey: Hispanic HANES. Retrieved from https://www.cdc.gov/nchs/nhanes/hhanes.htm

Nedjat-Haiem, F. R., Lorenz, K. A., Ell, K., Hamilton, A., & Palinkas, L. (2012). Experiences with advanced cancer among Latinas in a public health care system. *Journal of Pain and Symptom Management, 43*(6), 1013–1024.

Negi, N. J. (2013). Battling discrimination and social isolation: Psychological distress among Latino day laborers. *American Journal of Community Psychology, 51*, 164–174. doi:10.1007/s10464-012-9548-0

Nolen, A. L., Ball, R., Pinon, M., & Shepherd, M. (2002). Using medications purchased in Mexico: Position statement of the Texas Society of Health-System Pharmacists. *American Journal of Health-System Pharmacy, 59*(13), 1289–1290.

Nuno, T., Martinez, M. E., Harris, R., & Garcia, F. (2011). A Promotora-administered group education intervention to promote breast and cervical cancer screening in a rural community along the U.S.-Mexico border: A randomized controlled trial. *Cancer Causes & Control, 22*(3), 367–374. doi:10.1007/s10552-010–9705-4

Oboler, S. (2005). Introduction: Los Que Llegaron: 50 years of South American Immigration (1950–2000)—An overview. *Latino Studies, 3*(1), 42–52.

O'Brien, M. J., Perez, A., Alos, V. A., Whitaker, R. C., Ciolino, J. D., Mohr, D. C., & Ackermann, R. T. (2015). The feasibility, acceptability, and preliminary effectiveness of a Promotora-Led Diabetes Prevention Program (PL-DPP) in Latinas: A pilot study. *Diabetes Educator, 41*(4), 485–494.

O'Connor, K., Stoecklin-Marois, M., & Schenker, M. B. (2015). Examining nervios among immigrant male farmworkers in the MICASA study: Sociodemographics, housing conditions and psychosocial factors. *Journal of Immigrant and Minority Health, 17*(1), 198–207.

Office of Disease Prevention and Health Promotion. (2017). Social determinants of health. Retrieved from https://www.healthypeople.gov/2020/topics-objectives/social-determinants-of-health

Ogden, C. L., Carroll, M. D., Kit, B. K., & Flegal, K. M. (2014). Prevalence of childhood and adult obesity in the United States, 2011–2012. *Journal of the American Medical Association, 311*(8), 806–814.

Ojeda, V. D., Patterson, T., & Strathdee, S. A. (2008). The influence of perceived risk to health and immigration-related characteristics on substance use among Latino and other immigrants. *American Journal of Public Health, 98*(5), 862–868.

Okamoto, J., Ritt-Olson, A., Soto, D., Baezconde-Garbanati, L., & Unger, J. B. (2009). Perceived discrimination and substance use among Latino adolescents. *American Journal of Health Behavior, 33*, 718–727.

Organista, K. C. (2000). Latinos. In J. R. White, & A. Freeman (Eds.), *Cognitive behavioral group therapy: For specific problems and populations* (pp. 281–303). Washington, DC: American Psychological Association.

Organista, K. C. (2007). *Solving Latino psychosocial and health problems: Theory, practice, and populations.* Hoboken, NJ: Wiley.

Organista, K. C., & Muñoz, R. F. (1996). Cognitive-behavioral therapy with Latinos. *Cognitive and Behavioral Practice, 3,* 255–270.

Ortega, A. N., & Alegría, M. (2002). Self-reliance, mental health need, and the use of mental healthcare among island Puerto Ricans. *Mental Health Services Research, 4,* 131–140.

Ortega, A. N., Canino, P. G., & Alegría, M. (2008). Lifetime and 12-month intermittent explosive disorder in Latinos. *American Journal of Orthopsychiatry, 78,* 133–139. doi:10.1037/0002-9432.78.1.133

Ortega, A. N., Fang, H., Perez, V. H., Rizzo, J., Carter-Pokras, O., Wallace, S. P., & Gelberg, L. (2007). Health care access, use of services, and experiences among undocumented Mexicans and other Latinos. *Archives of Internal Medicine, 167*(21), 2354–2360.

Ortiz, B. I., Shields, K. M., Clauson, K. A., & Clay, P. G. (2007). Complementary and alternative medicine use among Hispanics in the United States. *Annals of Pharmacotherapy, 41*(6), 994–1004.

Ortiz, F. A., Davis, K. G., & McNeill, B. W. (2008). Curanderismo: Religious and spiritual worldviews and indigenous healing traditions. In B. W. McNeill & J. M. Cervantes (Eds.), *Latina/o healing practices: Mestizo and indigenous perspectives* (pp. 271–302). New York: Routledge.

Ortiz, I. E. M., & Torres, E. P. (2007). Curanderismo and the treatment of alcoholism: Findings from a focus group of Mexican curanderos. *Alcoholism Treatment Quarterly, 25,* 79–90. doi:10.1300/J020v25n04_06

Otiniano, A. D., Carroll-Scott, A., Toy, P., & Wallace, S. P. (2012). Supporting Latino communities' natural helpers: A case study of promotoras in a research capacity building course. *Journal of Immigrant & Minority Health, 14*(4), 657–663.

Otiniano Verissimo, A. D., Grella, C. E., Amaro, H., & Gee, G. C. (2014). Discrimination and substance use disorders among Latinos: The role of gender, nativity, and ethnicity. *American Journal of Public Health, 104*(8), 1421–1428.

O'Toole, T. P., Aaron, K. F., Chin, M. H., Horowitz, C., & Tyson, F. (2003). Community-based participatory research: Opportunities, challenges, and the need for a common language. *Journal of General Internal Medicine, 18*(7): 592–594.

Padilla, A. M. (1980). Notes on the history of Hispanic psychology. *Hispanic Journal of Behavioral Sciences, 2,* 109–128. doi:10.1177/0739986303251691

Padilla, A. M. (1984). Synopsis of the history of Chicano psychology. In J. L. Martinez & R. H. Mendoza (Eds.), *Chicano psychology* (2nd ed., pp. 1–19). San Diego, CA: Academic Press.

Padilla, R., Gomez, V., Biggerstaff, S. L., & Mehler, P. S. (2001). Use of curanderismo in a public health care system. *Archives of Internal Medicine, 161*(10), 1336–1340.

Paniagua, F. A. (2014). *Assessing and treating culturally diverse clients: A practical guide* (4th ed.). Thousand Oaks, CA: Sage.

Pantin, H., Schwartz, S. J., Sullivan, S., Coatsworth, J. D., & Szapocznik, J. (2003). Preventing substance abuse in Hispanic immigrant adolescents: An ecodevelopmental, parent-centered approach. *Hispanic Journal of Behavioral Sciences, 25*, 469–500.

Parasuraman, S. R., & Shi, L. (2015). Differences in access to care among students using school-based health centers. *Journal of School Nursing, 31*(4), 291–299.

Parks, F. M., Zea, M. C., & Mason, M. A. (2014). Psychotherapy with members of Latino/Latina churches and spiritual traditions. In P. S. Richards, A. E. Bergin, P. S. Richards, & A. E. Bergin (Eds.), *Handbook of psychotherapy and religious diversity* (pp. 399–421). Washington, DC: American Psychological Association.

Parra-Cardona, J. R., Escobar-Chew, A. R., Holtrop, K., Carpenter, G., Guzmán, R., Hernández, D., . . . & Ramírez, D. G. (2013). "En el grupo tomas conciencia (In group you become aware)": Latino immigrants' satisfaction with a culturally informed intervention for men who batter. *Violence against Women, 19*, 107–132. doi:10.1177/1077801212475338

Pasquali, E. A. (1994). Santería. *Journal of Holistic Nursing, 12*, 380–390.

Passel, J. S., & Cohn, D. V. (2014). *Unauthorized immigrant totals rise in 7 states, fall in 14: Decline in those from Mexico fuels most state decreases.* Washington, DC: Pew Research Center. Retrieved from http://www.pewhispanic.org/files/2014/11/2014-11-18_unauthorized-immigration.pdf

Pastrana, A. (2015). Being out to others: The relative importance of family support, identity and religion for LGBT Latina/os. *Latino Studies, 13*, 88–112. doi:10.1057/lst.2014.69

Pastrana, A., Battle, J., & Harris, A. (2017). *An examination of Latinx LGBT populations across the United States: Intersections of race and sexuality.* New York: Palgrave Macmillan.

Patten, E. (2016). *The nations' Latino population is defined by its youth.* Washington, DC: Pew Research Center. Retrieved from http://assets.pewresearch.org/wp-content/uploads/sites/7/2016/04/PH_2016-04-20_LatinoYouth-Final.pdf

Paymar, M., Pence, E., & Aravena Azócar, L. (2002). *Creando un proceso de cambio para hombres que maltratan* [Creating a process of change for men who abuse]. Duluth, MN: Domestic Abuse Intervention Programs.

Pearson, W. S., Ahluwalia, I. B., Ford, E. S., & Mokdad, A. H. (2008). Language preference as a predictor of access to and use of healthcare. *Ethnicity & Disease, 18*, 93–97.

Peifer, K. L., Hu, T., & Vega, W. (2000). Help seeking by persons of Mexican origin with functional impairments. *Psychiatric Services, 51*, 1293–1298.

Penedo, F. J., Yanez, B., Castañeda, S. F., Gallo, L., Wortman, K., Gouskova, N., . . . & Sanchez-Johnsen, L. (2016). Self-reported cancer prevalence among Hispanics in the US: Results from the Hispanic Community Health Study/Study of Latinos. *PLoS One, 11*(1), e0146268.

Perez, G., Della Valle, P., Paraghamian, S., Page, R., Ochoa, J., Palomo, F., . . . & Corbie-Smith, G. (2016). A community-engaged research approach to improve mental health among Latina immigrants: ALMA photovoice. *Health Promotion Practice, 17,* 429–439. doi:10.1177/1524839915593500

Pérez, M. C., & Fortuna, L. (2005). Chapter 6. Psychosocial stressors, psychiatric diagnoses and utilization of mental health services among undocumented immigrant Latinos. *Journal of Immigrant & Refugee Services, 3,* 107–123. doi:10.1300/J191v03n01_06

Perez, V., Fang, H., Inkelas, M., Kuo, A., & Ortega, A. (2009). Access to and utilization of health care by subgroups of Latino children. *Medical Care Research and Review, 47*(6), 695–699.

Perez-Escamilla, R. (2009). Health care access among Latinos: Implications for social and health care reforms. *Journal of Hispanic Higher Education, 9*(1), 43–60. doi:10.1177/1538192709349917

Pérez-Escamilla, R. (2011). Acculturation, nutrition, and health disparities in Latinos. *The American Journal of Clinical Nutrition, 93*(5), 1163S–1167S.

Perez-Escamilla, R., Garcia, J., & Song, D. (2010). Health care access among Hispanic immigrants: ¿Alguien está esuchando? [Is anybody listening?]. *NAPA Bulletin, 34*(1), 47–67. doi:10.1111/j.1556-4797.2010.01051.x

Perou, R., Bitsko, R. H., Blumberg, S. J., Pastor, P., Ghandour, R. M., Gfroerer, J. C., . . . & Schieve, L. A. (2013). Mental health surveillance among children—United States, 2005–2011. *MMWR Surveillance Summary, 62*(Suppl 2), 1–35.

Pew Research Center. (2014). The shifting religious identity of Latinos in the United States: Nearly one-in-four Latinos are former Catholics. Retrieved from http://www.pewforum.org/2014/05/07/the-shifting-religious-identity-of-latinos-in-the-united-states/

Pew Research Center. (2015a). Modern immigration wave brings 59 million to U.S., driving population growth and change through 2065: Views of immigration's impact on U.S. society mixed. Retrieved from http://www.pewhispanic.org/2015/09/28/modern-immigration-wave-brings-59-million-to-u-s-driving-population-growth-and-change-through-2065/

Pew Research Center. (2015b). More Mexicans leaving than coming to the US. Retrieved from http://www.pewhispanic.org/2015/11/19/more-mexicans-leaving-than-coming-to-the-u-s

Pimentel-Narez, D. (2017). *The effects of immigrant status, gender and years of U.S. residency on the acculturative stress and psychological symptomatology of Mexican immigrants.* Unpublished dissertation. University of La Verne, La Verne, CA.

Piña-Watson, B., Lorenzo-Blanco, E. I., Dornhecker, M., Martinez, A. J., & Nagoshi, J. L. (2016). Moving away from a cultural deficit to a holistic perspective: Traditional gender role values, academic attitudes, and educational goals for Mexican descent adolescents. *Journal of Counseling Psychology, 63*(3), 307.

Pinheiro, P. S., Sherman, R. L., Trapido, E. J., Fleming, L. E., Huang, Y., Gomez-Marin, O., & Lee, D. (2009). Cancer incidence in first generation US Hispanics: Cubans, Mexicans, Puerto Ricans, and new Latinos. *Cancer Epidemiology and Prevention Biomarkers, 18*(8), 2162–2169.

Pippins, J. R., Alegría, M., & Haas, J. S. (2007). Association between language proficiency and the quality of primary care among a national sample of insured Latinos. *Medical Care, 45*(11), 1020–1025. doi:10.1097/MLR.0b0 13e31814847be

Pleis, J. R., & Lethbridge-Çejku, M. (2006). Summary health statistics for US adults: National Health Interview Survey, 2005. *Vital and Health Statistics, 10, 232*, 1–153.

Polk, S., Carter-Pokras, O., Dover, G., & Cheng, T. L. (2013). A call to improve the health and healthcare of Latino children. *Journal of Pediatrics, 163*(5), 1240–1241. doi:10.1016/j.jpeds.2013.07.033

Poquiz, J. L., & Fite, P. J. (2016). The role of perceived peer substance use in the associations between community violence and lifetime substance abuse among Latino adolescents. *Journal of Community Psychology, 44*(7), 945–952.

Potochnick, S., & Perreira, K. M. (2010). Depression and anxiety among first-generation immigrant Latino youth: Key correlates and implications for future research. *Journal of Nervous and Mental Disease, 198*, 470–477.

Prezio, E. A., Cheng, D., Balasubramanian, B. A., Shuval, K., Kendzor, D. E., & Culica, D. (2013). Community Diabetes Education (CoDE) for uninsured Mexican Americans: A randomized controlled trial of a culturally tailored diabetes education and management program led by a community health worker. *Diabetes Research and Clinical Practice, 100*(1), 19–28. doi:10.1016/j .diabres.2013.01.027

Pumariega, A. J., Rogers, K., & Roth, E. (2005). Culturally competent systems of care for children's mental health: Advances and challenges. *Community Mental Health Journal, 41*, 539–555.

Purnell, L. D. (2014). *Guide to culturally competent health care.* Philadelphia: Davis.

Quandt, S. A., Sandberg, J. C., Graham, A., Mora, D. C., Stub, T., & Arcury, T. A. (2017). Mexican sobadores in North Carolina: Manual therapy in a new settlement context. *Journal of Immigrant & Minority Health, 19*, 1186–1195. doi:10.1007/s10903-016-0466-3

Ramirez, M. (1998). *Multicultural/multiracial psychology: Mestizo perspectives in personality and mental health.* Northvale, NJ: Aronson.

Ramos, Z., & Alegría, M. (2014). Cultural adaptation and health literacy refinement of a brief depression intervention for Latinos in a low-resource setting.

Cultural Diversity & Ethnic Minority Psychology, 20, 293–301. doi:10.1037/a0035021

Ransford, H. E., Carrillo, F. R., & Rivera, Y. (2010). Health care-seeking among Latino immigrants: Blocked access, use of traditional medicine, and the role of religion. *Journal of Health Care for the Poor & Underserved, 21*(3), 862–878.

Rastogi, M., Massey-Hastings, N., & Wieling, E. (2012). Barriers to seeking mental health services in the Latino/a community: A qualitative analysis. *Journal of Systemic Therapies, 31*(4), 1–17.

Rayle, A. D., Sand, J. K., Brucato, T., & Ortega, J. (2006). The "Comadre" group approach: A wellness-based group model for monolingual Mexican Women. *Journal for Specialists in Group Work, 31,* 5–24.

Reichard, R. (2015). Why we say Latinx: Trans & gender non-conforming people explain. Retrieved from http://www.latina.com/lifestyle/our-issues/why-we-say-latinx-trans-gender-non-conforming-people-explain

Reinschmidt, K. M., & Chong, J. (2005). *SONRISA: A curriculum toolbox for promotores/community health workers to address mental/emotional health issues associated with diabetes.* Southwest Center for Community Health Promotion, Mel and Enid Zuckerman College of Public Health, Tucson: University of Arizona.

Resnicow, K., Baranowski, T., Ahluwalia, J., & Braithwaite, R. (1998). Cultural sensitivity in public health: Defined and demystified. *Ethnicity & Disease, 9*(1), 10–21.

Reyes-Ortiz, C. A., Rodriguez, M., & Markides, K. S. (2009). The role of spirituality healing with perceptions of the medical encounter among Latinos. *Journal of General Internal Medicine, 24*(3), 542.

Rhodes, S. D., Foley, K. L., Zometa, C. S., & Bloom, F. R. (2007). Lay health advisor interventions among Hispanics/Latinos: A qualitative systematic review. *American Journal of Preventive Medicine, 33*(5), 418–427.

Rios-Ellis, B., Frates, J., D'Anna, L. H., Dwyer, M., Lopez-Zetina, J., & Ugarte, C. (2008). Addressing the need for access to culturally and linguistically appropriate HIV/AIDS prevention for Latinos. *Journal of Immigrant & Minority Health, 10*(5), 445–460. doi:10.1007/s10903-007-9105-3

Rivera, J. O., Ortiz, M., Lawson, M. E., & Verma, K. M. (2002). Evaluation of the use of complementary and alternative medicine in the largest United States-Mexico border city. *Pharmacotherapy: Journal of Human Pharmacology and Drug Therapy, 22*(2), 256–264.

Robinson, J. A., Bolton, J. M., Rasic, D., & Sareen, J. (2012). Exploring the relationship between religious service attendance, mental disorders, and suicidality among different ethnic groups: Results from a nationally representative survey. *Depression and Anxiety, 29,* 983–990. doi:10.1002/da.21978.

Rodriguez, C. J., Allison, M., Daviglus, M. L., Isasi, C. R., Keller, C., Leira, E. C., . . . & Rodriguez, B. (2014). Status of cardiovascular disease and stroke in Hispanics/Latinos in the United States. *Circulation, 130*(7), 593–625.

Rodriguez, M. A., Bustamante, A. V., & Ang, A. (2009). Perceived quality of care, receipt of preventive care, and usual source of health care among undocumented and other Latinos. *Journal of General Internal Medicine, 24*(Suppl 3), 508–513. doi:10.1007/s11606-009-1098-2

Rogers, A. T. (2010). Exploring health beliefs and care-seeking behaviors of older USA-dwelling Mexicans and Mexican-Americans. *Ethnicity & Health, 15*(6), 581–599.

Rogler, L. H., Malgady, R. G., Costantino, G., & Blumenthal, R. (1987). What do culturally sensitive mental health services mean? The case of Hispanics. *American Psychologist, 42*, 565–570.

Rojas-Vilches, A. P., Negy, C., & Reig-Ferrer, A. (2011). Attitudes toward seeking therapy among Puerto Rican and Cuban American young adults and their parents. *International Journal of Clinical and Health Psychology, 11*, 313–341.

Romero, A. J., Edwards, L. M., Bauman, S., & Ritter, M. K. (2014a). *Preventing adolescent depression and suicide among Latinas: Resilience research and theory*. New York: Springer.

Romero, A. J., Edwards, L. M., Fryberg, S. A., & Orduña, M. (2014b). Resilience to discrimination stress across ethnic identity stages of development. *Journal of Applied Social Psychology, 44*(1), 1–11.

Romero, A. J., Martinez, D., & Carvajal, S. C. (2007). Bicultural stress and adolescent risk behaviors in a community sample of Latinos and non-Latino European Americans. *Ethnicity & Health, 12*, 443–463. doi:10.1080/1355785070 1616854

Romero, A. J., Piña-Watson, B., & Toomey, R. B. (2017). When is bicultural stress associated with loss of hope and depressive symptoms? Variation by ethnic identity status among Mexican descent youth. *Journal of Latina/a Psychology*. Advance online publication. doi:10.1037/lat0000078

Romero, A. J., & Roberts, R. E. (2003). The impact of multiple dimensions of ethnic identity on discrimination and adolescents' self-esteem. *Journal of Applied Social Psychology, 33*, 2288–2305. doi:10.1111/j.1559-1816.2003.tb01885.x

Romero, M. (2011). Constructing Mexican Immigrant women as a threat to American families. *International Journal of Sociology of the Family, 37*, 49–68.

Rosales Meza, R., & Arellano-Morales (2014). Mental health disparities among Latina/os. In R. Gurung (Ed.), *Multicultural approaches to health and wellness in America* (Vol. 2., pp. 59–88). Santa Barbara, CA: Praeger.

Rosario, A. M., & De La Rosa, M. (2014). Santería as informal mental health support among U.S. Latinos with cancer. *Journal of Religion & Spirituality in Social Work, 33*, 4–18. doi:10.1080/15426432.2014.873294

Rosselló, J., Bernal, G., & Rivera-Medina, C. (2008). Individual and Group CBT and IPT for Puerto Rican adolescents with depressive symptoms. *Cultural Diversity & Ethnic Minority Psychology, 14*, 234–245. doi:10.1037/1099-9809 .14.3.234

Rubel, A., O'Nell, C., & Collado-Ardón, R. (1984). *Susto, a folk illness*. Berkeley, CA: University of California Press.

Rubens, S., Gudiño, O. G., Fite, P. J., & Grande, J. M. (2016). Individual and neighborhood stressors, sleep problems, and symptoms of anxiety and depression among Latino youth. *American Journal of Orthopsychiatry*. Advance online publication. doi:10.1037/ort0000234

Ryan, C., Huebner, D., Diaz, R. M., & Sanchez, J. (2009). Family rejection as a predictor of negative health outcomes in White and Latino lesbian, gay, and bisexual young adults. *Pediatrics, 123*, 346–353.

Sabina, C., Cuevas, C. A., & Zadnik, E. (2015). Intimate partner violence among Latino women: Rates and cultural correlates. *Journal of Family Violence, 30*, 35–47.

Sáenz, R., & Morales, M. C. (2015). *Latinos in the United States: Diversity and change*. Malden, MA: Polity.

Salgado De Snyder, V. N., de Jesus Diaz-Perez, M., & Ojeda, V. D. (2000). The prevalence of nervios and associated symptomatology among inhabitants of Mexican rural communities. *Culture, Medicine and Psychiatry, 24*(4), 453–470.

Sanchez, M., Dillon, F., Ruffin, B., & De La Rosa, M. (2012). The influence of religious coping on the acculturative stress of recent Latino immigrants. *Journal of Ethnic & Cultural Diversity in Social Work, 21*(3), 171–194. doi:10.1080/15313204.2012.700443

Sandoval, M. C. (1979). Santería as a mental health care system: An historical overview. *Social Science & Medicine, 13*, 137–151. doi:10.1016/0160-7987(79)90009-7

Santiago-Rivera, A. L., Arredondo, P., & Gallardo-Cooper, M. (2002). *Counseling Latinos and la familia: A practical guide* (Vol. 17). Thousand Oaks, CA: Sage.

Satcher, D. (2006). The role of government in minority mental health: A surgeon general's perspective. In D. Satcher & R. Palmies (Eds.), *Multicultural Medicine and Health Disparities* (pp. 547–556). New York: McGraw Hill.

Sauaia, A., Min, S.-J., Lack, D., Apodaca, C., Osuna, D., Stowe, A., . . . & Byers, T. (2007). Church-based breast cancer screening education: Impact of two approaches on Latinas enrolled in public and private health insurance plans. *Preventing Chronic Disease, 4*(4), A99.

Schinke, S., Hopkins, J., & Wahlstrom, L. (2016). Drug abuse risk and protective factors among Hispanic adolescents. *Preventive Medicine Reports, 3*, 185–188. doi:10.1016/j.pmedr.2016.01.012

Schneiderman, N., Llabre, M., Cowie, C. C., Barnhart, J., Carnethon, M., Gallo, L. C., . . . & LaVange, L. M. (2014). Prevalence of diabetes among Hispanics/Latinos from diverse backgrounds: The Hispanic Community Health Study/Study of Latinos (HCHS/SOL). *Diabetes Care, 37*(8), 2233–2239.

Schwingel, A., & Gálvez, P. (2016). Divine interventions: Faith-based approaches to health promotion programs for Latinos. *Journal of Religion and Health, 55*(6), 1891–1906.

Scott, S. M., Wallander, J. L., & Cameron, L. (2015). Protective mechanisms for depression among racial/ethnic minority youth: Empirical findings, issues, and recommendations. *Clinical Child and Family Psychology Review, 18,* 346–369. doi:10.1007/s10567-015-0188-4

Seid, M., Castaneda, D., Mize, R., Zivkovic, M., & Varni, J. W. (2003). Crossing the border for health care: Access and primary care characteristics for young children of Latino farm workers along the US-Mexico border. *Ambulatory Pediatrics, 3*(3), 121–130.

Sentell, T., Shumway, M., & Snowden, L. (2007). Access to mental health treatment by English language proficiency and race/ethnicity. *Journal of General Internal Medicine, 22*(Suppl 2), 2289–2293. doi:10.1007/S11606-007-0345-7

Serrano-Villar, M., & Calzada, E. J. (2016). Ethnic identity: Evidence of protective effects for young, Latino children. *Journal of Applied Developmental Psychology, 42,* 21–30. doi:10.1016/j.appdev.2015.11.002

Shah, M., Zhu, K., Wu, H., & Potter, J. (2006). Hispanic acculturation and utilization of cervical cancer screening in the US. *Preventive Medicine, 42*(2), 146–149. doi:10.1016/j.ypmed.2005.10.002

Shah, N. S., & Carrasquillo, O. (2006). Twelve-year trends in health insurance coverage among Latinos, by subgroup and immigration status. *Health Affairs* (Millwood), *25*(6), 1612–1619. doi:10.1377/hlthaff.25.6.1612

Shedlin, M. G., Anastasi, J. K., Decena, C. U., Rivera, J. O., Beltran, O., & Smith, K. (2013). Use of complementary and alternative medicines and supplements by Mexican-origin patients in a US–Mexico border HIV clinic. *Journal of the Association of Nurses in AIDS Care, 24*(5), 396–410.

Siegel, R., Naishadham, D., & Jemal, A. (2012). Cancer statistics for Hispanics/Latinos, 2012. *CA: A Cancer Journal for Clinicians, 62*(5), 283–298.

Siegel, R. L., Fedewa, S. A., Miller, K. D., Goding-Sauer, A., Pinheiro, P. S., Martinez-Tyson, D., & Jemal, A. (2015). Cancer statistics for Hispanics/Latinos, 2015. *CA: A Cancer Journal for Clinicians, 65*(6), 457–480.

Smith, L. (2001). Evaluation of an educational intervention to increase cultural competence among registered nurses. *Journal of Cultural Diversity, 8*(2), 50.

Smokowski, P. R., & Bacallao, M. L. (2006). Acculturation and aggression in Latino adolescents: A structural model focusing on cultural risk factors and assets. *Journal of Abnormal Child Psychology, 34,* 659–673. doi:10.1007/s10802-006-9049-4

Smokowski, P. R., & Bacallao, M.L. (2007). Acculturation, internalizing mental health symptoms, and self-esteem: Cultural experiences of Latino adolescents in North Carolina. *Child Psychiatry and Human Development, 37,* 273–292. doi:10.1007/s10578-006-0035-4

Smokowski, P. R., Chapman, M. V., & Bacallao, M. L. (2007). Acculturation risk and protective factors and mental health symptoms in immigrant Latino adolescents. *Journal of Human Behavior in the Social Environment, 16,* 33–55. doi:10.1080/10911350802107710

Sorlie, P. D., Avilés-Santa, L. M., Wassertheil-Smoller, S., Kaplan, R. C., Daviglus, M. L., Giachello, A. L., . . . & Allison, M. (2010). Design and implementation of the Hispanic community health study/study of Latinos. *Annals of Epidemiology, 20*(8), 629–641.

Sosa, E. T. (2012). Mexican American mothers' perceptions of childhood obesity: A theory-guided systematic literature review. *Health Education & Behavior, 39*(4), 396–404.

Sosa, E. T., McKyer, E. L. J., Goodson, P., & Castillo, L. (2014). Mexican American mothers' perceptions of their role in childhood obesity prevention: A qualitative study. *Journal of Research in Obesity, 2014,* 1–10.

Sosa, E. T., Parra-Medina, D., He, M., Trummer, V., & Yin, Z. (2016). ¡Miranos! (Look at Us! We Are Healthy!) home-based and parent peer–led childhood obesity prevention. *Health Promotion Practice, 17*(5), 675–681.

Soto Espinoza, J. (2014). Puerto Rican spiritism (Espiritismo): Social context, healing process, and mental health. In P. Sutherland, R. Moodley, & B. Chevannes (Eds.), *Caribbean healing traditions: Implications for health and mental health* (pp. 113–127). New York: Routledge

Spencer, M. S., Rosland, A. M., Kieffer, E. C., Sinco, B. R., Valerio, M., Palmisano, G., . . . & Heisler, M. (2011). Effectiveness of a community health worker intervention among African American and Latino adults with type 2 diabetes: A randomized controlled trial. *American Journal of Public Health, 101*(12), 2253–2260. doi:10.2105/AJPH.2010.300106

Stepler, R., & Brown, A. (2016). Statistical portrait of Hispanics in the United States, 2014. Washington, DC: Pew Hispanic Research Center. Retrieved from http://www.pewhispanic.org/2016/04/19/statistical-portrait-of-hispanics-in-the-united-states/

Stinchcomb, D., & Hershberg, E. (2014). *Unaccompanied migrant children from Central America: Context, causes, and responses.* CLALS Working Paper Series No. 7. Washington, DC: Center for Latin American & Latino Studies. American University. Retrieved from https://papers.ssrn.com/sol3/papers.cfm?abstract_id=2524001

Sue, D. W., & Sue, D. (1999). *Counseling the culturally different: Theory and practice.* Hoboken, NJ: Wiley.

Sue, D. W. (2001). Multidimensional facets of cultural competence. *The Counseling Psychologist, 29*(6), 790–821.

Sue, D. W., Arredondo, P., & McDavis, R. J. (1992). Multicultural counseling competencies: A call to the profession. *Journal of Counseling and Development, 70,* 477–486.

Sue, D. W., Bernier, J. E., Durran, A., Feinberg, L., Pedersen, P., Smith, E. J., & Vasquez-Nuttall, E. (1982). Position paper: Cross-cultural counseling competencies. *The Counseling Psychologist, 10*(2), 45–52.

Sue, D. W., & Sue, D. (2016). *Counseling the culturally different: Theory and practice* (7th ed.). Hoboken, NJ: Wiley.

Sue, S. (1998). In search of cultural competence in psychotherapy and counseling. *American Psychologist, 53*(4), 440.

Sullivan, M. M., & Rehm, R. (2005). Mental health of undocumented Mexican immigrants. *Advances in Nursing Science, 28*, 240–251.

Sutherland, P. (2014). The history, philosophy, and transformation of Caribbean healing traditions. In P. Sutherland, R. Moodley, & B. Chevannes (Eds.), *Caribbean healing traditions: Implications for health and mental health* (pp. 15–28). New York: Routledge.

Swider, S. M. (2002). Outcome effectiveness of community health workers: An integrative literature review. *Public Health Nursing, 19*(1), 11–20.

Szapocznik, J., Hervis, O., & Schwartz, S. (2003). *Brief Strategic Family Therapy for adolescent drug abuse*. Bethesda, MD: National Institute on Drug Abuse.

Szapocznik, J., & Kurtines, W. M. (1993). Family psychology and cultural diversity: Opportunities for theory, research, and application. *American Psychologist, 48*, 400–407.

Szapocznik, J., Kurtines, W. M., Santisteban, D. A. Pantín, H., Scopetta, M., Mancilla, Y., . . . & Coatsworth, J. D. (1997). The evolution of structural ecosystemic theory for working with Latino families. In J. G. Garcia & M. C. Zea (Eds.), *Psychological interventions and research with Latino populations* (pp. 166–190). Needham Heights, MA: Allyn & Bacon.

Szapocznik, J., Santisteban, D., Kurtines, W., Perez-Vidal, A., & Hervis, O. (1984). Bicultural Effectiveness Training: A treatment intervention for enhancing intercultural adjustment in Cuban American families. *Hispanic Journal of Behavioral Sciences, 6*, 317–344.

Szapocznik, J., Santisteban, D., Kurtines, W., Perez-Vidal, A., & Hervis, O. (1986). Bicultural Effectiveness Training (BET): An experimental test of an intervention modality for families experiencing intergenerational/intercultural conflict. *Hispanic Journal of Behavioral Sciences, 8*, 303–330.

Tafur, M. M., Crowe, T. K., & Torres, E. (2009). A review of curanderismo and healing practices among Mexicans and Mexican Americans. *Occupational Therapy International, 16*, 82–88. doi:10.1002/oti.265

Tello, J., Cervantes, R. C., Cordova, D., & Santos, S. M. (2010). Joven Noble: Evaluation of a culturally focused youth development program. *Journal of Community Psychology, 38*, 799–811. doi:10.1002/jcop.20396

The DREAM ACT: Good for our economy, good for our security, good for our nation. (n.d.). Retrieved from https://www.whitehouse.gov/sites/default/files/DREAM-Act-WhiteHouse-FactSheet.pdf

The Urban Institute. (2002). *Preventing homelessness: Meeting the challenge*. Washington, DC: The Urban Institute.

Thomson, M. D., & Hoffman-Goetz, L. (2009). Defining and measuring acculturation: A systematic review of public health studies with Hispanic populations in the United States. *Social Science & Medicine, 69*(7), 983–991.

Tienda, M., & Sánchez, S. M. (2013). Latin American immigration to the United States. *Daedalus, 142*(3), 48–64.

Titus, S. K. F. (2014). Seeking and utilizing a curandero in the United States: A literature review. *Journal of Holistic Nursing, 32*(3), 189–201.

Torres, J. B., Solberg, V. S. H., & Carlstrom, A. H. (2002). The myth of sameness among Latino men and their machismo. *American Journal of Orthopsychiatry, 72*(2), 163.

Tovar, M. R. (2017). *Mexican American psychology: Social, cultural, and clinical perspectives.* Santa Barbara, CA: Praeger.

Tran, A. N., Ornelas, I. J., Perez, G., Green, M. A., Lyn, M., & Corbie-Smith, G. (2014). Evaluation of Amigas Latinas Motivando El Alma (ALMA): A pilot promotora intervention focused on stress and coping among immigrant Latinas. *Journal of Immigrant and Minority Health, 16,* 280–289. doi:10.1007/s10903-012-9735-y

Trotter, R. T. (2001). Curanderismo: A picture of Mexican-American folk healing. *Journal of Alternative & Complementary Medicine, 7*(2), 129–131.

Trotter, R. T., & Chavira, J. A. (1997). *Curanderismo: Mexican American folk healing* (2nd ed.). Athens: University of Georgia Press.

Trotter, R. T., & Chavira, J. A. (2011). *Curanderismo: Mexican American folk healing.* Athens: University of Georgia Press.

Umaña-Taylor, A. J., Diversi, M., & Fine, M. A. (2002). Ethnic identity and self-esteem of Latino adolescents: Distinctions among the Latino populations. *Journal of Adolescent Research, 17,* 303–327.

Underwood, S. M. (2000). Minorities, women, and clinical cancer research: The charge, promise, and challenge. *Annals of Epidemiology, 10,* S3–S12.

Unger, J. B., Cabassa, L. J., Molina, G. B., Contreras, S., & Baron, M. (2013). Evaluation of a fotonovela to increase depression knowledge and reduce stigma among Hispanic adults. *Journal of Immigrant and Minority Health, 15,* 398–406. doi:10.1007/s10903-012-9623-5

U.S. Census Bureau. (2008). U.S. Census Bureau, 1970, 1980, 1990, and 2000 decennial census: Population projections, July 1, 2010, to July 1, 2050. Retrieved from https://www.census.gov/population/hispanic/files/hispanic2006/Internet_Hispanic_in_US_2006.pdf

U.S. Census Bureau. (2015). Projections of the size and composition of the U.S. population: 2014 to 2060. Retrieved from https://www.census.gov/content/dam/Census/library/publications/2015/demo/p25-1143.pdf

U.S. Census Bureau. (2016). Annual estimates of the resident population by sex, age, race, and Hispanic origin for the United States and states: April 1, 2010 to July 1, 2015. Retrieved from https://factfinder.census.gov/faces/tableservices/jsf/pages/productview.xhtml?src=bkmk

U.S. Department of Education—National Center for Educational Statistics. (2000). *Statistics in brief—March 2000: Home literacy activities and signs of children's emerging literacy, 1993–1999*. Washington, DC: U.S. Government Printing Office.

U.S. Department of Health & Human Services. (2001). *Mental health: Culture, race, and ethnicity-a supplement to mental health: A report of the surgeon general*. Rockville, MD: U.S. Department of Health and Human Services, Public Health Service, Office of the Surgeon General.

U.S. Department of Health & Human Services. (2011a). HHS announces new investment in school-based health centers. Retrieved from www.hhs.gov/news/press/2011pres/07/20110714a.html

U.S. Department of Health & Human Services. (2011b). HHS Action Plan to Reduce Racial and Ethnic Health Disparities: A nation free of disparities in health and health care. Retrieved from https://www.minorityhealth.hhs.gov/npa/files/Plans/HHS/HHS_Plan_complete.pdf

U.S. Department of Health & Human Services. (2015). Summary health statistics: National Health Interview Survey. Retrieved from https://ftp.cdc.gov/pub/Health_Statistics/NCHS/NHIS/SHS/2015_SHS_Table_P-11.pdf

Valdez, C. R., Dvorscek, M. J., Budge, S. L., & Esmond, S. (2011). Provider perspectives about Latino patients: Determinants of care and Implications for treatment. *The Counseling Psychologist, 39*(4), 497–526.

Valdez, J. N. (2014). Curanderismo: A complementary and alternative approach to Mexican American healing psychology. In R. Gurung (Ed.), *Multicultural approaches to health and wellness in America* (Vol. 1, pp. 227–258). Santa Barbara, CA: Praeger.

Valdez, J., & de Posada, D. R. G. (2006). Strategies for improving Latino healthcare in America. *The Latino Coalition*. Retrieved from http://www.borderhealth.org/files/res_642_es.pdf

Vandebroek, I., Balick, M. J., Ososki, A., Kronenberg, F., Yukes, J., Wade, C., . . . & Castillo, D. (2010). The importance of botellas and other plant mixtures in Dominican traditional medicine. *Journal of Ethnopharmacology, 128*(1), 20–41.

Varela, R. E., & Hensley-Maloney, L. (2009). The influence of culture on anxiety in Latino youth: A review. *Clinical Child and Family Psychology Review, 12*, 217–233. doi:10.1007/s10567-009-0044-5

Vargas, S. M., Cabassa, L. J., Nicasio, A., De La Cruz, A. A., Jackson, E., Rosario, M., . . . & Lewis-Fernández, R. (2015). Toward a cultural adaptation of pharmacotherapy: Latino views of depression and antidepressant therapy. *Transcultural Psychiatry, 52*(2), 244–273.

Vaughan, E. L., Gassman, R. A., Jun, M. C., & Seitz de Martinez, B. J. (2015). Gender differences in risk and protective factors for alcohol use and substance use problems among Hispanic adolescents. *Journal of Child & Adolescent Substance Abuse, 24*, 243–254. doi:10.1080/1067828X.2013.826609

Vega, W. A., Aguilar-Gaxiola, S., Andrade, L., Bijl, R., Borges, G., Caraveo-Anduaga, J. J., . . . & Hans-Ulrich, W. (2002). Prevalence and age of onset for drug use in seven international sites: Results from the International Consortium of Psychiatric Epidemiology. *Drug and Alcohol Dependence, 68,* 285–297. doi:10.1016/S0376-8716(02)00224-7

Vega, W. A., Kolody, B., Aguilar-Gaxiola, S., Alderete, E., Catalano, R., & Caraveo-Anduaga, J. (1998). Lifetime prevalence of DSM-III-R psychiatric disorders among urban and rural Mexican Americans in California. *Archives of General Psychiatry, 55*(9), 771–778.

Vega, W. A., & Lopez, S. R. (2001). Priority issues in Latino mental health services research. *Mental Health Services Research, 3*(4), 189–200.

Vega, W. A., Rodriguez, M. A., & Ang, A. (2010). Addressing stigma of depression in Latino primary care patients. *General Hospital Psychiatry, 32*(2), 182–191.

Vega, W. A., Rodriguez, M. A., & Gruskin, E. (2009). Health disparities in the Latino population. *Epidemiologic Reviews, 31*(1), 99–112.

Velez, B. L., Campos, I. D., & Moradi, B. (2015). Relations of sexual objectification and racist discrimination with Latina women's body image and mental health. *Counseling Psychologist, 43*(6), 906–935. doi:10.1177/0011000015591287

Victorson, D., Banas, J., Smith, J., Languido, L., Shen, E., Gutierrez, S., . . . & Flores, L. (2014). eSalud: Designing and implementing culturally competent eHealth research with Latino patient populations. *American Journal of Public Health, 104,* 2259–2265. doi:10.2105/AJPH.2014.302187

Viladrich, A., & Abraido-Lanza, A. F. (2009). Religion and mental health among minorities and immigrants in the U.S. In S. Loue & M. Sajatovic (Eds.), *Determinants of minority health and wellness* (pp. 149–174). New York: Springer.

Viladrich, A., Yeh, M.-C., Bruning, N., & Weiss, R. (2009). "Do real women have curves?" Paradoxical body images among Latinas in New York City. *Journal of Immigrant and Minority Health, 11*(1), 20–28.

Villagran, M., Hajek, C., Zhao, X., Peterson, E., & Wittenberg-Lyles, E. (2012). Communication and culture: Predictors of treatment adherence among Mexican immigrant patients. *Journal of Health Psychology, 17*(3), 443–452. doi:10.1177/1359105311417194

Viruell-Fuentes, E. A. (2007). Beyond acculturation: Immigration, discrimination, and health research among Mexicans in the United States. *Social Science & Medicine, 65*(7), 1524–1535.

Vontress, C. E. (2001). Cross-cultural counseling in the 21st century. *International Journal for the Advancement of Counselling, 23,* 83–97. doi:10.1023/A:1010677807232

Wadsworth, T., & Kubrin, C. E. (2007). Hispanic suicide in US metropolitan areas: Examining the effects of immigration, assimilation, affluence, and disadvantage. *American Journal of Sociology, 112*(6), 1848–1885.

Wahl, A. G., & Eitle, T. M. (2010). Gender, acculturation and alcohol use among Latina/o adolescents: A multi-ethnic comparison. *Journal of Immigrant and Minority Health, 12,* 153–65. doi:10.1007/s10903-008-9179-6

Walker, P. F., & Jaranson, J. (1999). Refugee and immigrant health care. *Medical Clinics of North America, 83*(4), 1103–1120.

Wallis, F., Amaro, H., & Cortés, D. E. (2012). Saber es poder: The cultural adaptation of a trauma intervention for Latina women. In G. Bernal & M. M. Domenech Rodríguez (Eds.), *Cultural adaptations: Tools for evidence-based practice with diverse populations* (pp. 157–178). Washington, DC: American Psychological Association.

Ward, D. S., Welker, E., Choate, A., Henderson, K. E., Lott, M., Tovar, A., ... & Sallis, J. F. (2017). Strength of obesity prevention interventions in early care and education settings: A systematic review. *Preventive Medicine, 95*, S37–S52.

Ware, J. E., & Davis, A. R. (1983). Behavioral consequences of consumer dissatisfaction with medical care. *Evaluation and Program Planning, 6*(3–4), 291–297.

Watson, M.-R., Kaltman, S., Townsend, T. G., Goode, T., & Campoli, M. (2013). A collaborative mental health research agenda in a community of poor and underserved Latinos. *Journal of Health Care Poor & Underserved, 24*(2), 671–687.

Waugh, I. M. (2010). Examining the sexual harassment experiences of Mexican immigrant farmworking women. *Violence against Women, 16*, 237–261. doi:10.1177/1077801209360857

Weick, A., Rapp, C., Sullivan, W. P., & Kisthardt, W. (1989). A strengths perspective for social work practice. *Social Work, 34*(4), 350–354.

Weller, S. C., Baer, R. D., de Alba Garcia, J. G., Glazer, M., Trotter, R., Pachter, L., & Klein, R. E. (2002). Regional variation in Latino descriptions of susto. *Culture, Medicine and Psychiatry, 26*, 449–472.

Weller, S. C., Baer, R. D., de Alba Garcia, J. G., & Rocha, A. L. S. (2008). Susto and nervios: Expressions for stress and depression. *Culture, Medicine, and Psychiatry, 32*(3), 406–420.

WestRasmus, E. K., Pineda-Reyes, F., Tamez, M., & Westfall, J. M. (2012). Promotores de salud and community health workers: An annotated bibliography. *Family & Community Health, 35*(2), 172–182.

Willerton, E., Dankoski, M. E., & Martir, J. F. S. (2008). Medical family therapy: A model for addressing mental health disparities among Latinos. *Families, Systems, & Health, 26*(2), 196.

Williams, D. R., Yu, Y., Jackson, J. S., & Anderson, N. B. (1997). Racial differences in physical and mental health: Socio-economic status, stress and discrimination. *Journal of Health Psychology, 2*(3), 335–351.

Williams, M. V., Derose, K. P., Aunon, F., Kanouse, D. E., Bogart, L, M., Griffin, B. A., ... & Collins, D. O. (2016). Church-based HIV screening in racial/ethnic minority communities of California, 2011–2012. *Public Health Reports, 131*(5), 676–684.

Woodruff, S. I., Talavera, G. A., & Elder, J. P. (2002). Evaluation of a culturally appropriate smoking cessation intervention for Latinos. *Tobacco Control, 11*, 361–367. doi:10.1136/tc.11.4.361

Wu, S., Ridgely, M. S., Escarce, J. J., & Morales, L. S. (2007). Language access services for Latinos with limited English proficiency: Lessons learned from Hablamos Juntos. *Journal of General Internal Medicine, 22*(Suppl 2), 350–355. doi:10.1007/s11606-007-0323-0

Yeh, C. J., Hunter, C. D., Madan-Bahel, A., Chiang, L., & Arora, A. K. (2004). Indigenous and interdependent perspectives of healing: Implications for counseling and research. *Journal of Counseling & Development, 82*, 410–419.

Yin, Z., Parra-Medina, D., Cordova, A., He, M., Trummer, V., Sosa, E., . . . & Wu, X. (2012). Miranos! Look at us, we are healthy! An environmental approach to early childhood obesity prevention. *Childhood Obesity, 8*(5), 429–439.

Zacharias, S. (2006). Mexican *curanderismo* as ethnopsychotherapy: A qualitative study on treatment practices, effectiveness, and mechanisms of change. *International Journal of Disability, Development and Education, 53*, 381–400. doi:10.1080/10349120601008522

Zayas, L. H., Aguilar-Gaxiola, S., Yoon, H., & Rey, G. N. (2015). The distress of citizen-children with detained and deported parents. *Journal of Child and Family Studies, 24*(11), 3213–3223.

Zayas, L. H., Lester, R. J., Cabassa, L. J., & Fortuna, L. R. (2005). Why do so many Latina teens attempt suicide? A conceptual model for research. *American Journal of Orthopsychiatry, 75*, 275–287

Zuckerman, H. S., Kaluzny, A. D., Ricketts, T. C. (1994). Alliances in health care: What we know, what we think we know, and what we should know. *Health Care Management Review, 20*, 54–64.

Zuñiga, M. E. (1992). Using metaphors in therapy: Dichos and Latino clients. *Social Work, 37*, 55–60.

Index

Page numbers followed by *t* indicate tables and *f* indicate figures.

About the Authors

LETICIA ARELLANO-MORALES, PhD, is an Associate Professor in the Department of Psychology at the University of La Verne (in La Verne, CA). Her research interests focus on the psychological and physical well-being of Latina/os, as well as on multiracial feminism, college students, and multicultural counseling competencies. She is co-editor of *Handbook of Chicana/o Psychology and Mental Health* and the upcoming *Mexican Psychology: Indigenous, Colonial, and Post-Modern Contributions*. She has made presentations to local, state, and national conferences and provided workshops and training on multicultural counseling competencies. She is also a Trainer and Consultant for the California Brief Multicultural Competence Scale (CBMCS) Multicultural Training Program.

ERICA T. SOSA, PhD, is an Associate Professor of Community & Public Health at the University of Texas at San Antonio. She has conducted intervention research to address public health issues that disproportionately impact Latina/o communities. Her research interests include examining structural, cultural, and psychosocial contributors to the onset of diabetes and obesity among minority populations. She investigates cultural factors influencing Mexican Americans' perceptions of health, health behaviors, and programs and assesses environmental correlates of physical activity and dietary behaviors among underserved communities. She is also Co-Director of the Center for Community-Based and Applied Health Research at the University of Texas at San Antonio.

About the Series Editor

REGAN A. R. GURUNG is Ben J. and Joyce Rosenberg Professor of Human Development and Psychology at the University of Wisconsin, Green Bay (UWGB). Born and raised in Bombay, India, Dr. Gurung received a BA in psychology at Carleton College (in Northfield, MN), and a Masters and PhD in social and personality psychology at the University of Washington (in Seattle). He then spent three years at UCLA as a National Institute of Mental Health Research fellow.

He has received numerous local, state, and national grants for his health psychological and social psychological research on cultural differences in stress, social support, smoking cessation, body image, and impression formation. He has published articles in a variety of scholarly journals, including *American Psychologist, Psychological Review, Personality and Social Psychology Bulletin*, and *Teaching of Psychology*. He has a textbook, *Health Psychology: A Cultural Approach*, that relates culture, development, and health published with Sage (now in its fourth edition) and is also the co-author/co-editor of 14 other books. He has made over 150 presentations and given workshops nationally and internationally (e.g., in Australia, India, Saudi Arabia, and New Zealand).

Gurung is also a dedicated teacher and has strong interests in enhancing faculty development and student understanding. He was Co-Director of the University of Wisconsin System Teaching Scholars Program, has been a UWGB Teaching Fellow and a UW System Teaching Scholar and is winner of the American Psychological Foundation's Charles L. Brewer Award for Distinguished Teaching, the CASE Wisconsin Professor of the Year, the UW

System Regents Teaching Award, the UWGB Founder's Award for Excellence in Teaching, as well as the Founder's Award for Scholarship, UW Teaching-at-its-Best, Creative Teaching, and Featured Faculty Awards.

He has strong interests in teaching and pedagogy and has organized statewide and national teaching conferences, is a Fellow of the American Psychological Association, the Association for Psychological Science and the Midwestern Psychological Association, and has served on the Division 2 (Teaching of Psychology) Taskforce for Diversity, as Chair of the Division 38 (Health Psychology) Education and Training Council, and as President of the Society for the Teaching of Psychology.